The Complete MRCGP *Blueprint* Casebook

This is the most comprehensive resource for GP registrars sitting the RCGP's new Simulated Consultation Assessment (SCA) exam, offering 60 role plays that can be practised in pairs or small groups.

With chapters seamlessly aligned to the new blueprint groups, our Third Edition of **The Complete MRCGP *Blueprint* Casebook** is designed to provide a 'HOW TO' approach and give you as much help as possible as you prepare for the SCA exam.

Whether using this book alone, to learn how to approach cases, or practising in pairs or small groups, **The Complete MRCGP *Blueprint* Casebook** is essential reading for preparation for the SCA exam and will remain an invaluable resource for best practice after qualification.

Emily Blount • Helen Kirby-Blount • Liz Moulton

The Complete MRCGP BLUEPRINT Casebook

Example consultations and how to pass the SCA exam

Third Edition

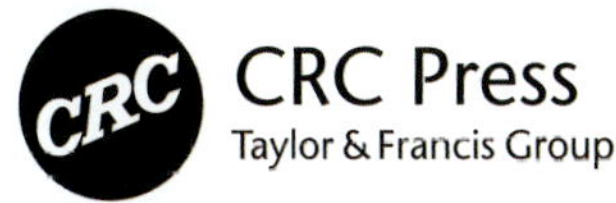

CRC Press is an imprint of the
Taylor & Francis Group, an **informa** business

Third edition published 2026
by CRC Press
2385 NW Executive Center Drive, Suite 320, Boca Raton, FL 33431

and by CRC Press
4 Park Square, Milton Park, Abingdon, Oxon, OX14 4RN
CRC Press is an imprint of Taylor & Francis Group, LLC

First edition published by CRC Press 2017
Second edition published by CRC Press 2020

Library of Congress Cataloging-in-Publication Data

Names: Blount, Emily, author. | Kirby-Blount, Helen, author. | Moulton, Liz, author.
Title: The complete MRCGP blueprint casebook : example consultations and how to pass the SCA exam / Emily Blount, Helen Kirby-Blount and Liz Moulton.
Other titles: Complete MRCGP casebook
Description: Third edition. | Boca Raton, FL : CRC Press, 2025. | Preceded by The complete MRCGP casebook / Emily Blount, Helen Kirby-Blount, Liz Moulton. Second edition. 2022. | Summary: "This is the most comprehensive resource for trainees sitting the RCGP's new Simulated Consultation Assessment (SCA) exam, offering 60 roleplays that can be practised in pairs or small groups. Why choose The Complete MRCGP Blueprint Casebook? With chapters seamlessly aligned to the new Blueprint groups, our 3rd edition of The Complete MRCGP Blueprint Casebook is designed to provide a "HOW TO" approach and give you as much help as possible as you prepare for the SCA exam. HOW TO approach cases from start to finish, with full example consultations. HOW TO demonstrate the skills within the Blueprint groups. HOW TO demonstrate skills within the marking scheme. HOW TO demonstrate your skills across a range of consultation challenges. HOW TO approach clinical assessment so you can complete data gathering in good time! HOW TO provide a comprehensive, patient centred, shared management plan. We include: Summaries of up-to-date NICE guidelines .Top tips from the authors' own experience of the RCGP exams – both as candidates and as teachers. Colour coding for easy reference. An easy way to mark each other's role plays. Whether using this book alone, to learn how to approach cases, or practising in pairs or small groups, The Complete MRCGP Blueprint Casebook is essential reading for preparation for the SCA Exam and will remain an invaluable resource for best practice after qualification. To complement your reading and put your skills into practice, join thousands of your colleagues who have already attended our Complete MRCGP SCA Course - delivered by the Authors and RCGP Examiners on Zoom with Professional Patient Simulators" — Provided by publisher.
Identifiers: LCCN 2024052514 | ISBN 9781032913094 (paperback)
Subjects: MESH: General Practice—methods | Physical Examination—methods | Clinical Competence | Diagnosis | United Kingdom | Case Reports | Study Guide
Classification: LCC RC78.7.D53 | NLM WB 18.2 | DDC 616.07/54—dc23/eng/20250303
LC record available at https://lccn.loc.gov/2024052514

ISBN: 9781032913094 (pbk)

Typeset in Minion Pro
by Evolution Design & Digital Ltd (Kent)

Dedication

In memory of our dear friend and neighbour Nick Hungerford, this book is dedicated to Elizabeth's Smile. This charity supports grieving children and their caregivers and empowers people to address grief and build resilience. www.elizabeth.org

Contents

Preface

Sixty example consultations are presented for the RCGP Simulated Consultation Assessment, fully aligned to the new 2025 RCGP curriculum. *The Complete MRCGP Blueprint Casebook* provides examples of **how to** overcome the challenges and demonstrate competence throughout the marking domains for all cases across the curriculum. For every case we provide 'Example Consultations' to demonstrate how each challenge could be achieved within 10–12 minutes, as well as 'Learning Points', which summarise up-to-date guidance. All RCGP curriculum modules are colour coded, helping you to keep the cases in order and stay organised.

Our FOCUS Consultation Model was created specifically for the RCGP consultation skills exam, to focus your preparation, provide structure and give you an easy-to-use tool to help you 'mark' your own consultations.

The authors are three experienced GP educators who have run CSA, RCA and SCA preparation courses for many years, working in collaboration with senior RCGP examiners. We have systematically condensed our experience into this comprehensive *Casebook* to help you complete your GP training and become a confident and independent practitioner.

Authors

Dr Emily Blount

MBBS (merit) DRCOG DFSRH MRCGP

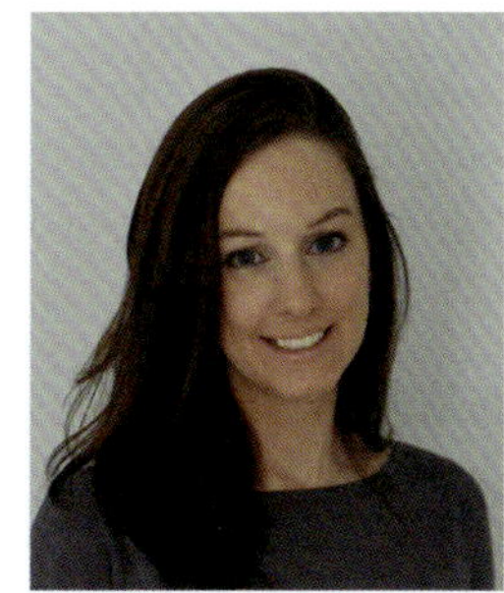

Emily is a mother, GP in Oxfordshire and Principal Safety Officer at www.Healthily.ai. With an interest in using technology to improve healthcare accessibility, she leads the clinical risk management and governance of the medical device product development. She graduated from Newcastle University and has since lived in Auckland, New Zealand, and Boston, Massachusetts. She is a former Oxford Training Programme Director and continues to enjoy medical education alongside her NHS and MedTech roles.

Dr Helen Kirby-Blount

MBChB (hons) DRCOG MRCGP PGCME

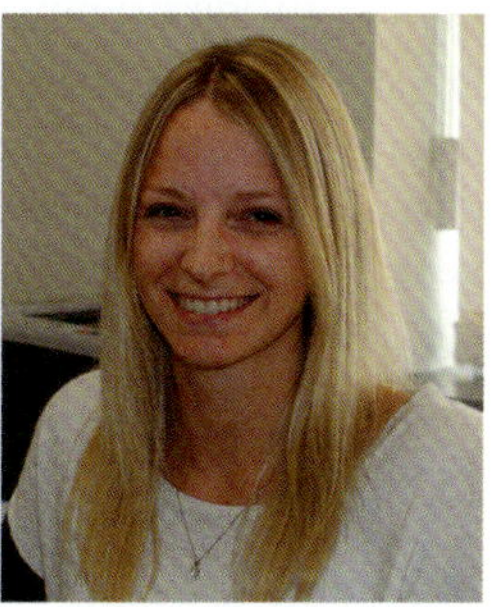

Helen graduated from Manchester University in 2009 and sat the CSA exam in 2013. Helen is now a GP partner, trainer and training programme director in the South Yorkshire–North Nottinghamshire borders. She facilitates teaching sessions on consultation skills for GP registrars on her scheme, where she also leads on differential attainment. She is a clinical director for her PCN. Helen created the FOCUS Consultation Model. In her 'spare time' she is a busy mother of two and loves all things 'sport'.

Dr Liz Moulton

MBE MB ChB DRCOG FRCGP MMEd (distinction)

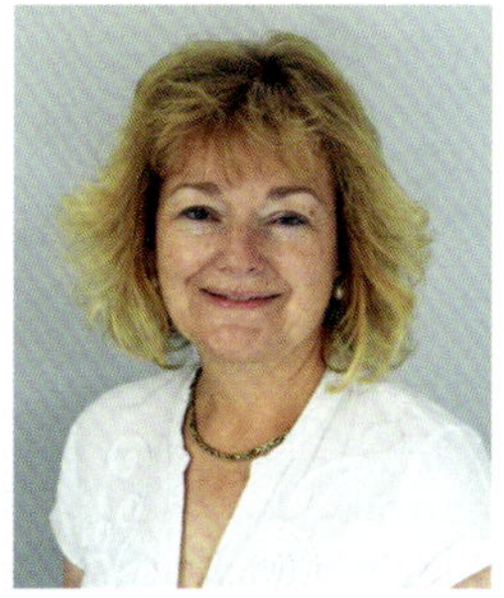

A GP trainer for more than 30 years, with a wealth of experience of preparing candidates for the MRCGP, Liz has also undertaken most roles within HEE Yorkshire and Humber and was Deputy Director of Postgraduate GP Education. Liz was a GP advisor to Leeds Health Authority and to the Department of Health, where she provided the GP input to the AAA screening programme and electronic transfer of prescriptions, amongst other areas. She currently works as a freelance consultation skills' teacher and GP and NHS England appraiser. Liz is the author of *The Naked Consultation* and co-author of *What Do I Say Next? Everyday Mental Health Conversations in Primary Care.* Liz has three grown-up children and four grandchildren.

Introduction

The Complete MRCGP Blueprint Casebook will help you with your exam preparation for the SCA. We provide examples of how to demonstrate skills in 60 cases covering all the blueprint groups and across the new RCGP curriculum.

The challenge of the SCA is to be able to synthesise 10 years of medical education competently, sensitively, quickly and safely, to manage any medical problem presented by any patient. This is also the challenge faced every day by busy GPs in clinical practice. To help show you what can be achieved, the Casebook breaks down the consultation into elements: important building blocks of the consultation which encourage demonstration of all the skills across the marking domains.

The more you practise these skills, the more likely it is that they will, both consciously and unconsciously, become an integral part of your consultation toolkit. When under exam pressure, remember that these elements are grouped into our FOCUS Consultation Model, an easy to remember acronym.

The Example Consultations may give you ideas about how to develop your consultation skills and meet the challenge of managing the presenting problem safely and effectively within 10–12 minutes. Our Learning Points provide a summary of guidance or a discussion around the topic.

Whatever consultation model(s) you use, we strongly advise that you use your own style for authenticity, have a fluid approach and adapt to meet the needs of each individual consultation. When you meet a new acquaintance or a friend in any setting, demonstrating courtesy and respect for that person and showing a genuine curiosity and interest in their life will enable rapport, storytelling and conversation to come naturally – there is no need to follow a rigid formula.

We appreciate that some readers may have specialist knowledge in particular areas and may well approach some problems differently. The authors are conscientious generalists and this is reflected in our approach to the cases. We hope you find our Example Consultations helpful – but would remind you that there are many ways to deliver a good consultation, and to pass your final RCGP assessment!

The Learning Points for each case include information from the relevant resources or guidance, and we strongly advise always referring to the full text of the most up-to-date guidelines.

See our website www.completeMRCGP.co.uk for dates for exam preparation courses created and run by the authors and RCGP examiners.

You may also wish to look at *The Naked Consultation: A Practical Guide to Primary Care Consultation Skills* which will help you develop and hone your consultation skills further.

When role playing cases, we encourage the doctor to remember this:

'Common things are common … But what mustn't I miss?'

Finally, the responsibility of making frequent and fast decisions while holding risk, the urge to always get it right (with the fear of getting it wrong), the pressure to not waste NHS resources, whilst managing complexity, with a high patient load and the medicolegal need to document it all within too little time can feel overwhelming. However, take every opportunity to remember your own loved ones and just do your best for the person looking to you for help. Keep faith in general practice and remember the unique, professional and supportive work ethos we share.

We wish you all the best.

Emily, Helen and Liz

CHAPTER 1

INTRODUCTION AND BACKGROUND TO THE EXAM

The Royal College of General Practitioners simulated consultation assessment (SCA) was introduced in November 2023, replacing the recorded consultation assessment (RCA) which was an interim exam introduced during the COVID pandemic. The College intends that, going forward, the SCA will be the 'forever' exam to assess consultation skills towards the end of GP training.

The Complete MRCGP Blueprint Casebook is designed to help you in your exam preparation, complementing your daily learning from consultations with patients, conversations with colleagues and team members and learning from your trainers and teachers.

In Chapter 1, we introduce and fully describe the new exam and explain how to use this book to help you prepare effectively.

- **Chapter 1A.** Here we describe the structure and process of the exam and how to use the case material in the book, whether you are working alone or, ideally, in a study group with colleagues.
- **Chapter 1B.** We define and explain some of the terminology and how different facets of the RCGP curriculum interrelate, for example the new term 'blueprint groups' and how these link with the curriculum, clinical topics, life stages, the core statement and capabilities. Finally, we describe some of the available consultation models and explore how these also fit with the exam.
- **Chapter 1C.** We describe the skills required for the exam, looking particularly at the FOCUS consultation model which we developed specifically for the exam. As well as discussing how to find out the patient's thoughts (ICE1), fears (ICE2) and hopes (ICE3), we describe how to make use of this knowledge as you complete data gathering, using the tool Summar**ICE** and in the second half of the consultation using the tool **I**n**C**lud**E**.

  We discuss how to demonstrate your skills in order to score marks in each of the domains, making use of our easy-to-use 'Generic Feedback' card.
- **Chapter 1D.** This section covers consultation structure, time management and how to optimise this – crucial to a good score in the exam! If the first half of the consultation is too long, it is difficult to score well in the domain of clinical management and medical complexity. We explore efficiency tools to ensure you have time for all aspects of the consultation, even those particularly tricky consultations where there are multiple problems.

  It can be challenging to demonstrate skills in the domain of relating to others and we describe our top tips for doing this. We also cover 'special' types of consultations such as those with child patients, or parents/carers talking about their children, and patients returning for test results.

  Our 'jargon switch' will remind you to use natural language when talking to patients and offers useful suggestions of alternative words that are patient-friendly, avoiding doctor-speak.

  In this section, we also explore what might have gone wrong if you are unfortunate enough to have not achieved the pass mark, including common problem areas and how to address them when you resit.
- **Chapter 1E.** Finally, we cover the 'nuts and bolts' of the exam – what must you have with you on the day? What are you not allowed to have? Our top tips will help to set you up for success.

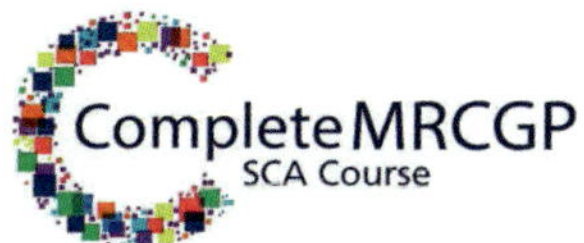

CHAPTER 1A INTRODUCTION AND HOW TO USE THE BOOK

Introduction

The SCA exam is designed to assess your ability to undertake a 12-minute primary care consultation, demonstrating your skills as a doctor performing at the level of a newly qualified GP, across the breadth of the curriculum.[1] The exam is marked against the following three domains and you will need to demonstrate your skills in each of these:

- **Data gathering and making a diagnosis** – mainly the skills you use in the first half of the consultation to make a holistic assessment of the patient's problem(s) and reach a working diagnosis or differential.
- **Clinical management and medical complexity** – this domain includes second-half skills as well as testing whether you have been able to uncover and manage the inherent complexity in a case.
- **Relating to others** – this domain used to be called 'interpersonal skills' and tested the communication skills you use during the consultation. It is now a broader domain and includes not only communication skills but also how you relate to **others** in the consultation (e.g. both a parent and a child, or others in the team who may be speaking to you about a patient, or others whom you might involve going forward, for example planning a referral to the district nurse). It follows from this that, as well as practising your communication skills, you also need to know about the various roles of members of the primary healthcare team and in secondary care.

How to Use the Book

You could work through the book alone; however, if you can, we recommend using the book in groups of two or three, taking the parts of: a doctor, a patient and an examiner. The more frequently you practise the consultation skills that you hope to demonstrate in your exam, the more likely you are to be able to use them fluently when under pressure.

Each case has one page for the doctor (**Doctor's Notes**). Once you've completed your consultation, turn over the page to find our suggested **Example Consultation**. You can also read the **Learning Points**, which cover the important facts or guidelines relevant to the case, on the flip side of the **Patient's Story**.

Where we have provided learning points from NICE or other sources, you should always refer to the latest version of the full guidance as this changes frequently, and please remember that this guidance is only applicable to UK patients.

When we suggest a medication, you should always refer to the most up-to-date version of the BNF, as well as NICE guidelines, as indications, dosages and other aspects may have changed.

Instructions for the patient

The presenting complaint (PC) is the *'opening gambit'*. Further information should be given only if the doctor asks relevant questions. In the exam, the simulated patient is likely to pause after the opening gambit, waiting for the doctor to ask a question and find out more. Remember that, although 'real' patients may deliver a 'speech' full of everything you need to know, if you are playing the role of 'patient' avoid this as it does not give the doctor the opportunity to showcase data-gathering skills. As the consultation progresses, you may freely give the doctor anything in quotation marks. Avoid over-sharing! The simulated patients in the exam will respond to questions and appropriate non-verbal skills, but will not spontaneously volunteer large amounts of information.

Instructions for the doctor

In the exam, you should assume that the correct patient is in front of you: there is no need to check the identity of the patient, other than briefly, and this can save precious seconds. Also remember that the simulated patient is unlikely to volunteer anything more than their opening gambit, so practise having different ways to respond to opening gambits that encourage a patient to tell you more. We suggest using our **FOCUS model**, which has been broken down into elements in each Example Consultation, as a guide. Include all these elements and you have an excellent consultation, but be flexible, so that the consultation is conversational.

Instructions for the examiner or time keeper

Remember that, in the SCA, the examination clock starts ticking at the first moment of the consultation (no longer after introductions) and stops at exactly 12 minutes, even if the doctor or patient is in the middle of a sentence. During and after the consultation, mark the 'Generic feedback' card. We have also provided tick boxes on each Example Consultation page and you could mark these as the consultation progresses.

Constructive criticism is essential.

Agree on the rules for constructive feedback before you start and always be honest with each other! For marking, you can use:

- The RCGP marking criteria – see 'How to Demonstrate Skills: The Marking Scheme Made Easy'.
- The 'Generic Feedback' card.
- The tick boxes within the Example Consultations.

Blueprint Groups for the SCA Exam

The SCA exam has introduced a new term – blueprint groups.[2] There are 12 of these and, between them, they ensure that the SCA exam covers as much of the curriculum as possible, within the constraints of a remote exam. Areas that the exam cannot cover, such as clinical skills in examining patients, are tested in other ways such as workplace-based assessment.

The 12 blueprint groups are:

1. Patient less than 19 years old
2. Gender, reproductive and sexual health, including women's, men's, LGBTQ+, gynae and breast
3. Long-term conditions, including cancer, multi-morbidity and disability
4. Older adults, including frailty and people at the end of life
5. Mental health, including addiction, smoking, alcohol and substance misuse
6. Urgent and unscheduled care
7. Health disadvantage and vulnerabilities, including veterans, mental capacity, safeguarding and communication difficulties
8. Ethnicity, culture, diversity and inclusivity
9. New presentation of undifferentiated disease
10. Prescribing
11. Investigation/results
12. Professional conversation/professional dilemma

RCGP Curriculum

The RCGP defines and describes the GP curriculum – the competencies and capabilities that you need to develop (and demonstrate through evidence) to become an effective and safe GP. You can find this on the RCGP website, but we describe it in this chapter for convenience and to explain which areas are tested by the exam and are therefore particularly relevant to this book.

The RCGP curriculum has different facets:

- The topic guides:
  - Professional topics
  - Life stages
  - Clinical topics
- The core statement – being a general practitioner

We will look first at how the topic guides are related to the blueprint groups of the exam, and then explore aspects of the core statement, **'Being a general practitioner'**, as these link well with the marking scheme.

The Curriculum Topic Guides and the Exam (Professional, Life Stages, Clinical)

How do the professional topics link with the exam?

There are six professional topics and the RCGP gives examples of how each may be tested in the SCA.

1. **Consulting in general practice.** Example: *An older woman asks about options for euthanasia when her condition worsens. A hospital letter confirms her diagnosis of motor neurone disease.*
2. **Equality, diversity and inclusion.** Example: *A Muslim man with insulin-dependent diabetes wishes to fast during Ramadan.*
3. **Evidence in practice, research, teaching and lifelong learning.** Example phone call: *A father wants to know why an antibiotic was not prescribed during an earlier consultation for his child, who now has acute otitis media.*
4. **Continuity and quality of care, safety and prescribing.** Example: *Your practice nurse sustains a needle-stick injury while taking blood from an intravenous drug user.*
5. **Leadership, management and administration.** Example: *A patient who is a receptionist in the practice requests sick leave because she is being bullied by the practice manager.*
6. **Population and planetary health.** Example: *A Bangladeshi man who is also overweight and smokes e-cigarettes attends for results of cardiovascular disease (CVD) assessment which show impaired fasting glycaemia.*

How do the life stages link with the exam?

There is clear overlap between the four life stages and the blueprint groups, with the blueprint group 'older adults' covering both 'older adults' and 'end of life':

1. **Children and young people**
2. **People with long-term conditions, including cancer**
3. **Older adults**
4. **End of life**

The table on the following page illustrates this.

The Curriculum Topic Guides and the Exam (Professional, Life Stages, Clinical)

How the blueprint groups relate to the life stages of the curriculum

	Blueprint groups 1–12											
Life stages	1. <19	2. Gender	3. LTC	4. Older	5. MH	6. Urgent	7. Vulnerable	8. Ethnicity	9. New problem	10. Rx	11. Ix, Mx	12. Prof. conversation
Children + young people	✓	⚠	⚠	✗	⚠	⚠	⚠	⚠	⚠	⚠	⚠	⚠
LTCs, including cancer	✗	⚠	✓	✓	⚠	⚠	⚠	⚠	✗	⚠	⚠	⚠
Older adults	✗	✗	⚠	✓	⚠	⚠	⚠	⚠	⚠	⚠	⚠	⚠
End of life	✗	⚠	⚠	✓	⚠	⚠	⚠	⚠	✗	⚠	⚠	⚠

Key:

✓ Clear connection between blueprint group and topic

⚠ Likely to be overlap – e.g. a young person or an older adult might have an ENT problem

✗ Although there may be an overlap, this is less likely – e.g. a young person is relatively unlikely to be at the end of life

How do the clinical topics link with the exam?

The 22 clinical topics cover all areas of the clinical curriculum from 'Allergy and clinical immunology' through to 'Urgent and unscheduled care'. Here is the complete list:

1. Allergy and clinical immunology
2. Cardiovascular health
3. Dermatology
4. ENT, speech and hearing
5. Eyes and vision
6. Gastroenterology
7. Genomic medicine
8. Gynaecology and breast health
9. Haematology
10. Infectious diseases and travel health
11. Learning disability
12. Maternity and reproductive health
13. Mental health
14. Metabolic problems and endocrinology
15. Musculoskeletal health
16. Neurodevelopmental conditions and neurodiversity
17. Neurology
18. Renal and urology
19. Respiratory health

The Curriculum Topic Guides and the Exam (Professional, Life Stages, Clinical)

20. Sexual health
21. Smoking, alcohol and substance misuse
22. Urgent and unscheduled care

Any of these may be tested in the SCA and clearly many could form part of several different blueprint groups. For example, the blueprint group *'Gender, reproductive and sexual health, including women's, men's, LGBTQ+, gynae and breast'* includes:

7. Genomic medicine
8. Gynaecology and breast health
10. Infectious diseases
20. Sexual health
22. Urgent and unscheduled care

The Core Statement

The RCGP **core statement 'Being a general practitioner'** is divided into five general areas of capability and each of these is subdivided, so there are 13 specific areas of capability for general practice:

1. **Knowing yourself and relating to others**
   a. Fitness to practise
   b. An ethical approach
   c. Communicating and consulting
2. **Applying clinical knowledge and skill**
   a. Data gathering and interpretation
   b. Clinical examination and procedural skills
   c. Making decisions
   d. Clinical management
3. **Managing complex and long-term care**
   a. Medical complexity
   b. Team working
4. **Working well in organisations and systems of care**
   a. Performance, learning and teaching
   b. Organisation, management and leadership
5. **Caring for the whole person and wider community and the environment**
   a. Holistic practice, health promotion and safeguarding
   b. Community health and environmental sustainability

The RCGP website gives detailed descriptions and explanations of each of these areas and can be accessed online.

RCGP Capabilities

The marking scheme for the exam relates to the RCGP capabilities, which fit within the three exam domains of data gathering and making a diagnosis, clinical management and medical complexity and relating to others.[3] When analysing your consultations, you might ask yourself which of the 13 capabilities you demonstrated and how you did this. Here are the 13 capabilities and the domains in which you may be able to demonstrate your skills. As a reminder, the three domains are:

- Data gathering and making a diagnosis (DG&D)
- Clinical management and medical complexity (CM&C)
- Relating to others (RTO)

The 13 capabilities are:

1. **Fitness to practise (DG&D, CM&C, RTO)**

   Demonstrate the attitudes and behaviours expected of a good doctor. Where a doctor is aware that their actions, behaviours or health, or those of others, may put patients at risk, they should take steps to protect them

2. **An ethical approach (RTO)**

   Treat others fairly and with respect, acting without discrimination or prejudice

   Provide care with compassion and kindness

   Promote an environment of inclusivity, safety, cultural humility and freedom to speak up

3. **Communicating and consulting (DG&D, CM&C, RTO)**

   Establish effective partnerships through a range of in-person and remote consulting modalities

   Manage the additional challenge of consultations with patients who have particular communication needs or who have different languages, cultures, beliefs and educational backgrounds, to your own

   Maintain continuing relationships with patients, carers and families

4. **Data gathering and interpretation (DG&D)**

   Apply an organised approach to data gathering and investigation

   Interpret findings accurately and appropriately

5. **Clinical examination and procedural skills (CEPS) (DG&D)**

   Demonstrate a proficient approach to clinical examination and procedural skills

6. **Decision making and diagnosis (DG&D)**

   Adopt appropriate decision-making principles based on shared understanding

   Use best available, current, valid and relevant evidence

7. **Clinical management (CM&C, RTO)**

   Provide collaborative clinical care to patients that supports their autonomy

   Use a reasoned approach to clinical management that includes supported self-care

   Make appropriate use of other professionals and services

   Provide urgent care when needed

8. **Medical complexity (DG&D, CM&C, RTO)**

   Enable people living with long-term conditions to optimise their health

   Use a personalised approach to manage and monitor concurrent health problems for individual patients

   Manage risk and uncertainty while adopting safe and effective approaches for patients with complex needs

   Coordinate and oversee patient care across healthcare systems

RCGP Capabilities

9. **Team working** (RTO)
   Work as an effective member of multiprofessional and diverse teams
   Lead and coordinate a team-based approach to patient care
10. **Performance, learning and teaching** (DG&D, CM&C, RTO)
   Continuously evaluate and improve the care you provide
   Adopt a safe and evidence-informed approach to improve quality of care
   Support the education and professional development of colleagues
11. **Organisation, management and leadership** (RTO)
   Advocate for medical generalism in healthcare
   Apply leadership skills to improve your organisation's performance
   Make effective use of data, technology and communication systems to provide better patient care
   Develop the financial and business skills required for your role
12. **Holistic practice, health promotion and safeguarding** (CM&C, RTO)
   Demonstrate the holistic mindset of a generalist medical practitioner
   Support people through their experiences of health, illness and recovery with a personalised approach
   Safeguard individuals, families and local populations
13. **Community health and environmental sustainability** (RTO)
   Understand the health service and your role within it
   Build relationships with the communities in which you work
   Promote population and planetary health

How the capability areas fit with the marking domains of the SCA exam

Capability area	DG&D	CM&C	RTO
Fitness to practise	✓	✓	✓
Ethical approach	✗	✗	✓
Communicating and consulting	✓	✓	✓
Data gathering and interpretation	✓	✗	✗
CEPS	✓	✗	✗
Decision making and diagnosis	✓	✗	✗
Clinical management	✗	✓	✓
Medical complexity	✓	✓	✓
Team working	✗	✗	✓
Performance, learning and teaching	✓	✓	✓
Organisation, management and leadership	✗	✗	✓
Holistic practice, health promotion and safeguarding	✗	✓	✓
Community health and environmental sustainability	✗	✗	✓

Key:

✓ Capability area is **likely** to be evidenced and marked in this domain

✗ Capability area is **unlikely** to be evidenced and marked in this domain

Consultation Models

You may well have been taught a framework or model for your consultations and this is one of the RCGP's 13 capabilities: **'Communicating and consulting'**. Using a tried and tested structure can help to ensure that you remember all the key phases and don't leave anything out. As we have described already, the exam is marked in three different domains, and we will explore how some of the common models fit with this and which skills contribute to each domain. Although the individual models differ in their detail, most conform broadly to the following five-stage structure:

- Find out why the patient has come
- Work out what's wrong
- Explain the problem(s) to the patient
- Develop a management plan and share this with the patient
- Use time well and efficiently

Some also have a sixth stage – take care of yourself. This is very important for both exam purposes and life beyond as an independent practitioner.

Remember that the exam marking domains are:

- **Data gathering and diagnosis:** Find out why the patient has come, work out what's wrong and make a diagnosis or state your impression.
- **Clinical management and medical complexity:** Explain the problem to the patient and develop and negotiate a management plan.
- **Relating to others:** Evidenced throughout the consultation from beginning to end.

It is vital to use your 12 minutes effectively and efficiently because if you run out of time before you get to the management plan you will score no marks in that area – a recipe for a disappointing outcome and particularly so with the potential 150% weighting of the domain 'Clinical management and medical complexity'.

Looking after yourself between each consultation is vital otherwise one 'bad' consultation will lead to another. In the exam, some people, after a difficult or dysfunctional simulated consultation, will use any time between patients to pore over the previous patient's notes or reflect on what they did or didn't do. They try to work out what went wrong, rather than putting the consultation out of their mind and spending precious moments reading and thinking about the next patient. Don't let this happen to you! Similarly, after a real consultation that may not have gone well, or has left you feeling strong emotions, it is important to regather your thoughts, 'housekeep' and focus before seeing the next patient, putting aside time later in the day to reflect on that difficult consultation, perhaps with the help of others.

Let's look at some common consultation models and see where the different stages fit within the exam marking structure.

Consultation Models

Pendleton (1984)[4]

This is one of the first patient-centred models, with seven tasks.

A. **Data gathering and diagnosis**

   1. Find out why the patient has come, including the problem (cause, effects, history) and the patient's ideas, concerns and expectations.
   2. Consider other problems.

B. **Clinical management and medical complexity**

   3. Choose (with the patient) an appropriate action for each problem.
   4. Achieve a shared understanding of the problems.
   5. Involve the patient in the management and encourage them to accept appropriate responsibility.
   6. Use time and resources appropriately.

C. **Relating to others**

   7. Establish or maintain a relationship with the patient that helps to achieve the other tasks.

Helman (1981)[5]

Although this isn't a model of consultation, Cecil Helman, a medical anthropologist, described six questions that any patient might have in their head when coming to see the doctor. It is well worth bearing these in mind when data gathering, particularly around ICE (ideas, concerns and expectations) and in clinical management, when you are explaining to the patient. Armed with the patient's own thoughts, fears and hopes, the answers to these questions could provide a useful framework for your explanation.

1. What has happened?
2. Why has it happened?
3. Why to me?
4. Why now?
5. What would happen if nothing was done about it?
6. What should I do about it or whom should I consult for further help?

Consultation Models

Neighbour (1987)[6]

This is a five-part model 'anchored' to the fingers of the left hand, so relatively easy to remember even when you are stressed.

A. **Data gathering and diagnosis**

1. **Connecting:** This stage is about rapport building (relating to others) as well as gathering data. 'Connection' starts the moment you first see, or hear, the patient. Look at the patient and listen to them, what do you notice? How do they seem? What is this telling you? Tune in to the patient to get on their wavelength. Explore their story until you have enough information to summarise.
2. **Summarising:** If you are unsure, or even in a consultation 'hole' where you are struggling, summarising is the best tool to get you back on track again.

B. **Clinical management and medical complexity**

3. **Handing over:** This is where the doctor and patient negotiate and agree a management plan and empower the patient by 'hand over' of control.
4. **Safety netting:** Safety netting ensures there are safe contingency plans. Neighbour describes a really robust structure for a three-point safety net. A vague '*come back if you're no better*' is unlikely to score you any marks in the RCGP consultation skills exam, so learn and use this structure for consultations that need a safety net (not all do):
   i. This is what I expect to happen.
   ii. This is how you [the patient] will know if I'm wrong.
   iii. If that happens, this is what you should do.

   Easy and safe!

C. **Relating to others**

5. As with other models, these interpersonal skills run as a thread from beginning to end of the consultation. Neighbour's fifth stage is 'Housekeeping'. In his book, he describes a number of quick and easy ways to deal with stress and negative feelings that have arisen during the consultation so that you can ensure you are in the best shape ready for the next patient. It is well worth a read. These techniques are easy to learn and applicable to all your future consultations.

Consultation Models

Calgary Cambridge[7]

This is a very comprehensive and evidence-based approach to the consultation – another five-stage model that includes specific detail of tools and techniques.

A. Data gathering and diagnosis

1. Initiating the session:

   Introductions

   Establishing rapport

   Finding out the reason for the consultation

2. Gathering information:

   Exploring the patient's perspective using a range of verbal and non-verbal communication skills including open and closed questions, ICE, clarification, summarising, etc. Finding out 'Why now?' – the universal question of the consultation is 'Why has this patient come today with this problem?' If you can't answer this by the end of the consultation, you may well have missed something important!

B. Clinical management and medical complexity

3. Explanation and planning:

   Finds out what the patient knows

   Asks what the patient wants to know

   'Chunks and checks' – information in digestible chunks

   Careful timing of explanations – not too soon

4. Closing the session:

   Safety nets and follow-up

C. Relating to others

5. Building the relationship:

   Developing rapport

   Accepting the patient's views as legitimate

   Using non-verbal behaviour

   Involving the patient (e.g. thinking aloud, explicitly describing examination process and findings)

Calgary Cambridge also explores the very important feature of providing structure to the consultation by approaching it logically, using mini-summaries and keeping to time. All very important – a messy disordered consultation is inefficient.

Consultation Models

6S for success[8]

This approach was developed in 2013 by Alex Watson using an alliterative, easy to remember '6S' model. Story, Summarising, Sharing, Securing, Status, Sanity.

A. **Data gathering and diagnosis**

1. **Story:** Connecting with the patient, being attentive, letting them tell their story, demonstrating verbally and non-verbally that you are listening to what they are saying. Find out thoughts, hopes and fears. Find the subplot if there is one.
2. **Summarising:** An opportunity to review what has been said so far, non-judgementally. The patient feels listened to and there is opportunity to clarify, add additional information and correct any misunderstandings before moving on.

B. **Clinical management and medical complexity**

3. **Sharing:** Moving from listening to discussion about management, including the patient's thoughts, fears and hopes and incorporating the doctor's view. Any risks can also be discussed and shared between doctor and patient.
4. **Securing:** Safety netting the consultation, securing the evidence by making notes. (Written notes are, of course, not currently assessed by the RCGP in the final clinical/consultation skills assessment exam!)

C. **Relating to others**

5. **Status:** Again, something that overarches and underpins the consultation: how we behave with others, how they perceive us and we perceive them and how this affects the consultation for good or bad. A mid-level point is the most helpful so that the clinician takes care to be warm, interested and on a level with the patient, avoiding the unhelpful extremes of arrogance/aloofness and timidity/being apologetic.
6. **Sanity:** Watson's sixth stage is 'Sanity' – similar to housekeeping described by Neighbour. Making sure that you are in good shape for the next patient and for your future in general practice.

CHAPTER 1C SKILLS REQUIRED FOR THIS EXAM AND MARKING THOSE SKILLS

FOCUS Consultation Model

We developed the FOCUS consultation model to help you demonstrate the skills required for the RCGP clinical and consultation skills exam. We don't expect you to learn and remember all the elements and a formulaic approach is not natural. We encourage you to find your own style – be flexible. However, the more you practise these elements, the more fluent you will become, so that you can use them with ease when you need to.

Consider how long you will allow yourself for each element. If an element is taking longer, keep bringing the patient back into the discussion, e.g. checking their understanding or reaction.

What does FOCUS represent?

F – Filter

O – Opportunity

C – Context

U – Unite

S – Safety

FILTER

Start your data gathering with many open questions, then group together closed questions (risk assessment and red flags) to focus the history as you formulate a potential hypothesis. If appropriate, check history, past medical history (PMH), drug history (DH), family history (FH) and social history (SH) – to look for relevant information that will ultimately affect diagnosis and management. When you make use of information from the notes, state this out loud so that you can discuss it with the patient if needed.

OPPORTUNITY

This is your opportunity to connect with the patient and demonstrate interpersonal skills, which are part of the relating to others (RTO) domain. Remember that these are not an assessment of being polite or articulate. Interpersonal skills are about making a connection, demonstrating a genuine interest in the person, and most importantly how you tailor the rest of the consultation to meet the patient's needs based on information they have shared. Use identified **cues** to give the patient the opportunity to discuss their ICE (ideas, concerns and expectations).

Be curious, sense how they are feeling and assess the impact of their symptoms on their life.

'Filter' and 'Opportunity' can be done in any order, and may well be interspersed. We would encourage trying to discover the 'Opportunity' information early in the consultation, particularly with vaguer presentations with no immediately clear clinical problem.

CONTEXT

This is where you question 'What is going on here?' and is the moment for the doctor and patient to come together on the same page. Think about how the information discovered in 'Filter' is affected by/relates to the information gathered in 'Opportunity'. The skill includes stating your impression regarding the potential diagnosis or differential diagnoses. Another important skill is referring to ICE within your explanation, and a statement of empathy reflects the challenges the patient is facing (problem + fears + social context).

FOCUS Consultation Model

UNITE

Share the management plan to unite doctor and patient. Discuss your recommendation as well as options: what can the patient do (demonstrating empowerment); what can I do; what can others (specialists/family) do; and finally what resources (websites, support groups, patient information leaflets) are available? Be specific regarding medicines, follow-up plans and logistics.

SAFETY

Always offer a specific safety net – What do they need to look out for? How long should they wait before returning? What should they do if they feel they are getting worse? What actions are required for both the doctor and patient? The safety net should not be overstated; think about what is realistic. A safety net rarely needs to include 999 and A&E as anticipated outcomes. It may be as simple as '*If you don't receive your appointment within 7 days, please let us know*' (e.g. urgent cancer referral but patient is well).

The diagrammatic model illustrates how the model links to the RCGP mark scheme.

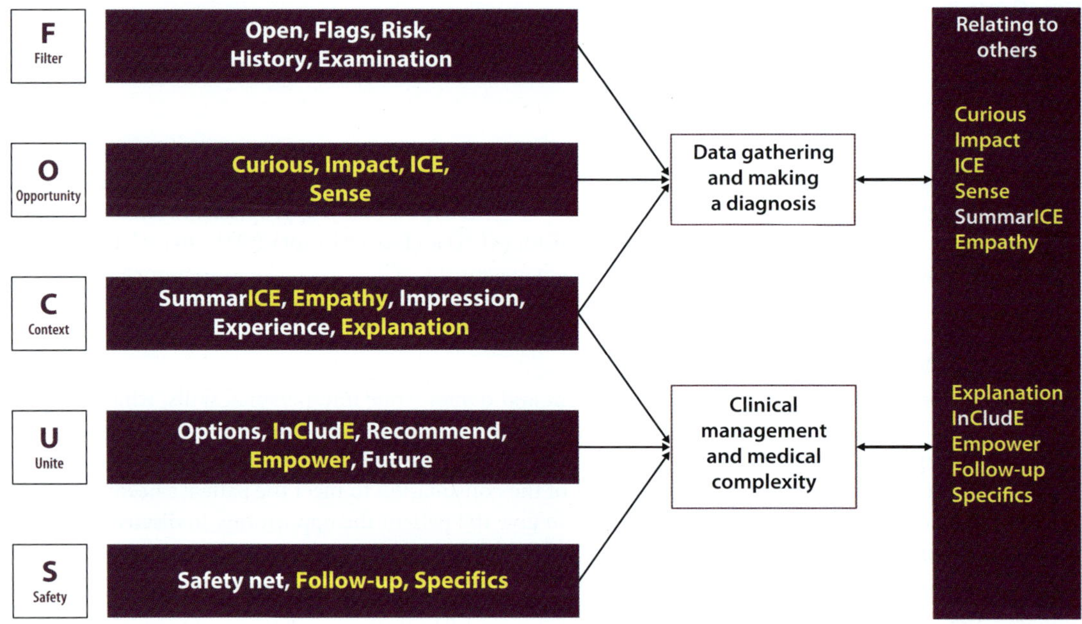

FOCUS Consultation Model

The **FOCUS consultation model** groups the key **elements** of the consultation.

FILTER

Open Ask as many open questions as possible to collect the story.

Flags Use focused questions. Check for red flags and whittle down differentials.

Risk Ask about risk factors for your suspected diagnosis.

History Take the history: past, systemic, family, medicines and social.

Examination Appropriate physical or mental examination, or both. In the SCA, the clinical examination findings may already be given on the doctor's notes. You may need to undertake mental health examination, for example to assess depression.

OPPORTUNITY

Curious Respond to verbal cues and explore.

E.g. *'You mentioned your friend. What is their experience of ...?'*

Impact Find out how the problem has affected the patient: open questions about impact can be very effective at the beginning of the consultation. Use this information to smoothly transition to ICE.

ICE Explore ideas, concerns and expectations. There is no need to ask these as a triad of questions – and the consultation may flow much better if you don't! If the patient tells you a thought they have had, use this opportunity to ask about other ideas or thoughts they may have had. If they express worries, or look anxious, use this moment to ask about concerns. Finally, 'expectations' is often much better asked just before you make a diagnosis and move into a plan.

Ideas – *'This is clearly affecting you a lot day to day. Have you had thoughts about what is going on?'*

Concerns – *'You said you were worried it might be pneumonia. What in particular worries you about that possibility? And did anything else go through your mind that worried you?'*

Expectations – *'I'm going to be making many suggestions but I am interested to know if there was anything specific you were hoping I might do?'*

Sense Reflect what you sense (feelings or emotions) from non-verbal cues.

E.g. *'I feel/can see that you are (fidgeting/breathless/distracted/in a rush) ...'*

FOCUS Consultation Model

CONTEXT

SummarICE Demonstrate that you have listened by summarising the ICE. This is a great tool for leading into management.

Empathy Show you have put the problem into the context of their life.

E.g. *'I can understand that your past experience of … could lead you to consider …'*

Impression State your impression! Make a diagnosis if you can, or state the likely differentials.

Experience Check their understanding or experience of what you have diagnosed. Incorporate what you have learnt from ICE.

Explanation Provide a concise and jargon-free explanation. Tell the patient what they need to know; don't bombard them with extra unnecessary detail, however much you know. Avoid being the 'clever doctor' who bamboozles the patient with jargon, acronyms and unsettling details they really don't need to know.

UNITE

Options Provide an organised list of options. Confirm their understanding and interest. A useful framework includes: *'Things that you can do …, I can do …, others can help with …'*

InCludE Incorporate what you have learnt from asking and listening to the patient's expectations.

Recommend As well as options, you should also help guide the patient's decision by stating your own recommendation for the way forward.

Empower Suggest what the patient can do themselves to help the problem.

Future Explain what you believe should or is likely to happen at the next steps.

E.g. *'Thinking ahead … Return to the GP in …'*

E.g. *'At the hospital you can expect to …'*

SAFETY

Safety net Give clear instructions about what to look out for and what the patient should do in these circumstances.

Follow-up Will you need to see the patient again? If so, when and how should they make this arrangement?

Specifics Remember to be specific about time intervals, for example who is booking an appointment, with whom, in what situation?

Remember to ask:

Paediatrics: gestation, delivery, postnatal, immunisations and development.

Women's health: last menstrual period, cycle, post-coital bleeding, intermenstrual bleeding, discharge, smears, parity and operations.

ICE, SummarICE and InCludE

Eliciting a patient's thoughts, fears and hopes can build rapport and address expectations. We recommend not just that you elicit ICE, but also that you make use of it! Many GP registrars forget to do this. We suggest the following easy to remember technique.

1. Elicit ICE – the questions that you ask to find out thoughts, fears and hopes are by nature **open** questions:
   - *'What do you think is happening?'* – Thoughts, open question.
   - *'What worries you about this?'* – Worries, open question.
   - *'Did you have anything in mind that you hoped we might do today?'* – Hopes, open question.

   We recommend you find out thoughts, worries and hopes about what might happen at appropriate times within the consultation. This may well mean separating them. It is very unnatural to ask the questions in succession and sounds formulaic.

   'What are you thinking? And what are you worried about? And what do you hope the outcome of today's consultation might be?' This series of questions, asked back to back, sounds unnatural – it would not happen in a conversation. In particular, 'hopes' are often best asked just before the midpoint.

   Therefore, you will see these elements displayed within our **Example Consultations** as:
   - **ICE1** – this represents 'Thoughts'. What the patient is thinking might be wrong.
   - **ICE2** – this represents 'Fears'. What the patient is worrying about, in respect of their symptoms. Is it going to get worse? Am I going to die? etc.
   - **ICE3** – this represents 'Hopes'. What the patient has in their mind for the future – for example aspects of the management plan. Do they need a referral, an X-ray, a prescription, etc?
2. Use this information in the midpoint summary – **SummarICE** – to demonstrate that you have heard the patient.
3. Include this information when negotiating a plan – **InCludE**.

Elicit ICE

With good rapport and attentive listening, any or all components of ICE may emerge naturally as the patient is talking to you, particularly if you use open questions. If they emerge readily, it is worth exploring deeper. For example, *'You said you were worried about X; what else worried you? Did any other possibilities go through your mind?'* If the components of ICE are not forthcoming, you may need to use some specific prompts.

Ideas/Thoughts

What does the patient think about their symptoms? In their eyes, what might the problem be? If it's not crystal clear, ask! If the patient says *'nothing'*, this is unlikely to be true: it's just that the patient has not yet felt able to tell you. Ask again, rephrase the question; show that you are interested in the patient's thoughts through rapport, such as eye contact, nodding, minimal encouragers, giving the patient your whole attention and allowing space to listen. Remember, their thoughts may have come from:

- Past experience
- Other people's experience – friends, work colleagues, neighbours
- The internet
- Newspaper articles, TV programmes – factual and fictional

There may be cues to follow – *'I read in the paper that …', 'John thinks …', 'I had this before and …'* or *'A friend at work …'*

ICE, SummarICE and InCludE

Concerns/Worries

What has worried the patient enough to make an appointment with you? You could try:

- '*I sense you are worried about this.*' (Pause and listen.) This is a statement used as a question, so is softer and less blunt than '*What are you worrying about?*' which may lead to the answer '*Nothing*' (unlikely to be true) or something that may not be directly relevant (my job/debt/the neighbours).
- '*Is there anything, however unlikely, that you are particularly worried this might be?*'
- If someone else has been mentioned (my friend, John, my husband/wife/daughter), make use of this and try '*Tell me what worries your friend/John, etc. about this.*'

Remember that you cannot second-guess what the patient's worries might be – they are unique to that person. If you try and guess, you may well be wrong. Their thoughts or worries may be incorrect or implausible, but they are the patient's reality – hold on to them so that you can use them later.

Expectations

Finding out what the patient is hoping for from you will potentially save you a lot of time later, whether or not it is a practical or appropriate way forward. Try:

- '*What did you have in mind that I might be able to do for you?*'
- '*When you booked the appointment/were sitting in the waiting room, was there anything in particular you were hoping for from today?*'
- '*From your reading/talking to ... about this problem, did you discover anything that you thought could be helpful?*'

Remember not to ask this too early, otherwise it might come across as if you don't know and are asking the patient for a clue to the way ahead. Try '*I've already got some thoughts myself about what we could do but I am interested to hear what you think.*'

SummarICE (Summarise ICE)

When you know you have enough information to formulate a diagnosis and a plan, including all three components of ICE, summarising is an excellent way to demonstrate to the patient that you have heard what they've said and to mark the transition from data gathering to clinical management.

Instead of summarising all the history, try summarising ICE, i.e. SummarICE. Perhaps also include impact – the way the problem is affecting the patient's life.

- '*You've had this cough for more than a week. You thought it might be a chest infection needing antibiotics, but at the back of your mind you are worried about cancer, given that you smoked until recently. It's been hard to sleep at night for coughing, so your husband's moved into the spare room.*'
- '*For a month or so you've had chest pain when you walk which you thought might be muscle strain from trimming the hedge, but you were also concerned about your heart and were hoping I might do a chest X-ray and heart tracing/refer you to the hospital.*'

This is a more time-efficient and tailored summary than going through all the symptoms again.

ICE, SummarICE and InCludE

InCludE (Include ICE)

The midpoint summary will remind you to include the patient's ideas and concerns when stating your 'Impression':

- *'You thought this might be a chest infection – having listened to your symptoms and examined you, I agree/I don't think it is.'*
- *'I don't think it's likely that the chest pain when you walk is connected with muscle strain from using the hedge trimmer. The fact that it comes on when you exercise and goes when you stop might suggest pain from the heart muscle, called angina.'*
- *'You were worried about cancer – although unlikely because you haven't lost weight or coughed up blood [red flags], I agree it is something we should exclude.'*

You can include expectations either here or a little later when negotiating the plan:

- *'As you've had the symptoms for a week, and I can hear signs of infection in your chest, I agree an antibiotic may well help.'*
- *'You mentioned a chest X-ray – I don't think that would add much at this stage but if you still have symptoms in a week, we should think about one then.'*

Practising the Skills within FOCUS

Recognise your strengths! Then consider which elements you find the most challenging.

Target your revision. Analyse and fine tune each microskill, a day at a time.

FILTER

Be assertive and sharpen your history.

Non-verbal Use videos to analyse non-verbal communication.

Open Concentrate on routinely asking a series of encouraging/open questions – at least three before you move to semi-closed or closed questions. Can you rephrase your questions? For example, *'When did it start?'* is a semi-closed question, but *'How did it start*?' is open and will yield much richer answers.

History Critique your consultations. Do you ask questions that actually change your management?

OPPORTUNITY

Use every opportunity to explore cues and find out ICE and impact.

Curious Work on reacting to those cues, e.g. repeating phrases back to patients.

ICE Ensure you have found the answers to all three questions. If a patient has already provided you with the information, to demonstrate you were listening, acknowledge this and consider asking questions to explore if there's more to be found. The way the questions are phrased can make or break a consultation. For example, '*What would you like me to do?*' may be received negatively, whereas *'I'm going to be making many suggestions, but was there anything specific you were hoping for today?*' enhances rapport and shared understanding.

Impact/Sense To find out impact, you need to know something about the patient's life as well as the problem and ask or explore how the two are related. Put a Post-it note on your desk at work to remind you to do this; write it on your whiteboard in the exam.

CONTEXT

The midpoint when you empathise, SummarICE, state your impression and explain.

Empathy and SummarICE With every patient you see, practise summarising their ICE followed by a statement that links the ICE to their background, experience or situation.

Impression and Experience Always ensure you state your impression/diagnosis at 5–6 minutes followed by a pause.

Explanation Practise giving clear and concise explanations for diagnoses and your recommendations.

Practising the Skills within FOCUS

UNITE

The negotiated and shared management plan.

Options Organise your thoughts and practise using a three-dimensional approach. Think about what you can do, what the patient can do (self-help) and where others (friends, family, referrals) could help. Using this framework will help you to produce a structured management plan for almost any presenting problem.

InCludE *'You were worried about … and thought we should do … However, what's going through my mind is … What would you like to do?'*

Recommend Have the confidence to state *'My recommendation is … Other options are …'*

Empower *'Things you may be interested in are … What are your thoughts?'*

Future *'We should catch up to discuss this again; how about in …'* Have you been specific? Is it clear to the patient what steps you and they are taking regarding any agreed logistics and management?

SAFETY

The essential safety net and good documentation.

Safety net Although you don't need to write up notes in the SCA exam, practise excellent documentation when consulting with patients in your clinics. Any safety net should be specific and watching recorded consultations can help you check how clear yours is. Remember the three-point safety net – *'This is what I expect to happen … This is how you will know if I'm wrong … This is what to do then.'* The safety net should of course always be tailored to the patient and the problem. It should flow naturally from what has been discussed in the consultation and should provide reassurance and empowerment for the patient, rather than baffling or scaring them unnecessarily. It is unhelpful and inappropriate to use *'Call 999'* as a backstop at the end of a safety net for a self-limiting and relatively minor problem.

Remember that few consultations need a catch-all safety net for every eventuality, however unlikely. For example: a 30-year-old female patient phones you and describes intermittent diarrhoea and vague abdominal pain for the last year. There are no red flag symptoms at all and she has had no symptoms of any sort for several days. You are planning to see her tomorrow to examine her and suspect she might have IBS. A 'safety net' that infers she might develop an acute abdomen before you see her, and need to go immediately to hospital, is inappropriate for this patient and her symptoms. It is likely to be confusing and unnecessarily increase any anxiety. A much simpler statement *'I'll see you tomorrow as we agreed. I don't imagine your symptoms will change between now and then but please phone the surgery if they do'* is all that is needed.

How to Demonstrate Skills: The Marking Scheme Made Easy

Data gathering and diagnosis is about uncovering the clinical information appropriate to the problem/s presented by the patient. This process should be efficient and logical, using appropriate open and closed questions, including finding out risk factors and red flags.

Acknowledging information from the notes may include the medical history, medications, investigations and colleagues' consultations and examination findings.

Sharing your diagnosis – skills of how to approach this are discussed later in this chapter.

Clinical management and medical complexity should reflect the differential diagnosis that you have made and be feasible and evidence based, taking account of any identified risks. In the exam, it is highly likely that you will already have been given all the relevant examination findings (e.g. the patient was seen by a colleague yesterday) and all examination is documented in the information that you have. Therefore, you should be able to use this to describe an actual management plan, even though the consultation is remote and you have not personally examined the patient.

When demonstrating skills in medical complexity, the first skill is to recognise the complexity that emerges through excellent data-gathering skills, and then the challenge is to manage the complexity.

Managing medical complexity in the SCA

For the first time in the consultation skills examination, managing medical complexity is explicitly mentioned in the marking domains. It has always been there but is now at the forefront of the mark scheme. Not only is it mentioned, but there is now weighting in the management domain adding to the importance of this skill. We believe this is due to an appreciation that the ability to manage medical complexity is fast becoming a GP's USP, or unique selling point to borrow from the marketing world.

So, what does it mean? Often when we ask GP registrars this question, the first thing that comes to mind is co-morbidity; managing a problem in the context of other illnesses, but then they get stuck. Co-morbidity is certainly an element of medical complexity, but it is only part of the story.

The definition of managing medical complexity given by the RCGP is *'Aspects of care beyond managing straight-forward problems including management of co-morbidity, uncertainty, risk and focusing on health rather than illness'*.

Breaking this down, there are four key areas:

1. Co-morbidity
2. Uncertainty
3. Risk
4. Health rather than illness

Another way of thinking about it is to consider building up different layers of complexity or adding in dilemmas. The layers and dilemmas begin to make a simple problem no longer seem so simple.

Let's look at each of the elements and how they may become apparent during your cases.

Co-morbidity

Co-morbidity adds to complexity by causing interactions between conditions themselves or the treatments we use. Co-morbidity is usually obvious – we can see long lists of significant problems and medications when we open the patient's medical record. In your exam, any significant co-morbidity will be identified in the case notes. Which conditions are listed? Which medications are prescribed? Can you see anything which may complicate care such as chronic kidney disease? What about the medication list? Are there any risky medications there such as ACE inhibitors, diuretics or immunosuppressives? Does anything jump out at you as not quite right, perhaps multiple stomach irritating medications and no gastroprotection? Medications which interact? Co-morbidity often leads to dilemmas. You may find yourself thinking 'normally I would do X but due to Y I can't'. This is an indication of complexity. It is useful to voice this dilemma when explaining to the patient their options: *'Normally I would suggest X but because of Y I think Z might be a better option for you. What do you think?'*

Uncertainty

Uncertainty occurs in two primary ways – firstly, uncertainty felt by the doctor, secondly, uncertainty felt by the patient. If there is uncertainty felt by the doctor, you are likely to be aware of this as you are wondering what approach to take or what the best next step is (in an exam setting your heart may be racing a bit faster than it was before) … here lie those dilemmas again. Uncertainty can develop because the diagnosis is unclear, or the management options don't fit the patient's circumstances as they normally would. Typically, we will manage uncertainty by either obtaining more information to make the diagnosis clearer (e.g. using time and follow-up, investigations, advice from colleagues or trial of treatment) or by exploring the possible management options with the patient. Doing this in an honest and shared way can help us work through the dilemma to determine the plan. Again, we may seek advice from a colleague to help identify the most appropriate and acceptable way forward. In your exam, there shouldn't be a case which you cannot manage without advice, so do try to work with the patient to agree a plan.

Uncertainty felt by the patient may be less clear. You may pick this up using the ICE triad or through more subtle clues in the way the patient responds to your suggestions. Managing this uncertainty will involve trying to understand why the uncertainty exists and then using clear explanations and reassurance to ensure the patient is happy and onboard with the plan. Again, using investigations, time or trial of treatment can help reduce uncertainty experienced by the patient. Perceived or actual lack of control can underpin uncertainty, but through your explanations and safety-netting you should aim to empower the patient, increasing their sense of control.

Risk

There are different areas of risk to consider. The most obvious type is physical risk. There is always risk in medicine; if we do nothing, the problem may worsen, if we do something, there could be side effects/consequences of that action. You may feel comfortable discussing the risks involved in prescribing a medication, or recommending a procedure, or what could happen if the patient doesn't go to hospital or declines the suspected cancer pathway referral, but what about other types of risk?

We often neglect or ignore social risk. This is most important for vulnerable groups, e.g. children, elderly, those with severe mental health problems, learning disability, dementia, patients struggling with substance misuse, those at risk of or experiencing domestic violence, people new to the country. Consider the social risks associated with the person's particular demographics, e.g. falls, ability to manage activities of daily living for the elderly, grooming and exploitation for teenagers. The risks involved vary with the type of vulnerability. In your exam cases, you can identify social risks by asking about impact, being 'nosey' and considering the social risks alongside the physical risks when asking red flag questions. Don't forget safeguarding – this comes up in virtually every exam diet.

Psychological risk is another area of concern. We will commonly consider this in our mental health consultations as part of the risk assessment around self-harm and suicide. But there can be other situations where psychological risk is present, such as when breaking bad news, how will the patient react to this news? Here, our best strategy is to ensure we leave enough time to deal with the consequences of the news and not rush the patient. Silence can be very helpful!

How to Demonstrate Skills: The Marking Scheme Made Easy

Health rather than illness

One definition of health is *'The state of complete physical, mental and social wellbeing, not just the absence of disease or infirmity'* (WHO), in other words, holistic care. To provide holistic care, the clinician must understand the context of the patient's experience. Again, being 'nosey' is a helpful attribute to gaining this understanding, alongside asking about the impact of the problem. By asking about the effect the problem is having, we can gain insight into the areas the patient may need support with. This is often where the 'layers' appear; the diagnosis may be straightforward but social problems are adding layers of complexity. Using the biopsychosocial model when considering interventions, think 'What can I do to help the physical issues, what can I do to support the patient's psychological wellbeing and is there anything I can do to help the patient with their social problems?' We can't always 'fix' everything, but there is often signposting and support we can offer patients to improve their overall health. Consider the role of your community team, social prescribers, social services, etc. to support the patient.

Solving the social problem

Many SCA cases contain a social problem which needs to be addressed to allow the GP registrar to gain enough marks to pass the case. For example, you may have a patient who has a condition which is causing significant impact on their home life (e.g. carer responsibility), their work life (e.g. manual job which they aren't able to do, leading to financial worries), or their hobbies (e.g. important sporting event coming up which they are desperate to be well for). In the exam, you will of course be expected to diagnose and treat the underlying problem but also should work with the patient to reduce the impact of the problem on their home/work/social life. Can you make any suggestions about adjustments at work, or provide extra support to the carer, or advise on fastest route to recovery to the sportsman?

There are also cases where the patient's personal circumstances are causing difficulties with the management plan. E.g. a patient requiring urgent investigations or referral who is currently or imminently travelling, or a patient requiring regular drug monitoring who can't attend the practice for blood tests as they work away during the week. In these examples, it is not enough to just tell the patient they need urgent tests but not address how/when these will happen, e.g. can you travel back? Can you cancel your holiday? Here explanation of risk is important for the patient to make an informed decision about whether they cancel their plans or not. For the patient requiring blood test monitoring, it's not enough to lecture the patient about the risks of not having the tests or refuse to prescribe the medication; you need to work with the patient to facilitate getting the blood tests done. Could they come during an extended access session? Could they get their bloods done at the hospital phlebotomy service at the weekend? Another example may be a patient declining hospital admission due to a caring responsibility (e.g. partner or even a pet), how can you help facilitate the patient to access the care they need?

How to manage medical complexity

In your management plan ensure you manage the physical problem in the context of co-morbidity (where it exists), link back to ICE as discussed before, use explanation to manage uncertainty, consider and explain risks which need addressing AND ***solve the social problem***.

Thinking about clinical management, there are several approaches here that may help:

- Structuring your management into solutions for physical, psychological and social problems.
- Structuring your management into:
  - What I the GP can do to help.
  - What other professionals can do to help.
  - What you the patient can do to help yourself.

How to Demonstrate Skills: The Marking Scheme Made Easy

There are many grey areas in general practice! Holding the responsibility of potential risk is the greatest challenge. Diagnoses and management plans don't always fit into boxes or guidelines. Use present **and** absent red flags to help direct your management or possible referral. It is usually helpful to verbalise the dilemma: if you explain clearly why the symptom or your management suggestion is atypical, the standard guidance and what details have led to your uncertainty, both the patient and the examiner will then understand your thought process.

The doctor should present their rationale using evidence-based medicine and provide a recommendation to empower the patient and enable an informed decision. Consider if you can tailor your recommendation to the important features of the history. Be organised with your explanations and ensure you are clear.

Relating to others (RTO) skills are the communication skills and collaboration with patients, including ethics, values and attitudes, that you demonstrate throughout the consultation.

Any plan should demonstrate that you have responded to the patient's feelings, preferences and hopes, including explaining risk effectively.

RTO skills also include demonstrating equality, responding positively to problems, admitting mistakes and being open and non-judgemental.

Demonstrating RTO as a GP requires proactive and reactive communication skills. Our FOCUS model (Filter, Opportunity, Context, Unite, Safety) reminds you to take the opportunity to connect with the patient and demonstrate these skills at every stage of the consultation.

Here are some specific examples of situations where social or other practical challenges may significantly influence your management, so that you need to adapt what you might normally do in order to best help the patient.

Homelessness

One of the social challenges you may come across in your cases is homelessness. This is challenging for several reasons, for example patients not being able to manage personal hygiene, access adequate nutrition, look after/store medication, afford prescriptions or receive important mail. To help patients access healthcare more effectively, there are a few things you could consider when working with the patient to formulate a plan.

- No postal address. Ask the patient if they have a friend/relative who would be happy to receive letters for the patient. Or do they attend a shelter for the homeless or a day centre? If none of these apply, you could suggest using the surgery address for the patient's medical correspondence, so that the practice will receive appointment/hospital letters which can either be passed on, or which the patient can call in and collect.
- Can't afford the prescription fee or can't safely store medication. Your social prescriber should be able to advise and help the patient regarding any benefits they may be entitled to, including access to free prescriptions. If the patient is concerned about storing or keeping the medication safe, giving small quantities of medication at a time may help.
- Most areas will have a healthcare outreach team to help homeless patients, including drug and alcohol services. Make sure you know how to contact yours.
- Most councils have teams dedicated to helping homeless people find accommodation and there are also charities that help. You could advise the patient about this or put them in touch with social prescribing. Consider access to foodbanks too.

How to Demonstrate Skills: The Marking Scheme Made Easy

Travelling communities

Healthcare for members of the travelling community can also be challenging. There are many barriers to healthcare including cultural differences and trust issues. As with homelessness, receipt of appointment information or letters may be inconsistent and erratic, resulting in missed appointments. Even if appointment information is received, the patient may no longer be in the area, making attending appointments impractical. Members of the travelling community may also have strong views about vaccination or screening tests and may be less likely to access these, resulting in health inequalities. Levels of education within the travelling community may also vary significantly and some patients may not be confident reading written information they receive, creating another barrier to access.

Things to consider:

- Could information be sent via phone text message instead of letter? If the person has reading difficulties, could the practice phone and speak to the patient instead of writing/texting?
- Are there elements of healthcare that could be accessed elsewhere, e.g. if the patient needs regular BPs, could they visit local pharmacies to obtain BP readings?
- Could you give the patient a printout of their record summary that they could show to other healthcare teams if they are temporarily registering elsewhere or attending a hospital out of area?
- There is a charity 'Friends, Families and Travellers' (https://www.gypsy-traveller.org/) who can help support access to healthcare for gypsies, Roma and travellers.

Communication difficulties

Problems with accessing and reading written information are, of course, not confined to people in travelling communities. Therefore, consider how you could help patients with poor vision or for whom English is an additional language who may lack fluent understanding. For example, voice messages, printed material in a larger font, text to speech apps, written materials in different languages or even translation apps such as Google translate.

Our useful Es for RTO skills

Encourage	Their contribution. Not only ask ICE, but also return to it during your explanations or recommendations.
Explore	Their cues or anything you sense from the patient. Explore ICE and the impact of the issue.
Empathy	Pulling together all the patient's challenges and collectively reflecting these back to them. We break this down to teach it as: Symptoms + fears + social challenges = impact + offer your support.
Explain	(i) Provide explanations of why your questions are important, e.g. you could do this with ICE questions. (ii) Share your thought process clearly, using language tailored to the individual patient.
Engage	Fully involve the patient in shared management and health promotion.
Empower	Share your knowledge to empower the patient and involve them at every step in the plan. Provide them with the opportunity to (i) make an informed decision and (ii) consider self-help strategies.
Elephants	E.g. issues either the patient or doctor is nervous to mention. Address them early in a sensitive way to allow time to deal with them.

This is not a finite list and you should carefully read the marking scheme available on the RCGP website for a more comprehensive description.

Easy-to-Use Generic Feedback Card

Below are some pointers that you can look for when marking each other's cases. On the next page there is a blank grid that you could photocopy to make marking easier. Look for what the doctor has done well and what could be improved in each domain.

Data gathering and diagnosis

- Was the main reason for attendance established? Were relevant red flags checked?
- Was an organised system used for gathering background information: PMH, DH, FH, SH?
- Was there an appropriate and slick examination where necessary (e.g. of mental health)?
- Did the doctor use information from the notes and was this made explicit and discussed?
- Was an appropriate working diagnosis made?

Clinical management and medical complexity

- Was the plan tailored to the patient?
- Did the doctor state their recommendation and other possibilities?
- Was an appropriate management plan discussed with the patient including appropriate tests, medication, referrals, follow-up, etc.?
- Were opportunities to tackle health promotion found and used?
- Did the doctor add an appropriate safety net?

Relating to others

- Were cues in the history picked up and addressed?
- Were ideas, concerns and expectations elicited?
- Did the doctor adopt a sensitive approach? Without prejudice, judgement and assumption?
- Did the doctor provide clear explanations using appropriate language?
- Did the doctor involve the patient in decisions?
- Did the doctor demonstrate active listening skills?
- Did the doctor demonstrate empathy through their communication skills?
- Did they find out how the patient's problem and individual psychosocial situation were intervolved?
- How did the doctor show that they were genuinely interested in the patient?
- Did the doctor empower the patient, and how?
- Did the doctor involve the patient in the plan?

Possible negative descriptors for feedback and to discuss

- The consultation appeared disorganised.
- Lack of structure – e.g. asking additional data-gathering questions during clinical management.
- A significant agenda, abnormal result or red flag was missed.
- Poor time management.
- The focus of the consultation was on the wrong agenda/complaint.
- The doctor provided little or no opportunity to involve the patient in management decisions.
- Cues were missed.

Easy-to-Use Generic Feedback Card

Case

Date Gathering and Diagnosis	
POSITIVE	NEGATIVE

Clinical Management and Medical Complexity	
POSITIVE	NEGATIVE

Relating to Others	
POSITIVE	NEGATIVE

CHAPTER 1D OUR USEFUL TIPS

Structure and Time Management

For every consultation, you need to find the answer to the question: 'Why has this patient presented today with this problem?'

How can we achieve this, every time, in a 12-minute consultation?

1. Be concise. Use as few words as possible and choose words carefully to ask concise, clear questions. Remember that open questions are most likely to reveal the detail you need.
2. In 'normal', non-exam consultations, the 'golden minute' is usually rich in important detail. In the exam, however, you should not expect a golden gift like this. Instead, the patient is likely to offer you a brief sentence, and you will then need to engage with this and explore using open, but focused questions. E.g. '*Tell me more about the chest pain, for example how did it start?*' '*Tell me more*' alone, will not elicit the information you need. The patient's conversational flow can be extended by using open questions. Choose questions that guide the patient to give information that is crucial to your assessment.
3. Repeat their words, with a rising inflexion so they sound like questions. '*Chest pain?*' '*Feeling low?*'
4. Absorb the answers that follow and don't ask questions where you already know the answers.
5. Be organised – ask lots of open questions first, then group your closed questions (red flags).
6. Aim for the important moment of the consultation at 5–6 minutes – where you state your impression.
7. Be systematic with how you present your management plan.
8. Be assertive. See next page.
9. Keep up momentum. Imagine you are on a ski slalom and quickly need to go around all the gates on the way down the hill. The gradient is the same throughout, so avoid being too slow at the start then speeding up in panic towards the end. Certainly don't turn around and go back up the hill to cover old ground!
10. Avoid wasting time with unnecessary phrases. Every second counts in a 12-minute consultation. We often hear '*May I ask you some questions?*' which is always followed by the patient's response ***'Yes of course'***. There's no need to say this unless you are signposting that you are about to ask some very personal questions – it is inefficient, wastes time and may halt the patient's narrative, so slowing the consultation.
11. Too much sympathy is neither helpful nor efficient. RTO skills require an assertive not just an empathetic doctor. However, always be sensitive. Continue to move the consultation forward and demonstrate you are empathetic by:
    - Asking thoughtful questions '*What is it like living with …?*'
    - Demonstrating an interest in the person '*What's this past year been like for you?*'
    - Connecting through exploring cues and ICE.

This information helps you to work towards demonstrating 'proactive empathy' (you've worked for it) which silently, yet powerfully, suggests to the patient '*I hear you*'.

Remember our empathy equation: Problem + fears + social context = an understanding and expression of how things are, e.g. '*really tough*'.

How to develop your time management skills

- Go back to basics. Write down a structure you hope to follow (allowing flexibility).
- Dissect your consultations in detail. Listen to your videos and be critical with your chosen words within questions. Could you have rephrased to ask more skilful questions that efficiently provide important answers?
- Practise going from the moment you give a diagnosis to how you present a recommended management plan and involve the patient in the decision-making process.
- Practise giving slick explanations of diagnoses to different patient groups, e.g. migraine to a lawyer, asthma to a 7 year old who just wants to play football.

Structure and Time Management

Remember you can be assertive and yet remain patient-centred. You can be assertive through having a structure, asking questions that demonstrate your curiosity and interest, reacting to the patient's needs, agenda and cues, being organised, using signposting and keeping the momentum of the consultation going. Encourage the patient's contributions, provide clear explanations to empower the patient and provide them with opportunities for informed decision making.

Signposting

This can be useful during data gathering and clinical management. It provides structure for both the doctor and patient and facilitates organisation of the consultation. Signposting is especially useful if the patient has questions that require answering or there are many problems. In both situations, the GP can propose an 'agenda' based on the patient's requests and any risk the doctor may have detected.

Managing the consultation with multiple problems

We expect most cases in your exam will have one presenting problem. However, sometimes the problems may be connected (e.g. symptoms of an underactive thyroid may manifest in many different areas – dry skin, tiredness, weight gain) or require management in parallel, e.g. a physical symptom and the psychological impact.

Phrases that may help: '*Tell me more about that*.' This gives you time to consider if they could be related (potentially a rare condition).

Risk assess! Ask them the red flags for both problems. Ensure you are safe with how you are using your consultation time.

You may decide the problems are indeed connected and need to be managed simultaneously. Or, if safe to do so and there is an additional aspect of health mentioned but not presented as the initial reason for the consultation, you could use your discussion about follow-up plans to explain how you can return to this problem and possibly briefly explain future options.

Structuring management plans

Here is a possible sequence to the latter half of a consultation. As we know, making a diagnosis is part of the data-gathering marking domain; however, **sharing** your diagnosis is an essential part of the discussion before clinical management so we will consider these together here. Remember, in order to also demonstrate RTO skills, after each point that you make, invite the patient into the conversation by pausing or asking for their thoughts.

1. **State your impression or differential diagnosis**. We refer to this as the pivotal moment. You share your thoughts with the patient and allow them a moment to absorb this information. The consultation is pivoting from data gathering to clinical management. Practise providing a differential diagnosis – i.e. not just the single most likely option, but also what is possible, even if less likely. Consider our mantra, 'Common things are common but what mustn't I miss?' You may find yourself in the following scenarios:
   - **i.** You believe that a worrying diagnosis (e.g. cancer) is low on your differential list, but still needs to be ruled out or discussed, to address the patient's fears or the potential 'elephant in the room'. Use a reassuring tone, explaining your suspected diagnosis. Use negative red flags to explain why you do not suspect cancer. Explain the importance of your recommendation of appropriate investigations to confirm your hypothesis and rule out a diagnosis of cancer.
   - **ii.** The cancer is at the top of your differential list. You therefore combine your breaking bad news skills as you sensitively approach the seriousness of the unconfirmed problem and the need for the suspected cancer referral.

2. **Pause**. Give the patient space to think or talk. If required, encourage their understanding or response to this information.
3. **Explanation (and empower)**. Consider incorporating the patient's ICE here so you haven't just asked it, you've woven their answers into the explanation to ensure you've addressed each health belief in turn. Ask yourself, 'Do I agree or disagree with the patient's thoughts? Do I share the patient's worries or can I reassure? Are the patient's expectations realistic or not?'
4. **Empathy**. This could be useful here if not already expressed.
5. **'My recommendation is** … What are your thoughts?'
6. **Aim for five appropriate things that you offer the patient to ensure you have provided a comprehensive management plan, which may include:**
   i. **Investigations** that may be needed to include or exclude differentials. Consider resources and avoid over-investigating. It is good practice to explain which tests you believe are necessary and why, and this also tells the examiner.
   ii. **Medications**. Use the five-point process – what the drug is, why you're recommending it, how to take it, potential problems and how they feel about this option. Leave the issuing of the prescription until the end.
   iii. **Referral**. The logistics of the referral process and what to expect from the referral.
   iv. **General health**. If there is more than one problem, or coexisting health issues, these should also be considered in the plan. Discuss what the patient can do through health promotion, disease prevention and rehabilitation (empowerment). A practical way of helping you do this is to consider the three dimensions of self, GP and others:
      - This is what you can do.
      - This is what I the GP can do.
      - This is what 'others' can do. Others may include other professionals, family members, exercises, resources such as educational material or leaflets.
   v. **Specifics** (who/what/when/how), when describing appropriate **follow-up** and a **safety net**.

Demonstrating Skills in the Domain of Relating to Others

Softening and normalising

If you ask formulaic questions this will not demonstrate your ability to **tailor** the questions to the information the patient has already provided. There are approaches that can soften questions and explanations and demonstrate that you are sensitive to the impact of your conclusions. We encourage you to find what feels authentic to you.

Here are some examples:

- '*Sometimes when people come to see me with acne, I find it is affecting their life in many different ways. I'm wondering how you are affected?*' (Normalising)
- '*What is it like living with this pain every day?*' (Exploring empathetically)
- '*Some people find X helpful.*' (Normalising)
- '*If I were to suggest you had X diagnosis, what would go through your mind?*'

How the patient should feel when they leave the consultation

- Understood.
- With a diagnosis or, as a minimum, the most likely explanation from a list of differentials.
- With an understanding of the plan and the specific actions required.
- Empowered – with the doctor's knowledge and involved in the plan.
- Feeling positive and reassured, if not from the diagnosis, from the comfort of receiving excellent care with a feeling of trust in their doctor.

Child consultation

You may be asked to discuss a child with their parent or carer, or have an actor who is playing the part of a teenager. Try to integrate both the child's and parent's perspectives, including ICE (think 'TwICE' – ICE twice), where possible. When speaking to a parent, remember there are essentially two patients to deal with – the child and their parent. The case may involve educating the parent or offering support to them, not just dealing with the underlying condition. Remember immunisation, development and, if appropriate, birth history. Ask about nursery or school interactions, feedback from teachers and consider their help in the management plan.

Connection and empathy

Rapport means connection with the patient. We avoid using the words '*I understand*', because we don't! These are empty words and sound hollow. Instead, we suggest you explore and absorb all the information and reflect it back to demonstrate '*I have heard you*'.

When we teach how to demonstrate empathy, we suggest using the following equation of challenges to reflect back to the patient:

Problem + Social context + ICE = What you sense (e.g. really tough, exhausting)

Demonstrating Skills in the Domain of Relating to Others

An example:

Susan, age 42, presents with painful hands and swollen joints

Symptoms:	Pains in hands + joint swelling
Ideas:	Mum had rheumatoid arthritis (RA) – ***'I think it's RA'***
Concerns:	Mum's hands became deformed – ***'Will this happen to me?'***
Expectations:	An X-ray to find out what's going on
Psychosocial:	Seamstress, works in a factory. Single mum of twins. Life is tough, only breadwinner

*'Given how **badly affected your mum was by rheumatoid arthritis** and how difficult life is for you just now as a **seamstress and single parent of twins**, I can understand why **these pains in your hands have worried you** and why **you hoped I might refer you for an X-ray**.'*

Follow this with silence and listen for a response.

Another very useful question to find out impact is *'What is it like living with X?'*

The good news is, the more challenging the case, the greater the opportunity to shine and overcome the challenge if you have skills to connect and empathise with the patient.

A useful approach to elicit the psychosocial context

This may include:

- *'Tell me about you … who is in your life?'*
- *'Do you work?'* Then either *'What does work involve?'* or *'What do you do in a typical day?'*
- *'What is home like at the moment?'*
- *'Have there been challenges or changes in your life?'*
- *'How have you been feeling with all this going on?'*

Avoiding assumptions

Avoid leading questions and make no assumptions. GP registrars may fall into this trap when they believe a patient has told them their concern. We recommend ensuring you acknowledge the concern you have heard and then ask explicitly about further thoughts, fears and hopes. If medication is potentially linked to the problem, don't assume compliance – ask about medication taken and doses.

Demonstrating Skills in the Domain of Relating to Others

Detecting and responding to verbal cues

Some of the consultations in the SCA will be on the phone rather than via video, in other words, audio consultations with no patient visible on the screen. In these situations, you need to work harder with your senses. Without visual cues, the doctor's ears need to be listening out for hesitations, changes and emotions within the voice. Remember we encourage you to make a statement about what you 'sense' (see FOCUS model).

Verbal cues are often expressions that are unique to the person, e.g. a description of a feeling (subjective rather than fact). A person may also be mentioned. Be curious; repeat the word they have chosen to find out why. Use your senses to also detect the non-verbal cues. Imagine you are opening a hyperlink to another page of information. Cues will be obvious to an examiner, but will require you to be receptive, remembering that you are in the 'hot seat' with the combined challenge of receiving, processing and formatting information. Do not fear that you may go down 'the wrong track'; you will soon discover if your hunch was wrong. Cues are clues to help us treat both the problem and the person.

Avoid 'parking' cues. We often hear doctors say '*We'll come back to that*' or state afterwards that they did hear the cue but feared going down the wrong path if they explored further. In a simulated case, an actor will normally 'shut you down' rather than fabricate an answer if you are on the wrong track. By responding to the cue, you may find out important information and are also demonstrating to the examiner that you have heard the cue. Always remember that cues are clues – for example leading you to important psychosocial factors which are affecting the patient.

Try repeating a word the patient has used, but in the style of asking a question – perhaps using a rising inflection in your voice. You may then discover that vital piece of information. In the exam, the simulators will quickly shut down any blind alleys and will not inappropriately lead you down the garden path.

Patients Returning for Test Results

In this book, there are some cases focused on patients returning for test results, for example in Chapter 12, and this is, of course, a normal part of everyday general practice. The pitfall here is that your data gathering may be curtailed or even non-existent, scoring no marks in this domain. Be careful to ensure that you take an appropriate and comprehensive history from the patient and that you have collected the information yourself rather than summarising what a colleague may have already discussed. This ensures that you give yourself the opportunity to score good marks.

When a patient consults for a test result, remember the following:

- To demonstrate skills in DG&D, ensure you actually elicit **new** information in the consultation. Summarising what you know so far does not demonstrate data-gathering skills.
- Put the investigation into context – why was the test performed and what is the patient expecting?
- There is a balance between keeping the patient waiting for the result but ensuring you have enough information to help you put the result into an appropriate context. You may need to collect some information, then provide the results, but of course remember to return to complete your data gathering.
- The result may be the 'elephant' in the room. Any result could be perceived by the patient as 'bad news,' so ensure you leave enough time to manage their feelings and expectations.
- If the patient tries to move the consultation ahead before you are ready, pressing you for the result, acknowledge their anxiety or question (e.g. blood test or diagnosis of CKD3) straight away and give them the answer. However, do not be pressured into immediately discussing management options, and go back to the beginning to take the history. It is difficult to score marks for data gathering if you gather no data!

  E.g. '*I can see you are keen for your results. The tests show your blood sugar is raised. I'm sure you are keen to know what that means and where we go from here but, to put this result into the context of you, I need to find out more about you and go through your medical history in more detail first, if that's OK please.*'

Vulnerable Patients

For vulnerable and elderly patients, the following questions may be helpful when speaking to them (e.g. teenager or a person with a learning disability):

- **Home**. Relationship with family? Any stress within the home? Are they a carer? Do they have any responsibilities (e.g. work to financially support the family)?
- **School**. Exams, stress with workload, relationships with friends and bullying?
- **Mental health**. Low self-esteem, mood, anxiety, self-harm or suicidal thoughts? Social habits. Alcohol, drugs and smoking?
- **Physical health**. Eating, exercise habits and weight changes?
- **Sexual health**. Are they sexually active? Who with? Discuss pregnancy and STI risk.
- **Vulnerability and abuse**. Which adults do they have time alone with? Use of social media? Does anyone upset them, hurt them, make them feel uncomfortable or encourage them to have sex?

And when consulting with an elderly patient:

- **Activities of daily living**. Shopping, meals, cleaning, washing.
- **Medications**. Compliance, polypharmacy and risks (e.g. anticholinergic burden). Is a dosette needed?
- **Memory and mood**.
- **Risk**. Leaving hob on/locking doors/wandering/falls/driving.
- **Isolation/loneliness**. When do they feel vulnerable?
- **Weight**. Are clothes loose? Are they eating?
- **Continence and bowels**.
- **Risk factors for AKI**.

Phrasing Your Questions

Top tips – when a case feels like it's going wrong or you have a brain freeze

There are ways to pull it back. Can you summarise ICE? Is there more information you need?

- '*What's been on your mind?*' is a good rescue question, especially if the patient has an unusual opening gambit.
- '*What's most important to you today?*' Or ask the patient if they have any questions.
- '*I'm going to be making suggestions, but was there anything you were particularly hoping for?*'

Can you empathise to reconnect with the patient?

Be honest. '*I feel I am not being as helpful as I could be. I'm sorry. Can we take a step back to … and go from there so I can do a better job?*'

FILTER

Clarify understanding – '*Can you describe what you mean by wheeze/palpitations?*'

Instead of the vague '*Tell me more*', which will waste time because the patient will ask you what exactly you want to know, try '*Tell me the story of (your headaches) from the beginning.*'

If they've had the symptom for months – '*What prompted you to come now?*'

Checking past history and investigations, etc. – '*As we haven't met before, would you mind telling me …*'

OPPORTUNITY

ICE, ICE, ICE. It is vital that these questions come across naturally and do not sound robotic, so consider what information you need. To understand a patient and, more importantly, for the patient to feel understood, the GP needs to explore their health beliefs; this means their thought process, what is on their mind, their fear, where this has come from, their experience of a 'similar' problem or what they have read, who they have spoken to and why they have presented now. Be **curious!** Being aware of what is going through the patient's mind will lead you towards what they may be assuming you will do.

If you miss any (or all!) of this, the patient may feel you have missed something crucial and they may be right.

Try variations on the following:

- '*Is there anything else that you have been wondering?*'
- '*Have you had any thoughts about what might be causing your symptoms?*'
- '*Is there anything else that has been on your mind?*'
- '*Do you have any thoughts about what you would like us to do?*'
- '*What is important to you when considering what needs to be done today?*'

CONTEXT

Summarise ICE – this is a powerful way to show you understand the patient. You could follow this with:

> '*Am I on the right track?*' or '*Have I understood you correctly so far?*'

ICE and empathy help address health beliefs in the context of the individual.

Incorporate their thoughts and experience together with their background (social history) to help you empathise.

> '*I can see that because your father had … you are worried this could be … and because you are under a lot of pressure at the moment with … I can see you have been frightened for what this could mean and had fears of … but I think what is going on here is …*'

Phrasing Your Questions

The result is:

- The patient feels listened to and understood.
- The doctor understands the patient's health beliefs and can educate.

You can only genuinely empathise when you have explored the person's experience.

Another example:

> *'You wonder if it could be … I see why you would think that, especially when you have experience of/have gone through/your mother has gone through … However, my impression is … which may have been caused by …'*

You could use the positive and negative red flags to help you here, explaining why you have reached that conclusion. Check **experience** (understanding): '*What do you know about …?*' Then educate: '*… is … and the cause of the problem is often …*'

UNITE

Rather than responding to an inappropriate request with a confrontational approach such as '*Have you thought about any problems with that?*' try being more collaborative, '*Let's think through this together*'.

Acknowledge their expectation before giving options. '*I understand you were hoping for … My suggestion of options for where we go from here include …*'

Remember you are the doctor – '*My recommendation would be …*'

But include the patient in the management plan, especially if there are a couple of appropriate options: '*What do you believe is best for you?*' or '*What is your preference?*'

Structure your management plan within your mind. What can the patient do (e.g. lifestyle factors), what can I do (e.g. medications, referrals) and what can others do (e.g. primary care team, charities, friends/family, specialists).

If you give a patient an information leaflet, you must explain its contents.

SAFETY

Remember to be specific – '*If you find your child is not able to keep down fluids, they are at risk of becoming dehydrated, so please contact us at the surgery. If the surgery is closed, dial 111 to speak to an on-call GP.*' '*If you find you require more than 10 puffs of your inhaler over 4 hours, please call the surgery. However, if you require 10 puffs at the same time, please call 999.*'

The motivational interview

Fantastic for health promotion cases:

- '*How is your general health do you think?*'
- '*What could be improved?*'
- '*Do you want … to change?*'
- '*Do you feel confident you can change …?*'
- '*How could you improve …?*'
- '*What challenges might you encounter with this?*'
- '*How could you overcome these obstacles?*'
- '*What steps do you think you may take?*'
- '*In what time frame should this change happen?*'
- '*When do you want to meet again to discuss this?*'

Jargon Switch

Consider the patient in front of you. You may need to change your language.

You may decide to tell your revision partner to tap their pen on the table whenever you use jargon.

For example:

Abdomen	Tummy
Acute	New symptom
Benign	Harmless
Cervix	The neck of the womb
Chronic	Symptoms you have had a long time
Cyst	Fluid-filled lump that is usually harmless
DNA	The genetic information passed down from our parents
ECG	Test where we put stickers on the chest to see a tracing of the heart, which we call an ECG
Fracture	Broken bone
Inflammation	Swelling/redness
Numbers	Heart rate, breathing rate, BP, temperature, etc.
Observations	Heart rate and blood pressure
Over the counter	From the pharmacy
Positive/Negative	Test result. Avoid using these words and explain exactly what the test shows. Patients may believe 'positive' means good, 'negative' means bad which may not actually be the case! 'Clear' can often be used to describe a normal result, e.g. your chest X-ray was clear, your urine sample was clear
Sinister	Significant
Ultrasound	Jelly scan called an ultrasound
Vital signs	Heart rate and blood pressure

Resitting the Exam

What may have gone wrong

- **Too slow – you do not reach the management plan.** Practise your time management. You may be spending too long on data gathering (for fear of missing something) but to the detriment of the rest of your case. Go back to basics, e.g. lots of well-chosen open questions that help you obtain lots of information quickly, then group the red flags.
- **The doctor talks more than the patient.** Consider the many opportunities within the FOCUS model to **engage** and involve your patient before giving information.
- **Missing the subtleties of the consultation and hence the reason for the patient's attendance.**
- **The patient leaves not knowing their diagnosis.** Even if you are unsure, you should reassure yourself and the patient with the important negatives, e.g. why it is not a sinister/serious diagnosis. Or share what you need to do to rule out the sinister/serious and how you will get more information (tests, referral, colleague advice) to make the diagnosis.
- **You do not produce a safe management plan.** Ask yourself if this is because you have not considered the sinister/serious causes of their symptoms.
- **Poor organisation.** Disorganised consultations don't give a good impression to the examiner or patient. Try to stick to your consultation model structure and don't jump between the story, the examination and information giving.

Still not sure? Think about the basics – whose needs aren't being met?

Patient's needs

- Wants to feel understood.
- Wants to share everything they have noticed.
  - To offload anxiety and hand over responsibility.
  - Just in case it may be relevant.
- Wants to know what is wrong.
- Wants reassurance.
- Wants to get better.

Doctor's needs

- To know the facts that will change management.
- Wants clear information so they can make the diagnosis and plan … within 12 minutes.
- Wants to fix the problem.
- Wants the patient to be satisfied with the plan.

Sometimes, after the exam results are out, GP registrars will speak to other GP registrars about what they did in their cases to try to understand what went wrong. If you discover you missed something major then this may provide the desired explanation; however, this might not always be the case. Comparisons can cause frustration or even anger as simplifying the cases down to 'What did you do in the management?' can result in GP registrars finding the outcome of the cases very similar in terms of advice and management yet the marks differ. As this exam focuses on overall consultation skills, it is often less about what you did but *how* you did it; more about the journey from A to B rather than the destination. Therefore, discussing what others did is not always helpful. If you feel your management plan was correct, think about how you got there. Did you tease out the relevant information subtly and skilfully using cues or useful insights? Did you explain the problem clearly and succinctly? Did you address ICE and impact? Did you involve the patient in the management plan or dictate what would happen next? Keep an open mind about how you may need to improve to be successful next time.

CHAPTER 1E THE NUTS AND BOLTS OF THE SCA

The SCA exam comprises 12 virtual cases and these include video consultations, where you and the patient can see each other, and audio calls, where you can hear but not see the patient. Typically, there are nine video consultations and three audio calls.

The 12 cases are spread across the blueprint groups:

1. Patient less than 19 years old
2. Gender, reproductive and sexual health, including women's, men's, LGBTQ+, gynae and breast
3. Long-term conditions, including cancer, multi-morbidity and disability
4. Older adults, including frailty and people at the end of life
5. Mental health, including addiction, smoking, alcohol and substance misuse
6. Urgent and unscheduled care
7. Health disadvantage and vulnerabilities, including veterans, mental capacity, safeguarding and communication difficulties
8. Ethnicity, culture, diversity and inclusivity
9. New presentation of undifferentiated disease
10. Prescribing
11. Investigation/results
12. Professional conversation/professional dilemma

Each chapter in this book focuses on one of the blueprint groups and provides five example cases.

Unless you have applied for reasonable adjustments, there are 12 minutes for each case from the moment the consultation starts, and 3 minutes between cases to prepare. We recommend this in-between time is used to carefully read the information about the case and keep an open mind about the problem.

The RCGP produces excellent online resources for candidates and we recommend you read these carefully.

What can you bring into the exam?

You can bring a whiteboard and water into the room with you. When reading the patient notes, you may wish to jot down any relevant details on your whiteboard. You are instructed to keep your phone on silent and out of reach. There is also an 'SCA comfort aid list' to address any personal medical or other needs that you may have. For example, you are allowed to bring a small snack and drink in addition to the water provided. If you need, for example, an Epipen, inhaler or eye drops with you, this is permitted without requesting prior permission. Please see the 'SCA comfort aid list' on the RCGP website for further details. Note that if you wear glasses, these must be removed for inspection prior to the exam.

SCA Marking Scheme

There are three domains within the marking scheme:

- Data gathering and diagnosis (DG&D)
- Clinical management and medical complexity (CM&C)
- Relating to others (RTO)

Each domain is marked against the following:

- **Pass (3 marks)** – Meets the standard of a newly qualified GP who is fit to consult (any omissions or errors are minor or trivial).
- **Bare pass (2 marks)** – Omissions or errors made, but candidate has done enough to demonstrate fitness to consult as an independent newly qualified GP.
- **Bare fail (1 mark)** – Presented some evidence, but insufficient for fitness to consult as an independent, newly qualified GP. Omissions or errors likely to impact on patient care/outcomes.
- **Clear fail (0 marks)** – Does not meet the standard for an independent newly qualified GP who is fit to consult. Minimal evidence presented and/or patient put at risk of harm.

The marking domains may be 'weighted' – in other words, the raw mark for a domain may be increased by a multiplying factor. In recent SCA exams, the CM&C domain has been weighted by +50%. The maximum mark awarded for this domain is still 3, but the mark is multiplied by 1.5. Therefore, the maximum total marks for each case were 10.5 (3 + 4.5 + 3). Note, therefore, that in recent sittings almost half the marks for each case (4.5/10.5) are awarded for clinical management. This means that your data gathering needs to be comprehensive and slick, in order to give enough time to generate an excellent and appropriate management plan.

Remember that you can 'fail a case' and continue to pass the exam. It is your overall score that leads to success.

When using this book, after you have watched or performed a consultation, it may be useful to reflect on the following skills within each marking domain. These are directly related to the RCGP 'feedback' statements, published on their website.

Data gathering

To pass this domain, you need to show that you have gathered enough relevant and targeted information to address the needs of the patient and their problem(s). For problem solving, that you have generated an appropriate list of differentials, or relied on first principles.

Specific capabilities that the examiners are looking for include:

- **Data gathering**
  - Being organised and systematic – your questioning was logical and you used targeted questions.
  - Safety – You found out enough information to make a safe assessment, including red flags.
  - Effective use of the information provided in the patient notes (including results and the wider context).
  - Physical, psychological and social aspects of the patient's health – you recognised, explored and responded to these.
- **Making a diagnosis**
  - Evidence based – you have shown that your reasoning is structured and based on evidence.
  - Probability – you have used your knowledge of incidence, prevalence and natural history to help decision making.
  - Revision of hypotheses – as new information emerges.
  - Undifferentiated problems – integration of all available information to help generate a reasonable working hypothesis.

SCA Marking Scheme

Pitfalls for DG&D

- Not making use of the information supplied – read **all** pages and make notes on your whiteboard.
- Being disorganised or unsystematic – there should be a logical flow to your questions.
- Not finding out enough to safely assess – remember red flags and risk factors. Always think, 'What mustn't I miss?'
- Failing to explore and make use of relevant psychological or social information. This is every bit as important as the clinical history.
- Prioritisation with multiple or complex problems. Ask yourself – 'What's most important?' Clinically? To the patient?
- Not recognising the implications of relevant findings identified during the data gathering. There is no point asking questions and then ignoring the answers!
- Didn't generate or test out relevant differentials or hypotheses. One diagnosis may appear to be the most likely, but have you tested out the others?
- For undifferentiated problems, have you integrated **all** information to reach a logical hypothesis?

Clinical management and medical complexity

To pass this domain, you need to show that you can generate safe and appropriate management options, taking into account effective prioritisation, continuity of care, how the problem may evolve over time and what the patient can do to help their own health. Also, that you are committed to providing optimum care, short and long term, whilst acknowledging the challenges.

Specific capabilities that the examiners are looking for include:

- **Clinical management**
  - Self-care – increasing the patient's health understanding, skills and confidence so that they can modify their lifestyle or improve their self-care.
  - Wait and see – considering this, if it is appropriate.
  - Prescribing – should be safe, cost-effective and in line with national or local guidelines.
  - Referrals – when appropriate and required, being mindful of resources.
  - Teamwork – showing that you can coordinate care with the practice team or other services, when appropriate.
  - Flexibility – being responsive to the circumstances and preferences of the patient and the priorities. Creating solutions that work for the patient.
- **Medical complexity**
  - Managing all health problems concurrently – i.e. acute and chronic, short and long term, and multi-morbidity, adjusting care as necessary, e.g. to take account of polypharmacy.
  - Prioritisation of management options based on risk.
  - Showing that you can manage uncertainty – yours and the patient's.
  - Health improvement, health promotion, rehabilitation and prevention.
- **Practising holistically, promoting health and safeguarding**
  - Offering support that is targeted to the patient's needs, or those of their family and carers.
  - Safeguarding – recognising concerns, responding to them and making appropriate referrals.

SCA Marking Scheme

Pitfalls for CM&C

- Poor time management meant that you did not have long enough to develop and share a holistic management plan.
- Knowledge gaps – the management plan relating to prescribing, investigations, health promotion or referral was inappropriate or not reflective of current practice.
- Risk management was inadequate or inappropriate.
- You didn't consider the patient's co-morbidities or polypharmacy.
- Uncertainty, including that experienced by the patient, was managed ineffectively.
- Safety net, follow-up and continuity of care was inappropriate or arrangements were inadequate.

Relating to others

To pass this domain, you need to be able to demonstrate ethical awareness, show that you can communicate in a way that is patient-centred, and demonstrate initiative and flexibility to overcome any communication barriers – for example the patient who is deaf, has sight loss or English as an additional language.

Specific capabilities that the examiners are looking for include:

- **Fitness to practise**
  - Respect for patients, treating all people fairly and without discrimination.
  - 'Owning' decisions, i.e. not offering the patient an unguided choice and asking them what they would prefer, when they do not have the skills, knowledge or tools to make an informed choice.
- **An ethical approach**
  - Demonstrate that you understand that everyone has their own values and beliefs, that there are cultural and personal differences in both patients and colleagues and act non-judgementally, with equity and fairness.
  - Whilst respecting people's autonomy, act with beneficence and in the patient's best interests.
  - Demonstrate that you understand medicolegal concepts such as informed consent, mental capacity and best interests.
- **Communication and consultation skills**
  - Use a range of communication skills – verbal, non-verbal, active listening.
  - Be empathetic, showing that you are trying to help and care for the patient.
  - Cues – spot them and use them!
  - Find out the patient's agenda, health beliefs and preferences and use these in your explanation.
  - Use comprehensible language (no jargon) and different communication techniques and materials to adapt your explanation to the patient.
  - Negotiate a clear, understandable plan that is acceptable to the patient and to you.
- **Working with colleagues**
  - Show that you understand what colleagues can do, treating them fairly and without discrimination, respecting their role and valuing their opinion (e.g. third-party consultation where a colleague is phoning you about a patient).
- **Practising holistically, promoting health and safeguarding**
  - Impact – recognising and acknowledging how a problem is affecting a person and their family and/or carers.
  - Challenge unhelpful behaviours or false health beliefs, whilst remaining respectful and maintaining the relationship.
  - Recognise what matters to the patient and work collaboratively to enhance their care.

SCA Marking Scheme

Pitfalls for RTO

- Weak communication skills, including non-verbal, failure to respond to cues and poor active listening.
- Not adequately exploring or considering or responding to the person's circumstances, agenda, relevant cultural differences, health beliefs and/or preferences.
- Explanations – inadequately sharing or adapting them to the person's needs.
- Being judgemental.
- Lack of respect or sensitivity to the person.
- Inadequate or inappropriate ownership or responsibility for decisions.
- Not showing that you understand teamwork and understand the roles of others in this.
- Missing or failing to deal with safeguarding concerns.

Top Tips for Success

Practise your technique

- Make sure you have a reasonably good quality webcam you can use for your exam.
- Ensure it works well with your PC before your exam.
- Make use of the RCGP 'onboarding' sessions, which allow you to test your connection and equipment as well as familiarise yourself with the platform.
- Think about the lighting in your room, ensure your face is well lit so that your facial expressions and non-verbal communication are clearly visible. Consider using a ring light to improve the lighting. Some webcams have a built-in ring light.

Case notes

- Ensure you read **all** the case notes. The notes may span more than one page and require you to scroll down. Sometimes, vital results or information are on a second page. Read until you see the 'end of notes' notification.
- Make a note of the patient demographics/physical attributes. The actor may not perfectly match the case patient, e.g. the notes may say the patient has a BMI of 35 – this is likely to be relevant to the case. However, the actor may have a much lower BMI so you may not get the visual cue to discuss weight. Perhaps write any key things like this on your whiteboard as a reminder.
- Pay attention to examination findings – normal or not? Accept these to be as described and use this information in your case. It is not generally necessary to repeat examinations.

Use your 3 minutes wisely

- The information in the case notes is there for a reason. Consider why the information may be included when reading the notes.
- Carefully check the drug history – are there any medications that you are not familiar with?
- Do the case notes give you a big hint about what is coming next, e.g. abnormal test result? Think about any key questions you may need to ask and consider what you may need to include in your management plan.
- Above all, resist the urge to look back at the previous patient's notes to work out why that consultation seemed difficult. Your full focus of attention should be on the next case, not the last one.

Your room and the run up to the exam

- You will have to ensure you have cleared your walls of posters/flowcharts that you normally use as reference points in day-to-day work. Doing this ahead of the exam can be helpful to get you used to the feel of the room, and also ensure that you can safely consult without needing to look at this information.
- Learn about drugs in your normal surgeries. Become as familiar as you can with common drugs and their doses. Remember, you will have no access to the BNF or drug databases during the exam but you are expected to be familiar with common drugs and how they are used.
- Practise with your whiteboard. During any telephone calls you have with patients, you could practise jotting key phrases/cues down to help you. Ensure you can do this without spending too much time looking down so when you have a patient on a video call, you are not breaking eye contact too frequently.

ABBREVIATIONS

#	fracture
°C	degrees centigrade
♀	female
♂	male
1/12	1 month
20/40	20 weeks' gestation
2°	secondary
2WW	2-week wait
3/7	3 days
αFP	alpha-fetoprotein
A&E	accident and emergency department
AA	Alcoholics Anonymous
AAA	abdominal aortic aneurysm
AAI	adrenaline autoinjector
ABC	airway, breathing, circulation
abdo	abdominal
ABPI	ankle brachial pressure index
ABPM	ambulatory blood pressure monitoring
Abx	antibiotics
AC	air conduction
ACE	angiotensin-converting enzyme
ACEI	angiotensin-converting enzyme inhibitor
ACL	anterior cruciate ligament
ACR	albumin creatinine ratio
ACS	acute coronary syndrome
ACT	acceptance and commitment therapy
ACTH	adrenocorticotropic hormone
ADHD	attention deficit hyperactivity disorder
ADL	activities of daily living
AF	atrial fibrillation
AKA	also known as
AKI	acute kidney injury (acute renal failure)
AKT	applied knowledge test
ALP	alkaline phosphatase
ALT	alanine aminotransferase
AMD	age-related macular degeneration
AMS	acute mountain sickness
AMTS	abbreviated mental test score
ANA	antinuclear antibody
ANP	advanced nurse practitioner
APC	adenomatous polyposis coli
APQ	alcohol problems questionnaire
APTT	activated partial thromboplastin time
ARB	angiotensin receptor blocker
AREDS2	vitamin C 500 mg, vitamin E 400 IU, lutein 10 mg, zeaxanthin 2 mg, zinc 25 mg and copper (cupric oxide) 2 mg
AS	ankylosing spondylitis
ASD	atrial septal defect
AST	aspartate transaminase
AUDIT	alcohol use disorders identification test
AUTI	atypical urinary tract infection
AV	arteriovenous
AVSD	atrioventricular septal defect
β-blockers	beta-blockers
β-hCG	beta-human chorionic gonadotropin
B12	vitamin B12
BAUS	British Association of Urological Surgeons
BC	bone conduction
BCC	basal-cell carcinoma
BCG	bacillus Calmette–Guerin
BD	twice daily
BDD	body dysmorphic disorder
BM	blood sugar level
BMD	bone mineral density
BMI	body mass index
BNF	British National Formulary
BNP	B-type natriuretic peptide
BP	blood pressure
BPH	benign prostatic hypertrophy
bpm	beats per minute
BPO	benzoyl peroxide
BPPV	benign paroxysmal positional vertigo
BRCA	breast cancer
BV	bacterial vaginosis
c/o	complaining of
Ca^{2+}	calcium
CA125	cancer antigen 125
CAMHS	Child and Adolescent Mental Health Services
CAPRIE	clopidogrel versus aspirin in patients at risk of ischaemic events
CAT	care assessment tool (RCGP)
CAT	COPD assessment tool
CBD	cannabidiol
CBD	case-based discussion
CBP	chronic bacterial prostatitis
CBT	cognitive behavioural therapy
CBT ED	cognitive behavioural therapy for eating disorders
CCB	calcium-channel blocker
CCB	coercive controlling behaviour
CCG	clinical commissioning group
CEA	carcinoembryonic antigen

CEPS clinical examination and procedural skills
CF cystic fibrosis
CFTR CF transmembrane conductance regulator
CHA_2DS_2 VASc clinical prediction calculator for estimating risk of stroke in patients with atrial fibrillation
CHC combined hormonal contraception
CHC continuing healthcare
CI contraindication(s)
CIBH change in bowel habit
CIDP chronic inflammatory demyelinating polyneuropathy
CK creatinine kinase
CKD chronic kidney disease
CKS Clinical Knowledge Summaries (NICE)
CM&C clinical management and medical complexity
CMHT community medical health team
CMV cytomegalovirus
CN cranial nerve
CNS central nervous system
COCP combined oral contraceptive pill
COPD chronic obstructive pulmonary disease
COT consultation observation tool
COVID coronavirus disease
CP chronic prostatitis
CPAP continuous positive airway pressure
CPPS chronic pelvic pain syndrome
CRB-65 confusion, respiratory rate, BP, age – assessment tool for community-acquired pneumonia
CRC Clinical Research Council
CrCl creatinine clearance
CRP C-reactive protein
CSA clinical skills assessment – the forerunner to the SCA exam
CT computed tomography
CT CAP CT chest abdomen and pelvis
CT KUB CT kidney, ureters and bladder
Cu-IUD copper coil
CURB confusion, urea, respiratory rate, blood pressure
CV cardiovascular
CVA cerebrovascular accident (stroke)
CVD cardiovascular disease
CXR chest X-ray

DAAT Drug and Alcohol Action Team
DBP diastolic blood pressure
DC direct current
DEET *N,N*-diethyl-meta-toluamide
DEXA dual energy X-ray absorptiometry
DG&D data gathering and diagnosis
DH drug history
DHEAS dehydroepiandrosterone sulfate
DKA diabetic ketoacidosis
DLA Disability Living Allowance
DM diabetes mellitus
DMPA depot-medroxyprogesterone acetate
DMSA dimercaptosuccinic acid
DNA did not attend (i.e. missed appointment)
DNACPR do not attempt cardiopulmonary resuscitation
DOAC direct oral anticoagulant
DOB date of birth
DPP4 dipeptidyl peptidase 4
DRE digital rectal exam
DSM-5-TR *Diagnostic and Statistical Manual of Mental Disorders*, 5th edition
DUB dysfunctional uterine bleeding
DV domestic violence
DVLA Driver and Vehicle Licensing Agency
DVT deep vein thrombosis

EBV Epstein–Barr virus
ECG electrocardiography
ECHO echocardiogram
ECP emergency contraceptive pill
ED erectile dysfunction
EEG electroencephalography
eGFR estimated glomerular filtration rate
eGFRcysC glomerular filtration rate (eGFR) by standardised cystatin C
ELISA enzyme-linked immunosorbent assay
ELSCS emergency lower segment caesarean section
ENT ear, nose and throat
ESR erythrocyte sedimentation rate
ETP essential thrombocytopenia

F female
F2F face-to-face
FAP familial adenomatous polyposis
FBC full blood count
FBG fasting blood glucose
FeNO fractional exhaled nitric oxide
FEV1 forced expiratory volume in 1 second
FH family history
FIT faecal immunochemical testing
FOB faecal occult blood
FOCUS Filter, Opportunity, Context, Unite, Safety

FODMAPs fermentable oligosaccharides, disaccharides, monosaccharides and polyols
FRAX fracture risk assessment tool
FSH follicle-stimulating hormone
FSRH Faculty of Sexual and Reproductive Healthcare
fT4 free thyroxine
FVC forced vital capacity

g grams
G6PD glucose-6-phosphate dehydrogenase
GAD general anxiety disorder
GAD-2 general anxiety disorder 2-item
GCS Glasgow Coma Scale
GCSE general certificate of secondary education
GF glandular fever
GFR glomerular filtration rate
GGT gamma-glutamyl transferase
GI gastrointestinal
GI glycaemic index
GINA Global Initiative for Asthma
GLP glucagon-like peptide
GMC General Medical Council
GnRH gonadotropin-releasing hormone
GOLD global obstructive lung disease
GORD gastro-oesophageal reflux disease
GP general practitioner
GQ gender-queer
GTN glyceryl trinitrate
GUM genitourinary medicine

h/o history of
HACE high-altitude cerebral oedema
HAPE high-altitude pulmonary oedema
HAS-BLED score for major bleeding risk
Hb haemoglobin
HbA1c glycated haemoglobin
HbeAg/Ab hepatitis B e antigen/antibody
HBsAg hepatitis B surface antigen
HBV DNA hepatitis B virus deoxyribonucleic acid
HCA healthcare assistant
HCM hypertrophic cardiomyopathy
Hct haematocrit
HCU homocystinuria
HCV RNA hepatitis C virus ribonucleic acid
HDL high-density lipoprotein
HDLC high-density lipoprotein cholesterol
HF heart failure
Hib *Haemophilus influenzae* type B (vaccine)
HIV human immunodeficiency virus
HLA B27 human leukocyte antigen B27
HMB heavy menstrual bleeding
HNPCC hereditary non-polyposis colorectal cancer
HOCM hypertrophic obstructive cardiomyopathy
HONK hyperosmolar non-ketotic acidosis
HPV human papillomavirus
HR heart rate
HRT hormone replacement therapy
HS heart sounds
HSP Henoch–Schönlein purpura
HTN hypertension

IBD inflammatory bowel disease
IBS inflammatory bowel syndrome
IBS-C IBS with constipation
IBS-D IBS with diarrhoea
IBS-M IBS with mixed bowel habits
IBS-U IBS unclassified
ICD-11 *International Classification of Diseases*, 11th Revision
ICE ideas, concerns and expectations
ICP intracranial pressure
ICS inhaled corticosteroids
ID intellectual disability
Ig immunoglobulin
IgG immunoglobulin G
IgM immunoglobulin M
IHD ischaemic heart disease
IM intramuscular
IMB intermenstrual bleeding
IMP progesterone-only implant
INR international normalised ratio
IPS interpersonal skills
IPSS International Prostate Symptom Score
IQ intelligence quotient
ISMN isosorbide mononitrate
IT information technology
ITU intensive treatment unit
IUD intrauterine device (copper coil)
IUS intrauterine system (e.g. Mirena)
IV intravenous
IVDU intravenous drug use
IVF in vitro fertilisation
Ix investigation

JVP jugular venous pressure

K potassium

LA local anaesthetic
LABA long-acting beta agonist

LAMA	long-acting muscarinic antagonist
LARC	long-acting reversible contraception
LBT	liver blood test
LD	learning disability
LDH	lactate dehydrogenase
LFT	liver function test (former name for LBT)
LGBTQ+	lesbian, gay, bisexual, transgender, queer or questioning +
LH	luteinising hormone
LIF	left iliac fossa
LMP	last menstrual period
LMWH	low molecular weight heparin
LNG-IUS	levonorgestrel-releasing intrauterine system
LOC	loss of consciousness
LRTI	lower respiratory tract infection
LTC	long-term condition/s
LTOT	long-term oxygen therapy
LUTS	lower urinary tract symptoms
LV	left ventricular
LVOT	left ventricular outflow tract
m	metres
M	male
M/R	modified release
MANTRA	Maudsley model of anorexia nervosa treatment for adults
MART	maintenance and reliever therapy
MASI	Melasma Area and Severity Index
MC&S	microscopy and culture
MCADD	medium chain acyl-CoA dehydrogenase deficiency
mcg	micrograms
MCS	multiple chemical sensitivity
MCUG	micturating cystourethrogram
MCV	mean corpuscular volume
MDI	metered dose inhaler
MDMA	3,4-methylenedioxymethamphetamine (ecstasy)
MDT	multidisciplinary team
MenC	meningitis C (vaccine)
MEWS score	modified early warning system score
mg	milligrams
MH	mental health
MI	myocardial infarction
mL	millilitres
MMR	measles, mumps and rubella
mMRC	modified Medical Research Council
MPLT	maintaining performance, learning and teaching
MRC	Medical Research Council
MRI	magnetic resonance imaging
MS	multiple sclerosis
MSK	musculoskeletal
MSU	mid-stream urine
MTP	metatarsophalangeal
MUSE	medicated urethral system for erections
Mx	results
N&V	nausea and vomiting
Na	sodium
NAD	no abnormality detected
NHS	National Health Service
NICE	National Institute for Health and Care Excellence
NIPT	non-invasive prenatal testing
NKDA	no known drug allergies
NOGG	National Osteoporosis Guideline Group
NOK	next of kin
NSAID	non-steroidal anti-inflammatory drug
NVD	normal vaginal delivery
NYHA	New York Heart Association
O/E	on examination
OA	osteoarthritis
OCD	obsessive-compulsive disorder
OCP	oral contraceptive pill
OD	once daily
Ofsted	Office for Standards in Children's Education, Children's Services and Skills
OGD	oesophago-gastroduodenoscopy
OGTT	oral glucose tolerance test
OM	once in the morning
ON	once at night
OOH	out-of-hours GP
ORBIT	score for atrial fibrillation to assess bleeding risk
ORBIT-AF	Outcomes Registry for Better Informed Treatment of Atrial Fibrillation
OSA	obstructive sleep apnoea
OSAHS	obstructive sleep apnoea/hypopnoea syndrome
OSAS	obstructive sleep apnoea syndrome
OSFED	other specified feeding or eating disorder
OTC	over the counter
PA	personal assistant
PC	presenting complaint
PCB	post-coital bleeding
PCDS	Primary Care Dermatology Society
PCKD	polycystic kidney disease

PCN	primary care network
PCOS	polycystic ovary syndrome
PCR	protein creatinine ratio
PCV	pneumococcal conjugate vaccine
PE	pulmonary embolus/embolism
PEF	peak expiratory flow
PEFR	peak expiratory flow rate
PERLA	pupils equal and react to light and accommodation
PF	plantar fasciitis
PID	pelvic inflammatory disease
PIL	patient information leaflet
PIP	Personal Independence Payment
PMB	post-menopausal bleeding
PMH	past medical history
PN	practice nurse
PND	paroxysmal nocturnal dyspnoea
POI	primary ovarian insufficiency
POP	progesterone-only contraception pill
PPI	proton pump inhibitors
PR	per rectum (rectal examination)
PRN	as required
PSA	prostate-specific antigen
PSC	primary sclerosing cholangitis
PSV	public service vehicle licence
PT	prothrombin time
PTH	parathyroid hormone
PTSD	post-traumatic stress disorder
PUD	peptic ulcer disease
PV	per vaginam (vaginal examination)
PVD	peripheral vascular disease
QDS	four times daily
QIP	quality improvement project
QOL	quality of life
QRISK4	algorithm for cardiovascular disease
RA	rheumatoid arthritis
RACPC	rapid-access chest pain clinic
RCA	recorded consultation assessment
RCGP	Royal College of General Practitioners
RCO	Royal College of Ophthalmologists
ReSPECT	recommended summary plan for emergency care and treatment
RFs	risk factors
RLQ	right lower quadrant
RNIB	Royal National Institute of Blind People
ROM	range of movement
RR	respiratory rate
RTO	relating to others
RUQ	right upper quadrant
RUTI	recurrent urinary tract infection
Rx	treatment
s/c	subcutaneous
SABA	short-acting beta-agonist
SADQ	severity of alcohol dependence questionnaire
Sats	oxygen saturation
SBP	systolic blood pressure
SCA	simulated consultation assessment
SCC	squamous cell carcinoma
SD	standard deviation
SGLT	sodium-glucose linked transporter
SH	social history
SHBG	sex hormone-binding globulin
SHIM	sexual health inventory for men
SI	sexual intercourse
SIGN	Scottish Intercollegiate Guidelines Network
SLE	systemic lupus erythematosus
SLR	straight leg raise
SMART	self-management and recovery training
SNHL	sensorineural hearing loss
SNRI	serotonin–norepinephrine reuptake inhibitors
SNT	soft and non-tender
SOB	shortness of breath
SOL	space-occupying lesion
SPC	summary of product characteristics
SSCM	specialist support for clinical management
SSRI	selective serotonin reuptake inhibitor
stat	immediately
STI	sexually transmitted infection
SUFE	subluxation of the upper femoral epiphysis
SVT	supraventricular tachycardia
T1DM	type 1 diabetes/diabetics
T2DM	type 2 diabetes/diabetics
T3	tri-iodothyronine level
T4	thyroxine level
TAH	total abdominal hysterectomy
TB	tuberculosis
TC	total cholesterol
TCA	tricyclic antidepressant
TCI	to come in
TDS	three times daily
TENS	transcutaneous electrical nerve stimulation
TFT	thyroid function test
THC	delta-9-tetrahydro cannabinol
TIA	transient ischaemic attack
TIBC	total iron-binding capacity
TSH	thyroid-stimulating hormone

TURP	transurethral resection of the prostate
TV	trichomonas vaginalis
TVUSS	transvaginal ultrasound
U&E	urea and electrolytes and eGFR
UC	ulcerative colitis
UKMEC	UK medical eligibility criteria for contraceptive use
ULT	urate lowering therapy
UMN	upper motor neurone
UO	urinary output
UPA	ulipristal acetate
UPSI	unprotected sexual intercourse
URTI	upper respiratory tract infection
USS	ultrasound scan
UTI	urinary tract infection
UV	ultraviolet
VA	visual acuity
VC	vital capacity
VEGF	vascular endothelial growth factor
VF	ventricular fibrillation
vs	versus
VT	ventricular tachycardia
VTE	venous thromboembolism
VZV	varicella-zoster virus
WCC	white cell count
WHO	World Health Organization
WPBA	workplace-based assessment

DISCLAIMER

The information or guidance contained in this book is intended for use by medical professionals (specifically general practitioners or general practitioner registrars) only and is provided strictly as a supplement to the reader's own judgement, their knowledge of the patient's medical history, relevant manufacturers' instructions and the appropriate best practice guidelines. The guidance we refer to within this book is specifically for general practitioners based in the UK, and international readers should refer to local guidance and advice. Because of the rapid advances in medical science, any information or advice on dosages, procedures or diagnoses should be independently verified. The reader should take into account that the information within this book is only part of any guidance mentioned and is strongly urged to consult the full text of up-to-date guidance. The text is not to replace specialist advice. The reader is strongly urged to consult the relevant national drug formulary and the drug companies' and device or material manufacturers' printed instructions, and their websites, before administering or utilising any of the drugs, devices or materials mentioned in this book. This book does not indicate whether a particular treatment is appropriate or suitable for a particular individual. Ultimately, it is the sole responsibility of the medical professional to make their own professional judgements, so as to advise and treat patients appropriately. We do not accept any liability or responsibility for any form of loss or any decision made by the reader.

CHAPTER 2
PATIENT LESS THAN 19 YEARS OLD

	Cases in this chapter	RCGP 2025 curriculum	Learning points
2.1	Anaemia	**Haematology** 'Common and important conditions – anaemia and its causes including iron, folate and vitamin B12 deficiency, sideroblastic, haemolytic, chronic disease' 'Communicate effectively and consider symptoms that are within the range of normal or self-limiting illness and differentiate them from underlying pathology such as anaemia'	Differential diagnosis of tiredness in children Management of anaemia in children
2.2	Eczema	**Dermatology** 'Dermatological disorders in childhood … atopic eczema' 'Common and important conditions – eczema: infantile, childhood, atopic' 'Prescribe appropriately and safely'	Information from the Primary Care Dermatology Society about the cause and management of eczema in children Red flags When to refer to specialist
2.3	Recurrent UTI	**Renal and urology** 'UTIs in children and adults including lower UTI, pyelonephritis and persistent or recurrent infection'	Urinary tract infection in under 16s: diagnosis and management
2.4	Eating Disorder	**Mental health** 'Eating disorders, including in those living with obesity, binge eating disorder, anorexia and bulimia nervosa'	Eating disorders, recognition and treatment
2.5	Asthma Diagnosis	**Respiratory health** 'Asthma: acute and chronic'	Asthma diagnosis and management in children Global Initiative for Asthma (GINA) guidelines Diagnosing asthma in <5 year olds

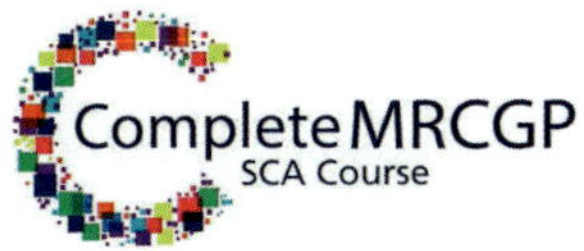

Links to the RCGP Curriculum

In this chapter, the cases are drawn from the following clinical topic guides:

- Haematology
- Dermatology
- Renal and urology
- Mental health
- Respiratory health

And the following life stages topic guide:

- Children and young people

Scope of Conditions

Remember that GPs are usually the first point of care for children and young people and provide the majority of the care. Children may have acute or chronic conditions, or both. GPs play a key role in coordinating holistic care, and this may involve the health, social and educational sectors. GPs should be able to identify and support vulnerable and at-risk young people, particularly with their mental health and always remembering that there may be safeguarding issues. The following curriculum areas may be particularly relevant to patients in this life stage group. Some case examples are included:

- Dermatology – eczema, pityriasis, molluscum
- Ear nose and throat, speech and hearing – glue ear, hearing loss, recurrent tonsillitis
- Eyes and vision – squint, conjunctivitis
- Gastroenterology – cow's milk protein allergy, reflux, appendicitis, cystic fibrosis
- Haematology – anaemia, lymphoma, leukaemia
- Infectious diseases – common childhood illnesses
- Renal and urology – urinary infections, reflux, enuresis
- Mental health – anxiety, depression, self-harm, OCD
- Sexual health – contraception (including Fraser competence), gender identity
- Metabolic problems – new type 1 diabetes
- Neurodevelopmental conditions and neurodiversity
- Respiratory health – asthma, chronic cough, cystic fibrosis
- Urgent and unscheduled care – e.g. acute asthma, fracture

Skills and Pitfalls

In addition to the information in Chapter 1 'How to Demonstrate Skills: The Marking Scheme Made Easy' consider the following challenges for this blueprint group:

- There may be two patients to consider – the child/young person and their care giver. You may be speaking to the patient or to a care giver. Consider how the problem impacts the wider family.
- Be able to demonstrate awareness of developmental milestones and assessment of any delay, which may be gross motor, fine motor, social or language.
- Knowledge and demonstration of the features of the acutely unwell child (traffic light chart). How will you assess this when not able to examine the child? Consider asking what the child is doing, how they are behaving and the usual questions around fluid intake and urine output, etc. The parent may be able to give information about temperature so you can ask this.

Know your team – demonstrate that you can coordinate care with other health professionals such as the practice nurse, health visitor, school nurse and children's social prescribers.

Doctor's Notes

Patient	Connor McGowen	12 years	M
PMH	None		
Medications	None		
Allergies	None		

Consultations 4 weeks ago by locum GP – mum noticed he looks a little pale and seems lethargic. Connor reporting feeling tired. No other symptoms other than occasional abdominal cramps, usually when he has been a little constipated. No red flags. Mum worried about coeliac disease due to family history (paternal cousin and grandfather). O/E looks pale. Chest clear, abdo NAD, no lymph nodes palpable, seems otherwise well. Agreed bloods, then review

Investigations 3 weeks ago

FBC: Hb 97 g/L
MCV 78 fL
WCC 7 × 10^9/L
Platelets 269 × 10^9/L

B12, folate – normal

Ferritin low

TFT normal

Coeliac screen normal

Household	Shona McGowen	42 years	F
	Patrick McGowen	43 years	M

Video consultation with mum – requests blood results.

Example Consultation

Anaemia

Open ☐ How can I help? Yes, we have the results. Please can you tell me what led to the tests?

ICE1 ☐ Was there anything particular you thought might be going on?

History ☐ You mentioned Connor had seemed tired and pale before. How is he now?

Impact ☐ How is the tiredness affecting him? Has it interfered with his hobbies or school work? Has it affected you as a family in any way?

Flags ☐ Have any new symptoms developed since you saw my colleague? Any diarrhoea? Any blood loss from anywhere such as nosebleeds or blood from his bottom? Any weight loss? Or fever? Any bruising? Or lumps/bumps?

ICE2 ☐ Have you been worrying about the results? What particularly worried you? How about Connor; is he concerned about anything?

Risk ☐ What does Connor like to eat? Does he eat meat? What about green leafy vegetables? Is he a fussy eater? I'm wondering if it is a struggle to give him a balanced diet? Does his diet cause you concern? Is there any family history of anaemia or blood problems?

ICE3 ☐ Other than going through the results, is there anything else you are hoping for today?

SummarICE ☐ So, to summarise, Connor has been more lethargic lately, just wanting to lie on the sofa after school, and has appeared a little pale for the last couple of months. You wondered about coeliac disease as two people on your husband's side have this. Have I got it so far? Anything you would like to add at all? OK, shall we talk through the results?

Impression ☐ Most of Connor's bloods were reassuring and his test for coeliac disease was negative. We did pick up one test result that wasn't quite right, though it's nothing serious and is something we sort out relatively easily. His blood count was a little low, something called anaemia.

Experience ☐ Have you heard of anaemia? You're right it is common in pregnancy and yes Connor's anaemia appears to be due to low iron.

Explanation ☐ When we are short of iron, our red blood cells can't carry as much oxygen around and this can make us feel tired. The red blood cells have less of a protein called haemoglobin which carries the oxygen. This protein also makes the blood red, so this is why some people with anaemia look pale. There are lots of reasons why someone can be short of iron. In Connor's case it is likely that he is not getting enough in his diet.

Empower ☐ There are things you and Connor can do to help. Eating foods rich in iron can boost his levels. Red meat, fish and green leafy vegetables all contain iron. Some cereals have iron added to them too. Increasing these foods will help Connor feel better and help reduce the chance of him becoming anaemic again. Do you think you could adjust the meals to increase iron-rich foods?

Options ☐ You could try increasing dietary iron alone …

Recommend ☐ … but I suggest we give Connor a course of iron to give his stores a boost and get him feeling better quicker. How does that sound? Is Connor able to swallow tablets?

Specifics ☐ I would suggest a 3-month course of a tablet called ferrous sulfate. He would need to take 1 × 200 mg tablet a day. These tablets can cause nausea and bowel upset – either constipation or diarrhoea – and do tend to turn poo black. However, most people tolerate them pretty well. Having vitamin C with the tablet, for example drinking a cup of orange juice, helps the iron be absorbed better and can reduce any side effects. What are your thoughts?

Future ☐ Great, we will need to repeat his blood test in 4 weeks to check he is responding and will check the test again at the end of the 3-month course.

Safety net ☐ If Connor has side effects from the tablets or develops new symptoms, particularly bleeding, bruising, weight loss, fever, sweats or bowel problems, please call me straight away.

Patient's Story

Anaemia

Doctor's notes Connor McGowen, 12 years. No PMH, medications or allergies.

Seen 4 weeks ago by locum GP – mum noticed he looks a little pale and seems lethargic. Connor reporting feeling tired. No other symptoms other than occasional abdominal cramps, usually when he has been a little constipated. No red flags. Mum worried about coeliac disease due to family history (paternal cousin and grandfather). O/E looks pale. Chest clear, abdo NAD, no lymph nodes palpable, seems otherwise well. Agreed bloods, then review.

Investigations 3 weeks ago. FBC: Hb 97 g/L, MCV 78 fL, WCC 7×10^9/L, platelets 269×10^9/L. B12, folate – normal. Ferritin low. TFT normal. Coeliac screen normal.

How to act Relaxed.

PC *'Hi. I was hoping to discuss Connor's recent blood test results.'*

History Connor has been more lethargic and tired for the last couple of months. He has been lying on the sofa after school and doesn't feel like going out to play football. You think he looks pale but is otherwise okay. He does get occasional abdominal pain but this usually coincides with when he becomes a little constipated. He doesn't eat a lot of fruit and vegetables. He prefers to eat chips and pizza if he has a choice. He has not suffered any weight loss, sweats, fevers, bruising, diarrhoea or significant abdominal pain. No blood loss from anywhere. You were anaemic during pregnancy but no other family history of blood problems.

Social Connor generally enjoys school and plays for a football team. He has had less energy and has been less enthusiastic about going to football training. Connor's dad is a builder and works long hours. You work in a supermarket, long hours too, so it is often tempting to make quick meals like pizza rather than cooking lots of meat and vegetable meals. You feel you should make more of an effort with the family's diet. You could pick up some healthier ingredients at work. Perhaps you could encourage Connor to cook with you.

ICE You aren't sure why Connor has been so tired but wonder about coeliac disease as his paternal grandfather and cousin have this. You just wish to discuss the results, though aren't impatient regarding this and are happy to discuss the background with the doctor. You have heard of anaemia – you had this whilst you were pregnant with Connor and took iron tablets for a month or two. You are happy for Connor to try tablets. You didn't have any problems with them when you took them, and you'd like him to be back to normal as soon as possible. You know he can swallow tablets because he has occasionally taken a paracetamol tablet when needed.

Anaemia

Haemoglobin concentration cut offs can vary between areas and laboratories but the accepted definition is a haemoglobin that is 2 standard deviations below the mean for age. The WHO defines anaemia for children[1]:

2–5 years: <110 g/L
5–11 years: <115 g/L
11–15 years: <120 g/L

Iron deficiency is most commonly due to inadequate dietary intake. Consider coeliac disease.

B12 and folate deficiency tend to cause megaloblastic anaemia. Again, usually dietary; rarely, pernicious anaemia can occur.

Consider inherited anaemias, particularly in certain ethnic groups, e.g. sickle cell and thalassaemia.

Other genetic causes, e.g. sideroblastic anaemia, hereditary spherocytosis, G6PD deficiency.

Where there are other abnormalities on the FBC consider conditions affecting the bone marrow such as leukaemia, secondary cancers or fibrosis.

Acquired haemolytic anaemias can be caused by infections, e.g. malaria, hypersplenism, toxins and auto-immune conditions.

Treatment

Depends on cause.

For deficiencies consult BNF for children[2] as doses vary with age and also whether medication is for prophylaxis or treatment. Both tablets and liquid forms are available. Sytron (sodium feredetate) is a commonly used oral solution for children unable to swallow tablets.

Children over 12 can have the same treatment as adults, i.e. one tablet a day of ferrous sulfate/fumarate/gluconate. NICE CKS guidelines now support once-a-day treatment after research showed that higher doses didn't have additional benefit but are associated with increased side effects.

Doctor's Notes

Patient	Arthur Miller	13 years	M
PMH	Eczema since age 5		
Medications	Eumovate ointment (clobetasone butyrate)		
	Oilatum cream		
Allergies	None		
Consultations	4 months ago, seen by GP colleague, mild–moderate eczema present at elbow and knee flexures. Flare diagnosed, Eumovate prescribed. 3 × Eumovate tubes issued since, practice pharmacist requesting a review		
Investigations	None		
Household	Anita Miller	45 years	F
	Gary Miller	49 years	M
	Sophie Miller	8 years	F

Video call with mum, Anita, to discuss Arthur's eczema.

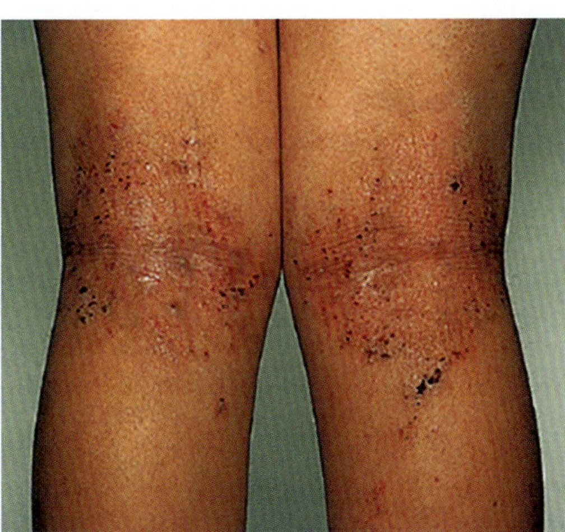

Reproduced from *Common Skin Diseases*, 18th edition, CRC Press. With thanks to the late Ronald Marks and Richard Motley.

Example Consultation

Eczema

Open ☐ Hello Anita. How can I help? We can certainly discuss putting that on repeat.

ICE1 ☐ I'm just wondering if we can improve things further. Are you/Arthur happy with how his skin is just now? Why not? What would you like to change?

Sense ☐ I can hear it is very important that you never run out of creams.

Curious ☐ What does Arthur use to wash? Does he wash his hair? Is his head itchy?

History ☐ Is he otherwise well? How often does he use the Eumovate cream? Is that once a day? And in between times how is his skin? Is it completely back to normal? How often does he use the Oilatum? Does he like it? Does anyone else in the family have eczema? Any other conditions which run in the family?

ICE2 ☐ What is the worst his skin has been? Can you describe that? What worried you both then? Do you or Arthur have any specific worries about his skin, now or for the future?

Risk ☐ Any allergies? Pets? How are things at school? Is anything making him unhappy?

Impact ☐ How does his skin affect his life? How about using his creams? How would he feel about using the Oilatum four times a day? Would that be possible? What would stop him?

ICE3 ☐ What did you think I may say today? And anything else you or Arthur would like?

SummarICE ☐ Arthur has long-standing eczema that requires frequent steroid use to keep on top of it. You would like the Eumovate on repeat to make it easier to get. Arthur is worried about the long-term effects of eczema, but is embarrassed to use his creams in front of his friends.

Impression ☐ As you're aware, eczema is a chronic problem which needs to be managed over time. Today we need to find a solution to help Arthur use more emollient and less steroid.

InCludE ☐ I hear that the eczema is rarely completely absent. I'd like to help prevent Arthur needing to use the Eumovate every 2 weeks. To reassure you both, it is most unlikely that there will be scarring; this very rarely happens with eczema.

Experience ☐ What have you been told about how to use the Oilatum cream? What about the Eumovate? Do you know why we don't suggest using the Eumovate every day?

Explanation ☐ Oilatum is a strong moisturiser. Used four times a day, it will stop the dryness, itching and flare-ups. Eumovate is a strong steroid cream. The emollient won't cause any harm so we can use lots of it, but the steroid creams can cause problems, for example thinner skin or bruising and weak bones or diabetes. It's unlikely Arthur has any of these complications but if we can reduce its use that would be great. Please use the steroid when it flares but let's try to reduce flares so it is less prone to cracks and infection. How does that sound?

Options ☐ It sounds like you're not really getting on well with the Oilatum; perhaps a change of emollient would be helpful? Some creams are designed to last longer so you don't need to use them so often. We could try an emollient which is also suitable for washing?

Recommend ☐ Doublebase Dayleve lasts longer so he could try this every morning. I suggest Dermol 500 for showering. Standard soaps/body wash irritate eczema-prone skin so should be avoided.

InCludE ☐ Regular use of emollients and reducing steroid will help prevent any permanent changes to his skin, which you said is important to Arthur.

Empathy ☐ No teenager wants to appear different and applying creams can be embarrassing.

Empower ☐ Could he put Dermol 500 in an empty shower gel bottle so it's not obvious he's using a moisturiser? If he can discreetly put another layer of Dermol on after a shower, e.g. in the toilet, then this would help. Shall I give him a small tube to keep in his bag? If you need Eumovate, use it once a day, before bed, to reduce side effects; what do you think?

Specifics ☐ Shall we catch up again in a month? I will add the creams to his repeat prescriptions.

Safety net ☐ If his skin ever looks red or oozing, please contact us as this may be a sign of infection.

Patient's Story

Eczema

Doctor's notes Arthur Miller, 13 years. PMH: eczema since age 5. Medications: Eumovate ointment (clobetasone butyrate), Oilatum cream.

4 months ago, seen by GP colleague, mild–moderate eczema present at elbow and knee flexures. Flare diagnosed, Eumovate prescribed. 3 × Eumovate tubes issued since, practice pharmacist requesting a review.

How to act Demanding, knowledgeable.

PC *'I need more steroid cream for Arthur but apparently he needs a medication review.'*

History Arthur is currently at school. He always responds well to the Eumovate, which he's been using for years. Arthur was born by NVD at term and had no antenatal or postnatal problems. He has had all his immunisations. There is no family history. Arthur has no other medical problems. At present, Arthur uses the Oilatum cream twice a day when the eczema is bad but doesn't use it the rest of the time. Every couple of weeks, Arthur has to use the Eumovate, twice a day, for a couple of days for his arms, wrists and legs. In between times his skin can be itchy but it doesn't always look red. Arthur uses shower gel and Head and Shoulders shampoo. In the past Arthur's skin has been cracked and painful and needed an antibiotic. Arthur's younger sister also has eczema and he has been using her hydrocortisone cream when he runs out of Eumovate.

Social Arthur lives with his parents and sister and is happy at school. Plays sports every day. No pets.

ICE **Mum:** You would like the prescription for the Eumovate to be on repeat so you don't have to keep coming back. You will tell the doctor if there is a problem. You have no concerns.

Arthur's ICE expressed to mum: Skin is itchy at times and this bothers him. He doesn't like using the emollient as it makes him feel sticky. He never takes it to school with him and he never applies it after showering following sport. He thinks his friends would laugh at him for putting moisturiser on but it does help. He thinks the creams work well when he uses them. Arthur is worried the eczema could leave scars that will last forever.

Learning Points

Atopic Eczema

Ask Atopy.

Family history.

Impact.

Compliance and regime with emollients and use of other soaps.

Stress.

Cause Genetic and environmental.

Mutation in the filaggrin gene in atopic eczema causing a defect in the skin barrier layer. 'Immunological changes are probably secondary to enhanced antigen penetration through a deficient epidermal barrier. The relevance of this finding is that it reinforces the importance of the regular use of emollients to help manage eczema.'[1]

Flags Sign of infection.

Overuse of steroids and underuse of emollients.

Arrange hospital admission if painful vesicular or ulcerated lesions, which may be eczema herpeticum.

Management **'Emollients are the mainstay of therapy and without them it is not possible to manage eczema effectively.'**[1] Moisturise '15–20 minutes before applying the topical steroid'.[1]

If compliance may be an issue, explore this and consider how to adapt the management plan for the individual to increase their emollient use.

'In both children and adults, it is more effective and safer to "hit hard" using more potent treatments for a few days than it is to use less potent treatments for longer periods of time.'[1]

Other Rxs Antihistamines for itch.

Advise emollients as soap substitutes.

Scalp preparations and shampoos.

Antibiotics – topical or oral.

Topical calcineurin inhibitors (immunomodulators) – tacrolimus and pimecrolimus. These have the advantage that they are not steroid based and so do not cause atrophy.[1]

Specialist referral[1] Diagnostic uncertainty.

Severe eczema.

Moderate–severe eczema but not responding to emollients/steroids/calcineurin inhibitors.

Signs of skin atrophy due to steroids.

Possible contact allergic dermatitis.

See the Primary Care Dermatology Society website for further information.[1]

Doctor's Notes

Patient	Kalpesh Khan	6 years	M
PMH	Urinary tract infection 6 weeks ago – *E. coli*, fully sensitive		
	Urinary tract infection 6 months ago – *E. coli*, fully sensitive		
Medications	No current medication		
	Past medication – two courses of trimethoprim		
Allergies	No information		
Consultations	Last appointment 2 days ago: attended with mum. Temperature 37.9°C, lower abdominal pain, dysuria, frequency and urgency		
	Abdominal examination – suprapubic tenderness, abdomen soft, no masses. No loin pains		
	Urine dip: protein +, blood +, leucocytes ++, nitrites ++		
	MSU sent		
	Trimethoprim prescription given		
	Weight 20 kg		
Investigations	MSU result from 2 days ago – *E. coli*, resistant to amoxicillin and trimethoprim, sensitive to nitrofurantoin and cefalosporin		
Household	Asaf Khan	43 years	M
	Yasmin Khan	41 years	F
	Ayub Khan	7 years	M
	Raja Khan	3 years	M
	Sabeen Khan	2 years	F

Mum, Yasmin, has booked an appointment to talk on the phone.

Example Consultation

Recurrent UTI

Open ☐ I'm sorry to hear that Kalpesh is no better. Could you tell me what has been happening over the last couple of days? How is he now? What is he doing at present?

History ☐ I see he has had two other urine infections in the past 6 months. In between his infections, how was he? And, generally, how is his health? I'm wondering if anyone in the family has experienced kidney problems?

ICE1 ☐ What is going through your mind about this?

Flags ☐ I need to find out how unwell he is just now. Do you know what Kalpesh's temperature is? Is he drinking well? When did he last pass urine? Do you know if his urine stream is normal? Have you seen any blood? Is he complaining of tummy or back pain? Has he vomited? Is he breathing normally? Is he drowsy, or able to concentrate on the TV?

ICE2 ☐ Is anything particularly worrying you about all of this?

Curious ☐ What is your experience of septicaemia? I'm sorry to hear that.

Empathy ☐ Infections must be worrying given what happened with your father.

Risk ☐ And Kalpesh's general health. Has he been growing and developing well? Were there any problems during your pregnancy? Does he ever struggle to open his bowels? Does he have any allergies? Has he had any tests at the hospital?

ICE3 ☐ Have you had any thoughts about what you would like to happen next? Was there anything specific you hoped I might suggest today?

InCludE ☐ You think Kalpesh has a urine infection but know that frequent urine infections in children aren't common. You are worried about septicaemia as this infection hasn't gone away.

Impression ☐ The laboratory sample confirms another urine infection, but unfortunately this one isn't sensitive to trimethoprim, which explains why he hasn't improved. The good news is that the laboratory has told us that a different antibiotic should work.

InCludE ☐ From your description of Kalpesh, it doesn't sound like he has septicaemia, but I agree this is a rare possibility if the infection isn't treated.

Experience ☐ Has another doctor talked to you about what tests we recommend with recurrent urine infections? Please tell me what you have read.

Explanation ☐ You are correct. Recurrent urine infections in children aren't that common, and usually need investigation. However, they do usually respond to antibiotic medicines.

Options ☐ Today I could either see Kalpesh in the surgery, if you feel he needs review, or send you a prescription for nitrofurantoin antibiotic which should kill the bacteria. Which would you prefer? Okay, I will do a prescription for nitrofurantoin. The dose is weight based so I will check this before sending the prescription.

Future ☐ As Kalpesh has now had three confirmed infections, I would like to refer him to see a specialist, would that be okay? May I order an urgent ultrasound scan to look at his kidneys and bladder, which will be done within 6 weeks? It is likely the specialist will want to do some other tests such as a special test that checks that his bladder empties properly and that urine doesn't flow back up into the tubes towards the kidneys, because this is one cause of recurrent urine infection in children.

Safety net ☐ Please monitor how much urine he passes. If significantly less, or he is more unwell, contact a doctor promptly. I will make the hospital referral; you should receive a letter within the next 2 weeks but please let us know if this doesn't happen.

Specifics ☐ If Kalpesh gets worse, please phone us promptly. I would expect him to improve within 48 hours, so if he is no better please let me know. If you're worried after 6 p.m. or at the weekend you can phone 111 for advice. Are you happy with the plan? Thank you.

Patient's Story

Recurrent UTI

Doctor's notes Mum calling to discuss Kalpesh Khan, 6 years. PMH: two UTIs – *E. coli*, fully sensitive, in past 6 months and further UTI confirmed on MSU, resistant to the recently prescribed trimethoprim.

How to act Concerned.

PC *'Hi Doctor, thanks for calling. I'm a bit worried about Kalpesh. He isn't responding to the antibiotics this time.'*

History You attended the surgery 2 days ago when Kalpesh had symptoms of a urinary tract infection. You were given antibiotics by the doctor and told to phone back if he didn't improve. Unfortunately, this time he hasn't improved with trimethoprim. This is his third urinary tract infection in the last 6 months. Kalpesh was born at term following a normal pregnancy. He has been developing normally and is getting on well at school. He is otherwise fit and well (including since his last infection). He opens his bowels daily. Currently Kalpesh is lying on the sofa watching TV but is alert and concentrating. He is still having a low-grade fever intermittently, has lower tummy pain and dysuria. His temperature is 37.2°C at present after paracetamol. He is eating and drinking okay and passing urine every 2–3 hours. You have seen no blood, and he has not complained of back pain. No vomiting. You have kept him off school for the last couple of days. There is no family history. He has no allergies.

Social You are a married full-time mum and have three other children. They are all well. Kalpesh's father is a mechanic during the day and works as a taxi driver in the evenings, so works long hours.

ICE You are worried that the antibiotics aren't working. You don't want Kalpesh to become really unwell. You are aware that infections can be serious – your father died of sepsis.

'I just don't want this to become a septicaemia.'

You have done some research and wonder if Kalpesh needs further tests. He has only had urine samples sent to date.

'I've read about tests he may need.'

Reading included an ultrasound scan and a kidney scan but this is all you understand. You would like to know what happens next. You are happy to accept antibiotics over the phone. You don't feel you could bring Kalpesh down to the surgery as you have no transport and the other children to look after. Resist any attempts to get you to attend the surgery, state *'He's really no worse than his last visit, it would be really difficult to get to you, can you not just treat him?'* You would like Kalpesh to be referred.

Learning Points

Most common signs and symptoms

- Infants (0–3 months): fever, vomiting, lethargy, irritability. Also, failure to thrive, poor feeding, jaundice, abdominal pain, haematuria, offensive urine.
- 3 months + (pre-verbal): fever. Also, abdominal pain, loin tenderness, vomiting, poor feeding, lethargy, irritability, haematuria, offensive urine, failure to thrive.
- 3 months + (verbal): frequency, dysuria, dysfunctional voiding, changes in continence, abdominal pain, loin tenderness, fever, malaise, vomiting, haematuria, offensive urine, cloudy urine.

Symptoms and signs that increase the likelihood that a UTI is present should be used to help decide if urine collection and testing is necessary.[1] Consider UTI in a baby or child under 5 with fever.[2]

Management of children with UTIs

Refer to NICE Guideline NG143 (2021) *Fever in under 5s: assessment and initial management.*[2]

Child's age	Testing	Management
3 months	Send urine for urgent MCS	Immediate admission to paediatrics for investigation and intravenous antibiotics in line with NICE Guideline NG143[2]
3 months–3 years	Dipstick testing	–ve nitrites and leucocytes = no antibiotic, no MCS +ve leucocytes and/or nitrites = start antibiotics and send urine for microscopy
3 years	'Dipstick testing for leucocyte esterase and nitrite is diagnostically as useful as microscopy and culture, and can safely be used'[1]	+ve nitrite and leucocytes = treat with antibiotics. Consider culture +ve nitrite, –ve leucocytes = treat (if urine sample was fresh) and send for culture –ve nitrite, +ve leucocytes = await MCS unless clinically UTI – may indicate infection outside urinary tract –ve nitrite and leucocytes = explore other causes of illness

Send an MSU if: suspected upper UTI (fever >38°C or loin pain), child <3 months, recurrent UTI, single positive for leucocytes or nitrites, no improvement within 24–48 hours (if sample not sent already),[1] child with intermediate–high-risk serious illness,[2] or when clinical symptoms and dipstick do not correlate.

For antibiotic choice: see your local antibiotic guidance and BNF.

Which investigations and should I refer?[1] Depends on the type of UTI and the child's age.

- **Typical UTI (UTI):** *E. coli* responding to treatment/48 hours, no other features of AUTI or RUTI.
- **Atypical UTI (AUTI):** seriously ill,[2] poor urine flow, abdominal or bladder mass, raised creatinine, non *E. coli* species, not responding to treatment within 48 hours or septicaemia. Admission often required.
- **Recurrent UTI (RUTI):** ≥2 UTIs (one must be upper) or ≥3 lower UTIs.

0–6 months
UTI: all require USS within 6 weeks, if abnormal consider MCUG.
AUTI: USS during acute infection **unless** * below. Also DMSA + MCUG.
RUTI: require urgent (during acute infection) USS,* DMSA + MCUG.

6 months–3 years
UTI: do not require investigation.
AUTI or RUTI: require USS (urgent for AUTI,* <6 weeks for RUTI) + DMSA ± MCUG.

Over 3 years
UTI: do not require investigation.
AUTI: urgent USS only **unless** * below.
RUTI: USS within 6 weeks and DMSA 4–6 months after the infection.

*__Unless__ in non-*E. coli* UTI, responding to antibiotics + no other features of AUTI – USS/6 weeks.

Doctor's Notes

Patient	Eleanor Cartwright	15 years	F
PMH	Constipation aged 4 years		
	Lower respiratory tract infection aged 11 years		
Medications	No current medications		
Allergies	No known allergies		
Consultations	Nurse minor illness clinic last week for URTI		
	'Looks thin.' Height 165 cm, weight 40 kg, BMI 14.7, pulse 58, BP 100/60, chest clear, abdo NAD, no neck lumps		
	Arranged routine bloods – FBC, U&E, LFT, glucose, TFT		
	Advised to book an appointment to speak with doctor'		
Investigations	All blood results normal		
Household	Brian Cartwright	55 years	M
	Faith Cartwright	54 years	F

Video consultation with Eleanor, 'Ellie'.

Triage note: Mum, Faith, booked this appointment. She is concerned about Ellie's weight and anger issues. Also heard vomiting when she was supposed to be showering.

Example Consultation

Eating Disorder

Open ☐ Hello Ellie, please tell me what led you to book the appointment today.

ICE1 ☐ How do you feel about your health? Have your parents commented on your eating?

History ☐ Please tell me about your family. How are things at home? How is school? Tell me what you like to do when you are not at school – hobbies and any socialising. Have you had any medical problems in the past? Do you take any medicines?

Impact ☐ Please tell me about any changes in your body you have noticed, for example going to the toilet, headaches or periods. Are you pleased or is that a worry? Have your parents noticed a change in you? And how about teachers at school – anything they have said?

Sense ☐ It sounds like your mum is worried about you. Can you tell me what you think she might be worried about? She mentioned vomiting?

ICE2 ☐ What have you noticed that worries you? What worries you most? Anything else?

Curious ☐ Ellie, your mum says you sometimes get angry. What makes you feel this way?

Risk ☐ Is anyone at school being horrible to you or bullying you? Because your periods have stopped, can I ask you some questions to make sure you are not pregnant? Do you have a boyfriend? Have you had sex? Has anyone made you feel uncomfortable or hurt you? Do you ever drink alcohol or take drugs?

Flags ☐ How is your mood? And your sleep? Can you concentrate on your schoolwork? A difficult question, but do you ever wish you were not alive? Have you tried to hurt yourself? Do you ever see or hear things that others can't? Or receive instructions that others are not aware of?

ICE3 ☐ When you were waiting for my call today, what did you think I might say? Is there anything specific you were hoping I would do today?

SummarICE ☐ To summarise, over the past 5 months you decided to change what foods you eat and exercise more. Since then, your parents and school teachers have been concerned about you and especially after your mum heard you being sick.

Experience ☐ Do you know the risks of losing too much weight? Have you known anyone who lost so much weight they became unwell?

Impression ☐ As your height is 165 cm and you weigh 40 kg, it means that your BMI is 14.7, so you are very underweight. Your blood results are normal, so I don't think there is any other illness causing weight loss. It sounds as if controlling your weight is really important to you. Sometimes, without realising it, a person can lose too much weight as they continue to focus on avoiding food and start to be sick to avoid absorbing food. This is called an eating disorder and your weight is now at a dangerous level. How do you feel, hearing me say that? What is going through your mind?

Explanation ☐ The body needs nutrition to work. Periods stopping is a sign your body is not healthy.

InCludE ☐ Exercise is unsafe at present as you may become very unwell if you lose more weight.

Recommend ☐ I would like to contact the children's psychiatry team who can help you be in control again at a safe and healthy level. You should see the dentist to check your teeth and gums as these may be affected by your diet and by vomiting. Would you be happy for me to refer you for help? The team can help monitor your weight and blood tests and provide talking therapy to help you eat again. I would like to arrange a heart tracing and some extra blood tests to check nutrients in your blood; would that be ok?

Specifics ☐ The children's team should see you in the next week. Please contact us if you don't receive an appointment. Would you mind me calling your mum to let her know what we have discussed?

Safety net ☐ If you feel dizzy or unwell, please speak to a doctor. Call 111 if we are closed.

Patient's Story

Eating Disorder

Doctor's notes Eleanor Cartwright, 15 years. PMH: constipation aged 4 years, LRTI aged 11 years. Medications/allergies: none.

Nurse minor illness clinic last week for URTI. 'Looks thin'. Height 165 cm, weight 40 kg, BMI 14.7, pulse 58, BP 100/60, chest clear, abdo NAD, no neck lumps. Arranged routine bloods – FBC, U&E, LFT, glucose, TFT; advised to book appointment to speak with doctor. All blood results normal.

Video consultation with Eleanor, 'Ellie'. Triage note: Mum, Faith, booked this appointment. She is concerned about Ellie's weight and anger issues. Also heard vomiting when she was supposed to be showering.

How to act Quiet, nervous.

PC *'Your nurse said I should talk to someone about my weight.'*

History You came to see the nurse for a bad cough last week (now better) and she weighed and measured you, said you were underweight and told you to book an appointment to speak with the doctor. You don't know what's wrong – you are just trying to eat healthily and look good. However, you are aware that your mum and dad are watching you eat and don't trust you. You deny losing your appetite or decreasing your meal size; you just eat healthier food. You are annoyed that your parents have stopped you from exercising when you return home from school. You just want to be healthy. It started when you realised that the other girls at swimming looked 'better' than you. You felt 'fat' so just decided to eat better and exercise – that's what everyone tells you is good for you anyway so you don't see the problem. You eat with your parents but feel annoyed if they try to sneak extra food onto your plate. You hope to lose more weight as you don't think anything has changed since you started being healthier 5 months ago. You do not use laxatives and do not disclose to the doctor that you have started vomiting unless specifically asked. You have always been well and there is no family history. Your periods stopped 4 months ago. You have never had sex. You sleep okay. You have no other symptoms and do not use drugs or alcohol and don't smoke. You have no thoughts of self-harm or suicide. Your form teacher asked if you were ok as you didn't seem well. You think they may have rung your mum. You are speaking to the doctor alone; your mum has gone out to the shops. You preferred to speak to the GP in confidence.

Social You are in all the top sets at the local school. Your mother is a journalist and you don't know what your father does exactly but he is always very busy. You get on 'fine'. You play the piano and the clarinet and have your grade 6 piano exam next month. You don't really like school anymore. You feel pressure to do well at everything and have a 'perfect' figure and life, like the people you follow on social media.

ICE You don't know why you had to come for this appointment but are not worried and expect the doctor will tell you to eat more. You don't like periods and you are thrilled they have stopped. You are cross that your mum has stopped you from exercising. You like running and going to the gym but tend to do this alone now rather than with friends. You are aware of eating disorders, but have never thought this applies to you; you just want to be healthy. You are willing to see a specialist if the GP explains well. You agree to the doctor ringing your mum to explain what has been discussed.

Learning Points

Information taken from NICE Guideline NG69 (2020) *Eating disorders: recognition and treatment.*[1] Please refer to full guidance.

As well as an unusually low BMI or body weight for age, other factors should raise suspicion:[1]

- Rapid weight loss
- Weight concerns despite not being overweight
- Menstrual disturbances
- Atypical dental wear (e.g. erosion)
- Gastrointestinal symptoms

Diagnosis

'Do not use single measures such as BMI or duration of illness to determine whether to offer treatment for an eating disorder.'[1]

Assessment, including Obs/investigations

Physical.

Psychological.

Social.

Possibility of alcohol or substance abuse.

Risk to self and risk of abuse.

Suicide risk or physical health compromised – emergency care.

Heart rate, BP, weight.

Be vigilant for refeeding syndrome, bradycardia and hypotension.

Management

Refer **immediately** to and be guided by your local community eating disorder team. Watchful waiting not appropriate for suspected eating disorders.

Consider emergency admission if: 'severe electrolyte imbalance, severe malnutrition, severe dehydration or signs of incipient organ failure.'[1]

For adults, consider psychological treatment such as:

> 'Individual eating-disorder-focused cognitive behavioural therapy (CBT-ED)
> Maudsley Anorexia Nervosa Treatment for Adults (MANTRA)
> Specialist supportive clinical management (SSCM)'.[1]

'Advise people with an eating disorder who are misusing laxatives or diuretics that [these] do not reduce calorie absorption and so do not help with weight loss [and] to gradually reduce and stop laxative or diuretic use.'[1]

Regular medical and dental reviews if vomiting.[1]

Osteoporosis risk – 'Advise people with anorexia nervosa and osteoporosis or related bone disorders to avoid high-impact physical activities and activities that significantly increase the chance of falls or fractures.'[1]

'Advise people with an eating disorder who are exercising excessively to stop doing so.'[1]

'Monitor growth and development in children and young people with anorexia nervosa who have not completed puberty (e.g. not reached menarche or final height).'[1]

At least annual review if stable/remission.

Confidentiality

Hold discussions in places where confidentiality, privacy and dignity can be respected but explain the limits of confidentiality, i.e. which professionals have access to information and when this may be shared. For children or young people <16, respect Gillick competence.

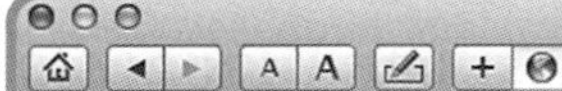

Doctor's Notes

Patient	Peter Atkins	9 years	M
PMH	Eczema		
	Hay fever		
	Viral-induced wheeze		
Medications	Current medication: Oilatum cream PRN		
	Previous medication: Salbutamol inhaler with spacer PRN Loratadine 10 mg once daily		
Allergies	No information		
Consultations	3 months ago – mild eczema. Emollients encouraged		
	1 week ago – nurse minor illness clinic. Mum reports dry cough present for months; worse when playing football		
Examination	Temp 36.6°C, height 140 cm, peak flow 270 L/min (expected 327 L/min). Chest clear and no wheeze, HS normal, Sats 98%, RR 17, HR 80 bpm regular		
Investigations	No information		
Household	Rachel Atkins	40 years	F
	Alexander Atkins	40 years	M

Mum (Rachel) is phoning you about her son Peter, age 9 years.

Example Consultation

Open ☐ How can I help today? Can you tell me more about Peter's cough? Have you noticed any problems with his breathing? What does Peter say about his breathing? Is he feeling unwell?

Flags ☐ Has he had a cold? Any phlegm? Does it hurt anywhere? When he is with his friends, can he run around like they do or does he need to stop more?

ICE1 ☐ What do you think may be causing his cough? You could be right. What led you to think that?

Risk ☐ I see Peter has hay fever and eczema. Has any other family member had asthma at all?

History ☐ Any other medical history? Any complications when Peter was born? Or any other medical problems afterwards? And the medicines that he takes at the moment? Any allergies?

Curious ☐ Why was Peter given the inhaler? And how often was he told to use it? When did he last use it?

Curious ☐ What has Peter said about his friend?

Sense ☐ I can hear you are concerned.

ICE2 ☐ What worries you about Peter's breathing? Are you worried about anything in particular?

ICE3 ☐ Today, what did you hope we would do?

SummarICE ☐ So, Peter has been coughing for months but otherwise feels fine. You are worried he could have asthma like his friend and would like an inhaler. Many doctors have told you that this is viral wheeze, not asthma, but you think this cough may be an infection. Is that correct?

Impression ☐ Viral wheeze is very common in young children but Peter is older now, and the breathing issues are affecting him frequently, so this sounds more like asthma. Coughing can be the only symptom, but Peter thinks he has been wheezy at times too. Asthma is also more likely if you suffer with hay fever or eczema.

Experience ☐ How much do you know about asthma?

Explanation ☐ In asthma the air tubes in your lungs become inflamed and narrow so there is less space for the air. This can happen with different triggers, such as allergies, infection or exercise.

Empathy ☐ I appreciate this may worry you, after you heard John went to hospital.

InCludE ☐ We can use inhalers to prevent breathing from getting worse. Due to the pattern of breathing problems and lack of fever and phlegm, I don't think there is likely to be infection present at the moment.

Options ☐ Firstly, to confirm asthma our nurse can do some special blowing tests. In the meantime, may I give him a new blue inhaler, called salbutamol, and a spacer to use it with? Do you remember how to use it? It's likely he will need a preventer inhaler too, but ideally we should do the tests before starting this so the results are more accurate. What do you think? The blue inhaler relaxes the airways so more air can get in, but ultimately we want to stop the airways reacting in this way by using a preventer to settle them down. Ask Peter to use the blue inhaler whenever he feels wheezy, breathless or coughs a lot. If this is happening frequently, call me and we can discuss starting the preventer straight away. I would also like Peter to complete a peak flow diary. This tells us how his lungs behave at different times of day. I will prescribe a peak flow meter and send you a link for the diary and video on how to use it from the Asthma UK website. I'll also send a link to a video on how to use the blue inhaler (salbutamol) and spacer device as a reminder.

Empower ☐ I'll write the details down in an asthma plan. Any questions so far?

Future ☐ Please book Peter with the nurse and bring him back a week later so we can discuss his results. If asthma is diagnosed, we can start the new inhaler. We can use this for prevention and treatment of asthma symptoms if this would be easier for Peter. Next time, I will update the asthma action plan so it tells you what to do if his asthma gets worse. Acting at the right time should prevent him getting poorly enough for hospital.

Safety net ☐ If he ever struggles with his breathing and needs more than 10 puffs of his inhaler at once, then this is when an ambulance should be called. Because ibuprofen can make asthma worse, it's best to avoid this and use paracetamol for colds/pains instead.

Patient's Story

Asthma Diagnosis

Doctor's notes Peter Atkins, 9 years. PMH: eczema, hay fever and viral-induced wheeze. Medications: Oilatum cream. Past medication: salbutamol inhaler with spacer PRN, loratadine 10 mg once daily.

How to act Concerned about your son. Wanting answers about his breathing, particularly whether it is an infection.

PC *'Doctor, Peter keeps coughing every night and it has been going on for months. We saw the nurse last week and she said to call you.'*

History Peter has had a dry cough for months, especially at night and it keeps you and your husband, Peter's father, awake.

He is not breathless and has no sputum or fever. He has not complained of pain.

He is well and you have not heard him wheeze.

He has had no other symptoms for a long time and has not used his (very) old inhaler for months, since the winter. It was prescribed during an episode of viral wheeze when he was 4 years old and you were told to stop using it once he was better.

He was born around his due date and was always well. Immunisations are up to date.

No FH. Eczema is mild and controlled with Oilatum.

History Peter has complained that when he plays football, he feels wheezy and out of breath. His friends can run around for longer. He has had no pain, no fever and no sputum. He does not have an itchy nose at present.

Social Pet rabbit. Only child. Non-smoking houshold.

ICE You know that Peter has *'viral wheeze'* after multiple doctors have said so.

You are not worried but have rung up in case he needs checking for infection.

Peter has told you about his friend John who has asthma. You remember when he came round for tea, John needed to use an inhaler after playing with your rabbit. Peter told you John was rushed to hospital one day at school as his breathing became really bad during sports.

You think he needs an inhaler like John. You don't want his breathing to get so bad he has to go to hospital.

Learning Points

Asthma Diagnosis[1–3]

Symptoms	Wheeze, cough, difficulty breathing and chest tightness. Especially at night or in the morning. Variability in symptoms.
Triggers	Exertion, weather, emotion, pets and hay fever. Screen for occupational asthma.
	Minus features that lower the probability: only with a cold, no interval symptoms, moist cough, dizziness, light-headedness, no wheeze.
	Also in adults: smoking history, cardiac disease, voice change.
Atopy	PMH or FH of hay fever, eczema or asthma.
Medications	Symptoms with aspirin, NSAID or beta-blockers.
Examination	May be normal or findings may include expiratory polyphonic wheeze, reduced air entry, low saturations and reduced peak flow levels.
Investigations	Spirometry and fractional exhaled nitric oxide (FeNO) testing are first-line tests for all people >5 years of age.
	If ongoing uncertainty, peak expiratory flow variability testing for 2–4 weeks.
	Specialist tests may include bronchial challenge test with histamine or methacholine.
	For older children and adults, do not rely on history alone.

Supporting the diagnosis

Symptoms:

- Positive FeNO level (positive levels according to age). Check prior to initiation of inhaled corticosteroids when possible (FeNO suppressed by ICS).
- Bronchodilator reversibility should be offered to adults (>17 years) and considered for children (5–16 years) where there is obstructive spirometry (FEV1/FVC <0.7). (Increase from FEV1 baseline of >12% (children and adults) and, additionally, in adults a 200 mL volume increase is a positive result.)
- Positive peak flow variability (>20%).

Criteria and algorithms for diagnosis according to age are available from NICE.

Aim of treatment

Control of disease with no day- or night-time symptoms, no asthma attacks, no limitations on exercise, normal lung function and minimal exercise.

GINA guidelines[3]

GINA guidelines move away from SABA + ICS use; over-reliance on SABA is linked with asthma deaths. GINA recommend maintenance and reliever therapy (MART) to manage asthma in adults and children >6 years. Lone SABA no longer recommended as only treats symptoms, not underlying cause. If mild, infrequent symptoms, use PRN LAMA/ICS (must contain formotorol as this LAMA is both fast acting and long acting). SABA + ICS can be used in children 6–11 years but consider compliance with ICS when SABA also used. Some LAMA/ICS inhalers are licensed for MART therapy. Advise these patients to take extra doses of LAMA/ICS when symptomatic. Not all inhalers suitable - check guidance/BNF.

Making a diagnosis in a child <5 years	Will be based on symptoms, judgement and observation following treatment.
Once >5 years	Repeat tests every 6–12 months until a diagnosis is confirmed.
Education	Provide a written asthma self-management plan, training in use of inhalers and information about how to seek help. Regular monitoring according to symptoms and control.
Allergy	Consider allergy screening. Skin prick testing or IgE tests may be helpful.

Patient Less Than 19 Years – 2.5

CHAPTER 3

GENDER, REPRODUCTIVE AND SEXUAL HEALTH, INCLUDING WOMEN'S, MEN'S, LGBTQ+, GYNAE AND BREAST

	Cases in this chapter	RCGP 2025 curriculum	Learning points
3.1	Varicella in Pregnancy	**Infectious diseases and travel health** **Maternity and reproductive health** 'Antenatal complications ... Infections, for example chickenpox'	Varicella in pregnancy Risks to mother Risks to fetus Assessing 'significant exposure'
3.2	Post-Menopausal Bleeding	**Gynaecology and breast health** 'Post-menopausal bleeding'	CA125 test Cervical, ovarian, endometrial, vulval and vaginal cancers
3.3	Genetic Testing	**Genomic medicine** 'Take and consider family histories in order to identify families with, or at risk of, genetic conditions' 'Principles of assessing genetic risk, including principles of risk estimates for family members of patients with single gene disorders'	Genetic testing Cystic fibrosis risk factors, diagnosis and management
3.4	Erectile Dysfunction	**Sexual health** 'Male sexual dysfunction, including erectile dysfunction due to organic causes (such as diabetes, drug induced (including smoking), neurological disease and vascular disease) and psychological causes'	ED causes, investigations and management The Well Man check
3.5	Gender Dysphoria	**Sexual health** 'Recognises that gender, gender identity, gender dysphoria and sexual orientation are all different facets of a person's health and that issues relating to these may present in childhood, adolescence or adulthood and have a wide influence on wellbeing' 'Feelings and behaviours related to gender dysphoria'	Terminology Helping patients with gender identity issues How parents can help their children with gender identity issues

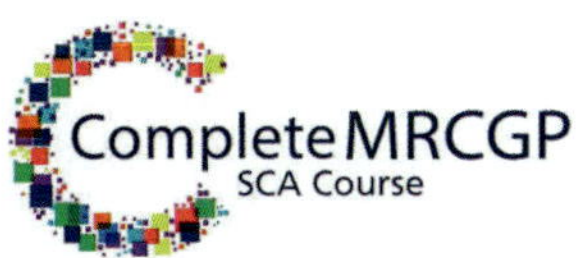

Links to the RCGP Curriculum

In this chapter, the cases are drawn from the following clinical topic guides:

- Infectious diseases and travel health
- Maternity and reproductive health
- Gynaecology and breast health
- Genomic medicine
- Sexual health

Scope of Conditions

Here are some examples of cases – this is not a complete list of all possibilities.

This is a broad area of the curriculum encompassing women's health, and sexual and breast health for people of all genders. It provides an excellent opportunity to demonstrate teamwork – for example working with midwives to provide antenatal and postnatal care, and health promotion such as prenatal care, as well as liaising with sexual health clinics. People who are pregnant may also have pre-existing medical conditions such as diabetes or hypertension and may enable you to demonstrate how you can manage medical complexity. There may also be ethical dimensions – for example the patient who is under the age of 16 years. At all times, remember to demonstrate that you are patient-centred and non-judgemental.

As well as the above clinical topics, the following areas of the curriculum may also be particularly relevant and be intertwined in the clinical presentation:

- Infectious diseases
- Mental health
- Metabolic problems
- Urgent and unscheduled care

Skills and Pitfalls

In addition to the information in Chapter 1 'How to Demonstrate Skills: The Marking Scheme Made Easy' consider the following challenges for this blueprint group:

- Some women may find discussing intimate issues difficult and may need empathy and encouragement.
- Remember that many gynaecological conditions may adversely impact all areas of a woman's life – physical, psychological and social wellbeing.
- Breast cancer is one of the commonest cancers in the UK so many will be living with the consequences.
- Ovarian cancer is easily missed and may present with vague symptoms that need to be explored and investigated.
- This area of the curriculum includes both women and men and people of all gender identities and expressions.
- Remember legal and ethical areas, particularly if a patient is <16 years.

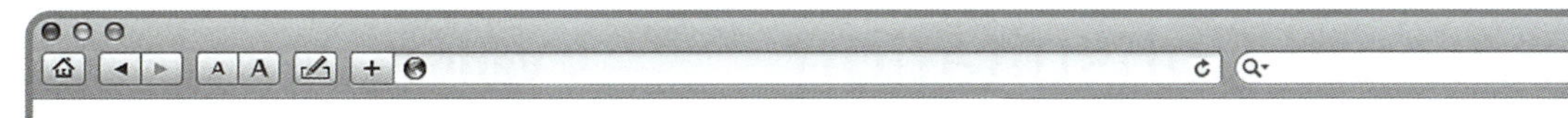

Doctor's Notes

Patient	Jennifer Adeyemi	27 years	F
PMH	No information		
Medications	No current medications		
Allergies	No information		
Consultations	Nil		
Investigations	No information		
Household	Amire Adeyemi	29 years	M

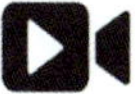

Example Consultation

Varicella in Pregnancy

Open ☐ How can I help? That must be worrying for you. What has led you to worry about chickenpox?

ICE1 ☐ What has been going through your mind about getting chickenpox whilst pregnant?

Risk/History ☐ When did you spend time with your niece? Would you say you were in close contact with her for more than 15 minutes? When did she become unwell? Do you know if you have had chickenpox before? How are you feeling? Have you felt unwell? How has your pregnancy been going so far? Is this your first baby?

ICE2 ☐ What specific worries do you have about this?

Sense ☐ I sense you are very worried about miscarriage. Is this something you have experienced before? Or did you have difficulty conceiving?

Impact ☐ How have all these worries been affecting you?

Curious ☐ How are things at home? Please tell me who you live with. Are you working?

ICE3 ☐ Was there anything in your mind you were hoping I might do today?

SummarICE ☐ So you are 16 weeks' pregnant with your first baby and have been exposed to chickenpox after babysitting your niece. You struggled to conceive so are frightened about any complications, in particular worrying about miscarriage or the baby being born with deformities. You don't think you've had chickenpox before but aren't certain. You hoped I could arrange a test and possibly a scan to check the baby is okay.

Empathy ☐ I can tell this baby is very precious so this must be very worrying for you.

Explanation ☐ Chickenpox in pregnancy can cause problems, particularly if the mother hasn't had it before. The chickenpox may make the mother more poorly with complications like pneumonia and, rarely, the baby can be affected. However, because you have contacted us so quickly, there are things we can do to try to prevent you getting chickenpox and therefore prevent your baby being affected.

InCludE ☐ Reassuringly, even in babies who are affected by the chickenpox virus, very few develop problems like deformity and there doesn't appear to be an increased risk of miscarriage.

Recommend ☐ Usually the first step would be to check the mother's immunity to chickenpox with a simple blood test. If it shows that you are immune, i.e. your body has fought chickenpox before and is ready to act, we don't need to worry – it is unlikely you will develop chickenpox again. If you aren't immune, we would refer you to the hospital to have a special protective injection. This should help prevent infection developing. How does this sound? As long as you don't develop any symptoms, you won't need extra scans.

Future ☐ You will get your detailed scan as normal in 4 weeks. If you did develop a rash or symptoms you should let us know straight away. We would then need to discuss with a specialist about giving you a medication to help treat the virus. The rash usually develops about 2 weeks after exposure so although this seems a while to wait to see if you have caught it, it does give us time to act.

Empower ☐ To help protect yourself, it would be a good idea to avoid seeing your niece until all her spots have scabbed over. This usually takes about 5 days. It's important to avoid anyone with shingles too, which is caused by the same virus.

Specifics ☐ I will ask our nurse to fit you in for the blood test this morning. The lab should send us the result in the next 48 hours. I will call you then to explain the next step. Is there anything that I can clarify or explain in more detail for you?

Safety net ☐ In the meantime, if you feel unwell with a fever or flu-like symptoms or develop a rash, please get in touch straight away.

Patient's Story

Varicella in Pregnancy

Doctor's notes Jennifer Adeyemi, 27 years.

How to act Anxious.

PC *'I'm worried I may have caught chickenpox from my niece. I'm 16 weeks' pregnant.'*

History You are 16 weeks' pregnant. Two days ago, you were babysitting your 2-year-old niece. You spent the whole day together and were playing together on the floor a lot. Your sister-in-law has called this morning to say your niece has come out in a chickenpox rash. You don't know if you have had chickenpox or not, but are aware it can be harmful to babies. You want to know what to do – will the baby be okay? You are anxious about the pregnancy because you struggled to conceive. You are worried the baby may be born with a disability if affected by chickenpox or that it may even cause a miscarriage. So far you have had an uneventful pregnancy – all seemed well at the dating scan. You feel well at present and haven't noticed any symptoms.

Social You moved to the UK from Nigeria when you were 18. You came to the UK to study history and English literature. You met your husband at a Nigerian Students Society dinner at university. You are very happy and have a good relationship with your husband. You got married 5 years ago. You were keen to start a family straight away but have struggled to conceive so your current (first) pregnancy is very precious to you. Your husband grew up in the UK and has a lot of family around. They are supportive. You do not smoke or drink. You are currently not working. Since your research role at the university came to an end, you have been a housewife. Your husband works in pharmaceuticals and so has a little medical knowledge. He encouraged you to get checked out.

ICE *Ideas*: you have probably caught chickenpox from your niece.

Concerns: your baby may be harmed or you may have a miscarriage. You worry your child may have deformities; you don't know how you would cope with a disabled child.

Expectations: you hope the doctor can do a test and maybe even arrange a scan to check the baby is okay. You would like to know how quickly the rash will come out if you have caught chickenpox.

Learning Points

Varicella in pregnancy[1] can be serious with consequences for both mother and baby. In Europe, most women have been exposed to chickenpox and so are less likely to be seronegative, whereas women from the tropics and subtropics have a higher chance of being seronegative. A clear history of previous chickenpox infection, or two doses of a varicella-containing vaccine, is reassuring. If there is doubt, a blood test for VZV IgG can be done to check immunity – but this is only useful, for potential prevention of infection developing, if results can be available within 24–48 hours of the exposure.

Risk to mother:

- Severe infection resulting in increased risk of pneumonia, hepatitis, encephalitis and even death.

Risk to fetus:

- Scarring of skin, eye and limb deformity, neurological problems, e.g. learning disability, microcephaly.
- Even in infected fetuses, the risk of fetal varicella syndrome is small, although it has been reported to occur in gestations from 3 to 28 weeks.
- Post-exposure prophylaxis in seronegative women is protective for the fetus – recommended from 20 weeks' gestation.
- There is no apparent link to miscarriage in the first trimester.

What is significant exposure? Take into account the ***type of varicella rash (e.g. exposed lesions), timing of exposure (e.g. between 48 hours prior to onset of rash to crusting of lesions)*** and ***closeness (e.g. in the same room for 15 minutes, face-to-face contact or in a large open hospital ward)***.[1]

Management[2]

- Clear history of previous infection; already received two doses of vaccine; or proven immunity on testing – reassure.
- No previous history of chickenpox or doubt – check VZV IgG (if result available within 48 hours).
- If seronegative or unable to get result within 48 hours – discuss with specialist about immunoglobulin prophylaxis.
- If not immune to VZV and significant exposure, specialist may offer post-exposure prophylaxis (PEP). UKHSA recommends oral antiviral therapy, i.e. aciclovir (or valaciclovir) as first choice. Day 7 to 14 post-exposure.
- Aciclovir and valaciclovir are not licensed for use in pregnancy but can be prescribed in the best interest of the woman, on the basis of available evidence, in consultation with her.
- If seropositive – can reassure.
- If chickenpox develops, discuss treatment with a specialist. Consider antivirals if woman presents within 24 hours of the rash and is >20 weeks' pregnant. Discuss with obstetrician first; informed consent and off-label use so discussion should include risks and benefits.

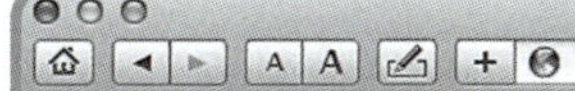

Doctor's Notes

Patient	Hilda Rowland	53 years	F
PMH	Mirena coil inserted aged 48 years		
	Menorrhagia		
Medications	No current medications		
Allergies	No information		
Consultations	Saw practice nurse 3 days ago for smear. Notes read: 'Patient requesting IUS removal. Mentioned irregular bleeding. Called duty GP. Abdomen examined NAD. PV examination – normal size uterus – cervix visualised, looked normal and IUS threads were seen. IUS not removed. Swabs taken for chlamydia and infection screen. BMI 24.'		
Investigations	Swabs – no infection, normal flora only. Smear not back yet		
Household	Brian Rowland	55 years	M

Follow-up appointment with GP to discuss further.

Example Consultation **Post-Menopausal Bleeding**

Open ☐ Hello. I'm sorry you've been having problems. What led to your decision about the coil? Tell me more about the bleeding? Any pattern? And your periods prior to this?

History ☐ Have you had any menopausal symptoms, for example hot flushes, night sweats or mood swings? Is your general health good? Any other medical problems? Do you take any medicines? Do you have children?

Impact ☐ How has this bleeding affected you? At work? Or leisure activities?

ICE1 ☐ You mentioned you think the bleeding is likely to be due to the coil. Tell me what makes you think that? Has anything else crossed your mind?

Flags ☐ It is helpful to know if you are sexually active and, if so, if there is bleeding after intercourse. May I ask if you have a sexual partner? Any bleeding after sex? Sometimes infection may cause bleeding – have you suspected this or had any discharge? Any weight loss?

ICE2 ☐ With the bleeding, are you concerned about anything that might be wrong? Did anything worrying cross your mind?

Risk ☐ Any family history? You've just had your smear; have you had any abnormal smears?

Sense ☐ You seem unconcerned about this bleeding.

ICE3 ☐ What did you think we may decide today?

SummarICE ☐ To summarise, you were warned that the coil, which is usually in for 5 years, may cause abnormal bleeding. Therefore, this bleeding, although a nuisance, has not come as a shock. You don't want a return of heavy periods but hope to try without the coil.

Impression ☐ My concern is that you may have gone through the menopause. I say 'may have' because we don't know whether the absence of bleeding until now is due to your coil. Bleeding after the menopause can be common but needs investigation. I don't think we should plan to remove the coil just yet as we don't know the cause of the problem.

Explanation ☐ There are many possible reasons for the bleeding: a fibroid which is a harmless lump in the womb; a polyp which may be harmless but could potentially become a cancer; it may be from the coil, but the coil's hormone usually lasts for 7 years; the bleeding may be coming from the cervix or vaginal walls which become more fragile as we age, but they looked fine when the you were examined. The swabs you had taken have ruled out infection. The priority is ruling out a cancer, which can cause abnormal bleeding.

Options ☐ We refer all women who bleed after the menopause urgently for an USS, which is a jelly scan to check the womb shows no sign of a cancer. What are your thoughts?

Empathy ☐ I appreciate the possibility of cancer may come as a shock, especially when bleeding at the 5-year mark makes sense from what previous doctors have said. Usually, nothing serious is found; however, I am sorry if this is upsetting and causes worry whilst we consider the possibility.

Future ☐ At the USS they will insert a probe into the vagina to look at the womb. Depending on what's found, you may need to see a specialist for a camera test and biopsy of a sample of the womb. If they don't remove the coil at the hospital, we can do this afterwards. Please make a follow-up appointment with me to discuss what they have found, a few days after the ultrasound. If they do find a womb cancer, this is usually very treatable.

Safety net ☐ If your bleeding becomes heavier or you have pain, please let a GP know.

Specifics ☐ You should be seen within 2 weeks from today. If you haven't received an appointment within 10 days let me know. If you have any questions inform reception and I'll phone you. Try not to worry – remember we are being thorough.

Patient's Story

Post-Menopausal Bleeding

Doctor's notes Hilda Rowland, 53 years. PMH: menorrhagia. Mirena coil inserted aged 48 years.

Medications: none.

Saw practice nurse 3 days ago for smear. 'Patient requesting IUS removal. Mentioned irregular bleeding. Called duty GP. Abdomen examined NAD. PV examination – normal size uterus – cervix visualised, looked normal and IUS threads were seen. IUS not removed. Swabs taken for chlamydia and infection screen. BMI 24.'

Swabs – no infection, normal flora only. Smear not back yet.

How to act Relaxed.

PC *'I went for my smear yesterday and they said I should talk to you. I just want my coil removed.'*

History You had the coil inserted 5 years ago for heavy bleeding. Your last period was 3 years ago, your smears are up to date, but over the last 3 months you have started bleeding. Prior to that, there was no spotting at all. The bleeding is random with no pattern. You don't take HRT and never have. Otherwise, you are well with no abdominal pain or weight loss and no urinary or bowel symptoms. You had hot flushes for a couple of years but these stopped a year ago. The bleeding is annoying because you have to remember to take sanitary towels with you. Brian is your only sexual partner. You have had no bleeding after intercourse and no discharge.

Social You are a headmistress for the local primary school.

You enjoy walking and you are a well-known member of the community, living a busy lifestyle with the school and church group charity events.

You have never smoked and enjoy a sherry on weekends but otherwise don't drink alcohol.

ICE You believe your coil has started to run out which is why you would like it out.

You are not worried, as you were told you may bleed at random times and that the coil usually lasts for 5 years, so this makes sense to you.

You expect the doctor will arrange to remove it very soon and then it will be sorted.

Another possibility is that you could have another one. You just worry about the heavy bleeding coming back but wonder if you could try without it first.

If the doctor mentions that this could be cancer, react to this: *'You think I have cancer? You've got me worried now!'*

Suspected Gynaecological Cancer

Always refer to the full text of the latest version of NICE Guideline NG12 (2023) *Suspected cancer: recognition and referral.*[1]

Cervical

When to examine the vagina and cervix with a speculum and palpate the uterus/ovaries:

- Every woman with abnormal or post-coital bleeding or pelvic pain.
- Do not rely on recent smear tests.
- Do not wait for the result of a smear test if there is any abnormality on the cervix. Make an urgent suspected cancer referral.

Ovarian

When to request CA125 testing for possible ovarian cancer:

- Be suspicious in any woman, particularly those over 50 with symptoms of bloating, feeling full, loss of appetite, abdominal or pelvic pain or frequency/urgency in urination especially if these symptoms occur more than 12 times a month.[1]
- Consider also if 'unexplained weight loss, fatigue or changes in bowel habit'.[1]
- Be aware that IBS rarely presents in women for the first time over the age of 50.

CA125 is ≥35 IU/mL:

- Urgently (within 2 weeks) 'arrange an ultrasound scan of the abdomen and pelvis'.[1] If this suggested to be a cancer, the patient would then require an urgent suspected cancer gynaecology referral.

CA125 is <35 IU/mL or ≥35 IU/mL and the USS is normal:

- Reassess for other conditions, then safety net for more frequent/persistent or new symptoms.[1]

Endometrial

Urgent suspected cancer referral to gynaecology if ≥55 years with PMB. Also consider if <55 years with PMB.[1]

Many GPs have direct access (urgent suspected cancer referral) to ultrasound (85% sensitivity) as a first-line investigation for PMB.

Consider a direct access USS for women ≥55 years with unexplained vaginal discharge if first presentation of this, have thrombocytosis or have macro/microscopic haematuria and low Hb or high platelets or raised blood glucose.[1]

Reasons to send an urgent suspected cancer gynaecology referral:

- Ascites and/or pelvic or abdominal mass.[1]
- If an ultrasound suggests cancer.
- Women with PMB – see above and your local guidelines.
- Consider if there is abnormal appearance of the cervix, vagina or vulva (e.g. lump, ulceration or bleeding).[1]

Vulval

In women with an unexplained vulval lump, ulceration or bleeding, consider an urgent suspected cancer referral pathway.[1]

Vaginal

In women with an unexplained palpable mass in or at the entrance to the vagina, consider an urgent suspected cancer referral pathway.[1]

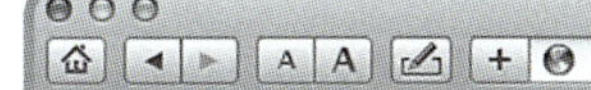

Doctor's Notes

Patient	Olivia Wales	29 years	F
PMH	No information		
Medications	No current medications		
Allergies	No information		
Consultations	No recent consultations		
Investigations	No recent investigations		
Household	No household members registered		

Example Consultation

Open ☐ I'm sorry to hear about your niece. Please tell me about her experience. How is she?

Impact ☐ How has her diagnosis affected your family? And you, what impact has it had on you?

Sense ☐ I can hear this has raised very important issues for you.

ICE 1 ☐ Apart from genetic testing, what other thoughts have gone through your mind?

Curious ☐ I'm wondering if you have discussed this with your sister and what she thinks you should do. You mentioned your husband. What does he think about whether you should have the test?

ICE 2 ☐ What do you fear the most? Do you have any other questions?

History ☐ Looking at your notes, I think you have always been well, is that correct? Do you take any medicines? Please tell me about your work.

ICE3 ☐ You were hoping we could arrange a genetic test for yourself. Is there anything else that is important to you for us to do today? What would it mean to you if you did have a gene that put you at increased risk of having a child with cystic fibrosis – how would this impact you and your life?

SummarICE ☐ To summarise what you have said so far, your sister's daughter, Grace, has had multiple chest infections and requires medication to help maintain her nutrition. You have watched the amount of stress your sister has had to go through and this has made you question whether you would like children. You are upset by the arguments you have had with your husband. You feel the test may help you to make the choice whether to have a child.

Empathy ☐ It sounds as if you have watched your sister through many sad and difficult times when Grace has been admitted to hospital. That must be hard.

Experience ☐ What is your understanding of CF? What do you know about what causes CF?

Explanation ☐ In cystic fibrosis there is a build-up of mucus in the chest and difficulty absorbing all the nutrients from food because an organ next to the stomach, called the pancreas, is not producing the chemicals needed to break food down so it can be absorbed. Unfortunately, it can also cause infertility.

Risk ☐ When a child is conceived, information from both parents is passed to the child. This information is coded in genes, one from each parent. Both parents need to pass on a faulty gene for a child to have cystic fibrosis. Everyone has a 1 in 25 chance of carrying the gene for cystic fibrosis. Your sister must have inherited one faulty gene from your parents, which she unfortunately passed on. You may or may not have a faulty gene. If we take the worst case scenario and assume that you did inherit the faulty gene too, your chance of passing on the faulty gene would be 1 in 2. However, your child would also need to inherit a faulty gene from your husband, who has the background risk of 1 in 25 and then a 1 in 2 chance of passing it on. So, based on this, your risk would be 1 in 100 of having a child with cystic fibrosis.

InCLudE ☐ We don't know that you have inherited the faulty gene; if either you or your husband doesn't have a faulty gene, there is almost no risk of having a child with cystic fibrosis.

Options ☐ How would you feel about speaking to a genetic counsellor about this?

Specifics ☐ I can write to the genetics team and explain what impact this has had, and we can be guided by them. They may offer a consultation for you to discuss what options are available. I suspect they will offer to test you or your husband for the faulty gene. Relationship counselling is another option if you think this may be helpful.

Future ☐ If you decide to start trying for a family, do phone again and we can discuss this in more detail. We can make sure that you are as healthy as you can be before any pregnancy, for example checking that you are immune to rubella and are taking folic acid.

Patient's Story

Genetic Testing

Doctor's notes Olivia Wales, 29 years. PMH: nil. Medications: none.

How to act Polite and quiet.

PC ***'My husband and I would like to start a family but my niece has cystic fibrosis. I'm wondering if there are any special tests we could have?'***

History You are well, take no medicines and have been happily married for 2 years. Your sister gave birth to Grace 10 years ago and soon afterwards they were told that she has cystic fibrosis. Your sister decided not to have another child. There have been no other members of the family with this condition. This includes your sister's husband's family. Your sister's spirit seems to have gone over the years. The more Grace attends hospital the more sadness your sister has to go through. You believe the stress of the situation led to the breakdown of your sister's marriage. You worry that your sister will be alone if Grace dies.

Social You are a teacher. You drink no alcohol and have never smoked.

ICE You have seen your niece have lots of chest physiotherapy and she has had multiple lung infections requiring hospital admissions. She has to take medicines to help absorb her food.

A charity is taking her to Disney World. You are aware that Grace may not live long.

What is your risk of having a baby with cystic fibrosis?

Is there a test you can have done to make sure you don't have the faulty gene?

You don't know if you want a child if there is a high risk of bringing a child into the world who has to go through Grace's experience. Your husband is desperate for children. He does not want you to have genetic testing. He believes your chances are low and you should just start trying. This has led to arguments within your relationship. You were very excited when Grace was first born but now, watching your sister's life, you don't think you ever want children. You have not told your husband this.

It was your sister's idea for you to have the genetic test.

CF is the most common inherited disease in people of White ethnicity, caused by mutations in the CF trans-membrane conductance regulator (*CFTR*) gene, on chromosome 7. This affects sodium transport across the cell membrane and antibacterial defences.[1]

Risk factors Positive FH is the only risk factor.

Carrier frequency 1:25.

Systems affected Respiratory and digestive – pancreatic insufficiency and biliary disease.

Presentation Usually recurrent LRTI with chronic sputum production. Digestive presentations less common as only 5% pancreatic function is necessary for normal digestive function.

Diagnosis[2]

Positive test result in people with no symptoms (e.g. infants screened with blood spot immunoreactive trypsin test) followed by sweat and gene tests for confirmation.

Clinical manifestations, supported by sweat or gene test results for confirmation.

Clinical manifestations alone, in the rare case of people with symptoms who have normal sweat or gene test results.

See NICE guidelines for a full list of who to assess for CF, but list includes the following:[1]

- Family history.
- Meconium ileus.
- Symptoms and signs that suggest distal intestinal obstruction.
- Faltering growth in infants and young children.
- Recurrent and chronic pulmonary disease.
- Acute or chronic pancreatitis.
- Malabsorption.

Management

Patients with CF will be managed in a specialist centre by MDTs. There may be implications for school, education and career planning, and they may require GP and/or specialist psychological support particularly at difficult times such as:

- Transition to adult care.
- Foreign travel.
- Contraception and pregnancy and becoming parents.
- Organ transplantation.
- End of life.

GPs can also help as follows:

- Prescribing cystic fibrosis medicines:
  - In batches of at least 1 month at a time for routine medicines.
  - For longer periods if advised by the specialist team.
  - Following guidance on arrangements for prescriptions of unlicensed medicines.
- Providing routine annual immunisation, including any alterations for people with CF.
- Flu vaccinations for family members and carers.
- Managing health problems unrelated to cystic fibrosis.
- Providing FIT notes as appropriate.
- End-of-life care, working in partnership with cystic fibrosis homecare teams.
- Caring for the person's family members or carers.

Doctor's Notes

Patient Kevin Barton 57 years M

PMH Hypertension

Medications Indapamide 2.5 mg OD

Allergies No information

Consultations Recent consultation (2 days ago) – hypertension review with practice nurse. BP 134/78, BMI 24

Investigations No recent investigations

Household No household members registered

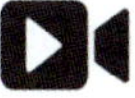

Example Consultation

Erectile Dysfunction

Open ☐ Tell me what made you ask for a Well Man check. What did you hope we might include?

Sense ☐ Are there changes in your body you have noticed or are worried about?

ICE1 ☐ What has been going through your mind?

History ☐ I see you have high BP but a recent reading was fine. Are you otherwise well? Do you live alone? Work? Any stress in your life? How is your mood?

ICE2 ☐ Do you worry about your health? What is your biggest fear?

Risk ☐ Do you smoke? How much alcohol do you drink? Any family history?

Flags ☐ Any pain in your chest, legs or breathing problems? Any problems going to the toilet? Do you get up to wee at night? Does the flow seem normal or slower than normal? Any dribbling at the end or needing to go again soon afterwards? Any testicular lumps? Any problems with erections? What have you noticed? Is this a problem maintaining erections or do you struggle to get an erection? Are you worried about anything else, e.g. when you ejaculate? Do you have any erections on your own or in the morning?

Impact ☐ How has the impotence affected you or your relationship?

Curious ☐ How is your relationship? What does your husband think? Have you had any other sexual partners? When was this? Tell me more about this person? Male or female?

Impact ☐ Has anything else in your life changed since? Your mood? How are you and David?

Curious ☐ You mentioned David encouraged you to attend – is he worried about you?

Flags ☐ Do you have any symptoms that may suggest an infection, for example a discharge from your penis, a rash or any lumps in the groin area?

SummarICE ☐ To summarise, you are troubled with impotence and you worry you may have an infection. You are feeling low in mood and fear this may affect your marriage.

Empathy ☐ Impotence can often be frustrating and can increase the stress in your life.

Experience ☐ Have you read or heard about anything that may cause impotence?

ICE3 ☐ Did you have anything specific in mind you were hoping we might be able to offer today?

Explanation ☐ Stress or low mood or conditions that affect the vessels can cause impotence. For an erection, blood needs to flow into the vessels in the penis.

Impression ☐ Either your BP or indapamide may contribute to impotence. But I think it's most likely due to your recent worries, because you are sometimes able to have erections. What do you think?

InCludE ☐ Infections don't usually cause impotence but worry certainly can.

Options ☐ We could check for infections here at the surgery or you could visit the GUM clinic which can quickly and thoroughly assess you. There is a walk-in clinic this afternoon. Shall I give you the details? We could try stopping indapamide to see if this helps. You could also talk to a relationship counsellor or try sildenafil (Viagra), which increases the blood flow to the penis. What would suit you best? Would you like information on Relate, the relationship counsellors?

Empower ☐ We can check your cholesterol and blood sugar, as both affect vessels, and there may also be lifestyle changes you could make. You have no prostate symptoms, but we offer a blood test for prostate cancer to anyone attending with impotence. Would you like to explore that? Okay, let's discuss this when you next come in.

Recommend ☐ I recommend waiting to have sex until your sexual health screen is clear and, if you do need treatment, both you and David should complete this before you have sex. I'll send a prescription for 50 mg sildenafil to your pharmacy. Take one an hour before you plan to have sex. It works for hours, so no rush. It will only cause an erection when you become aroused. Unfortunately, some men may get a headache.

Specifics ☐ Please book in to speak to me in a month to discuss your results and catch up.

Safety net ☐ If your mood deteriorates or anything else worries you, please phone me sooner.

Patient's Story

Erectile Dysfunction

Doctor's notes Kevin Barton, 57 years. PMH: HTN. Medications: indapamide 2.5 mg OD. BP 2 weeks ago 134/78. BMI 24.

How to act Embarrassed. You do not give much away unless pushed. You do not mention you have a problem with ED until the doctor asks directly. Then call it impotence.

PC *'I would like to know if I can have a Well Man check please.'*

History Your friends have had a Well Man check and although you are unsure what this is exactly, it sounds a good idea because you have had problems with ED. If asked, you have no symptoms of bladder outflow obstruction, do have morning erections and find masturbation easier. Your general health is good and you take regular exercise – twice weekly sessions at the local squash club. You have never smoked and drink 1 pint of lager a night. You have no other medical history and no family history. You work in finance. David is a social worker.

Social You married your male partner, David, 3 years ago. He has encouraged you to go to the GP to sort yourself out. Your relationship has been under strain because you had an affair a year ago with a male friend from the squash club, for which you feel guilty. You do not disclose this until the doctor explores your sexual history. You no longer see this friend but you do continue to play squash.

ICE You are worried that you have an STI and that one day your husband will discover this. In your mind, this would be the end of your relationship. The affair, and your guilt, are preying on your mind and you feel you have let him down.

You would like blood tests for a general check-up but don't insist on a prostate test and you would prefer time to think about prostate tests if this is mentioned.

You would like to try Viagra.

Learning Points

Causes of ED

Vascular disease Risk factors include HTN, smoking, hypercholesterolaemia and diabetes mellitus.

Structural Surgery within the pelvis. Peyronie's disease.

Skin disorders Foreskin problems such as lichen sclerosus (balanitis xerotica obliterans).

Neurological Tumour, spinal cord disease, MS, Parkinson's, stroke, peripheral neuropathy.

Hormonal Hypogonadism, Cushing's, thyroid, hyperprolactinaemia.

Drug induced Diuretics, SSRIs, GnRH analogues and antagonists, antipsychotics.

Alcohol and recreational drugs E.g. heroin, cocaine, amphetamines, MDMA (ecstasy).

Psychological causes Stress, depression, anxiety, relationship difficulties, performance anxiety.

SHIM Sexual Health Inventory for Men (SHIM) score may be useful. Available on BAUS website to download.[1]

Tailor investigations to the likely cause depending on symptoms, age and risk factors.

The patient may have their own terminology in a sexual health history. Use words they have chosen.

Make no assumptions. Ask about other sexual partners and confirm their partner's gender.

Management options

Sildenafil Generic available on NHS prescription. CI include: already on a nitrate, unstable angina, recent MI or stroke, optic neuropathy.

Side effects: headaches, flushing, N&V, dizziness and visual disturbances.

Interactions: no alpha-blocker within 4 hours.

Other options Second-line tadalafil (Cialis) with a longer duration of effect.

Vacuum pumps. MUSE (alfraprostadil per urethra) and Caverject.[2]

Relationship counselling[3] or a referral to psychosexual medicine may be helpful.

Show you have recognised the opportunity for health screening and promotion.

Well Man check CVD risk factors, prostate and testicular screening, weight and bowel changes, stress/mood.

PSA screening Offer all men with ED PSA screening.[4]

NICE CKS has a comprehensive overview of the assessment and management of ED.[5]

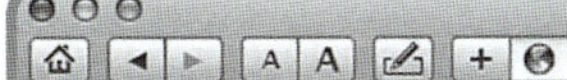

Doctor's Notes

Patient	Florence Wriggley	15 years	F
PMH	None		
Medications	None		
Allergies	NKDA		
Consultations	None		
Investigations	None		
Household	Michael Wriggley	40 years	M
	Veronica Wriggley	39 years	F

Veronica, Florence's mum, is phoning about Florence. There is written consent in the notes from Florence, giving permission for her medical records and health to be discussed with Veronica.

Example Consultation

Open ☐ I'm sorry you have been worried; what changes have you noticed?

ICE1 ☐ What thoughts have you had about what may be going on?

Impact ☐ This sounds like a challenging time. Has it been affecting the family?

ICE2 ☐ What worries you most?

History ☐ Did there seem to be any trigger to her change in behaviour? How are things at home generally? How has she been at school? Have you spoken to Flo about your worries? Have you noticed changes in her mood? Does she have a boyfriend or girlfriend?

Risk ☐ Are you aware of any bullying at school or over the internet? Has she struggled with her mood in the past? Has she mentioned feeling very low?

Flags ☐ Any concerns about self-harm? Has she expressed any suicidal thoughts? Does she use drugs or alcohol? Does she smoke?

Empathy ☐ This must be a confusing and worrying time for you and Flo. Nobody wants to see their child unhappy.

Sense ☐ Emotionally, how do you feel?

ICE3 ☐ Did you have any specific thoughts about how I could help?

Experience ☐ Have you come across gender identity issues before?

SummarICE ☐ So for the last year or so, Flo's behaviour has changed, for example wearing baggy clothes and getting rid of anything girly. She seems to be self-conscious about her body and she told you that she feels that she should have been born a boy. You wonder if she is gay or possibly transgender. You were hoping I could provide some information about this and how to support her.

Impression ☐ It sounds as if Flo may be struggling with her gender identity, or this could be a sign of a mental health problem, or possibly a mixture of both.

InCludE ☐ Being gay is a term which means you are romantically or sexually interested in people of the same sex. Transgender is different; this means that the person feels like they are a different gender from the one they were given at birth – as if the body is one gender but the mind is another. Gender is now thought of as a spectrum, with male and female at opposite ends but everything in between does exist.

Explanation ☐ It is completely normal for children and adolescents to explore gender and thoughts can change with time. However, if thoughts are persistent into adolescence, then help may be needed to explore the person's gender identity more formally.

Options ☐ Initially it would be really helpful if I could meet Flo so we can chat about her feelings and I can see if there are any signs of significant anxiety or depression. It may be that she needs help from our counselling team or even our children's mental health team. If needed, we could refer her to the gender identity team. We also have a counselling team set up specifically for LGBTQ+ persons.

Empower ☐ In the meantime you can support her by reminding her she is normal, that you love her and that it is fine for her to take her time in discovering who she is. It may be helpful to speak to school so they can be sure to support her too. The website of the National Gender Incongruence Service for children and young people has lots of information you and Flo may find helpful.

Future ☐ Would it be possible for us to meet up in person with Flo in the next couple of weeks?

Specifics ☐ Please arrange an appointment with me through reception.

Safety net ☐ Great, let's meet soon but if you notice any signs of self-harm, have concerns about suicidal thoughts or any other worries, please get in touch with us straight away.

Patient's Story

Gender Dysphoria

Doctor's notes Florence Wriggley, 15 years.

How to act You are her mother – Veronica Wriggley. Concerned.

PC *'I'm worried about Flo; she's been acting oddly recently and seems unhappy.'*

History Florence was always a happy child but over the last year or so she seems unhappy. Initially you thought that it was just the challenges of growing up but now you're not so sure. She has always been a 'tomboy' but last week you caught her wrapping a bandage around her chest. When you asked her what she was doing she looked embarrassed but then told you she 'should have been a boy'. Looking back, you feel that her mood changed about a year ago. Flo seems anxious a lot of the time and worries over small things. She has started refusing to do sports at school and says it's because she doesn't want to get changed in front of the other girls. She's cleared out her wardrobe and replaced anything even slightly girly with baggy T-shirts and jeans. She's started wearing trousers to school. Flo has been spending more and more time in her room. She has become distant from her friends and keeps saying that she no longer fits in. You are worried and don't know what to do.

Social Florence is attending school and still plays football but seems less enthusiastic about going now. You are not aware of any bullying at school. Her teachers have noticed a drop in the quality of her schoolwork. She doesn't smoke, drink alcohol or use drugs and she doesn't have a boyfriend or girlfriend. She is bright – but not attaining at present. You work as a nail technician and Florence's dad is a builder. You are open minded about gender/sexual identity issues but come from a traditional family and you worry what Flo's grandparents will say.

ICE You think Florence may be gay or possibly transgender but you aren't really sure what the difference is. You are worried that she is having a difficult time and will become depressed. You want information from the GP and advice about support and how to talk to Flo. You would like the GP to explain the difference between being gay and transgender.

Learning Points

Gender Dysphoria

Terminology[1]

Trans – an umbrella term to describe people whose gender is not the same as, or does not sit comfortably with, the sex they were assigned at birth.

Trans people may describe themselves using one or more of a wide variety of terms, including (but not limited to) transgender, transsexual, gender-queer (GQ), gender-fluid, non-binary, gender-variant, cross-dresser, genderless, agender, non-gender, third gender, bi-gender, trans man, trans woman, trans masculine, trans feminine and neutrois.

Transgender man – a person who was assigned female at birth but now lives and identifies as a man.

Transgender woman – a person who was assigned male at birth but now lives and identifies as a woman.

Non-binary – an umbrella term for people whose gender identity does not sit comfortably with 'man' or 'woman'.

Gender dysphoria – when a person experiences discomfort or distress because there is a mismatch between their gender assigned at birth and their gender identity.

Pansexual – a person whose romantic and/or sexual attraction towards others is not limited by sex or gender.

Body dysmorphia – body dysmorphic disorder (BDD), or body dysmorphia, is a mental health condition where a person spends a lot of time worrying about flaws in their appearance. These flaws are often unnoticeable to others.[2]

Helping patients with gender identity issues

Gender is now believed to be a spectrum with male on one end and female on the other. It is normal for children to explore gender and they may demonstrate preferences across the spectrum. Not all these preferences will remain with the child through adolescence. However, some will continue to identify with a different gender from that they were assigned at birth. In children and adults experiencing this, it is common for mental health problems to coexist, e.g. anxiety or depression. Helping patients will need to incorporate both gender identity needs and mental health needs. Specialist gender clinics exist, though these are currently being reconfigured due to recent controversies. There is a national referral service[3] where patients can be assessed by a specialist, and where appropriate, can be guided through gender reassignment treatments. Hormone blockers (GnRH analogues) can be used in adolescents followed by hormone treatments (testosterone or oestrogen). Ultimately, surgery can be performed to change a person's sexual characteristics. This usually takes place after 'social gender role transition' where a person is living as their chosen gender (e.g. changed name, etc.) and they have taken hormone treatments.

Ways parents can help[4]

- Remind young people that they are normal. It is normal to explore gender.
- Consider how gender identity is expressed in their family – does the child fit in? If not, they may need extra support to feel accepted. Try to avoid overtly masculine or feminine roles.
- Encourage the young person to talk about their feelings.
- Accept uncertainty about what the future holds. Encourage exploration and keep options open.
- Consider where sources of anxiety are coming from.

CHAPTER 4

LONG-TERM CONDITIONS, INCLUDING CANCER, MULTI-MORBIDITY AND DISABILITY

	Cases in this chapter	RCGP 2025 curriculum	Learning points
4.1	Down Syndrome	**Neurodevelopmental conditions and neurodiversity** **Learning disability** 'Onset before birth … Down syndrome' 'Annual health checks' 'Awareness of conditions that are more likely to develop … dementia'	Annual health check for people with learning disabilities Issues specific to the condition/life stage, i.e. prenatal, childhood, adolescence, later life and ongoing
4.2	Hyperthyroidism	**Metabolic problems and endocrinology** 'Thyroid diseases including … hyperthyroidism'	'Managing hyperthyroidism' flow diagram
4.3	Prostatitis	**Renal and urology** 'Prostatic problems such as acute and chronic prostatitis'	Acute and chronic prostatitis
4.4	Psoriasis	**Dermatology** 'Recognise the importance of the psychosocial impact of skin problems' 'Appreciate the complexity of care that is needed with some skin problems' 'Examination of the rest of the skin, nails, scalp, hair and systems such as joints when appropriate'	Management of psoriasis in adults, including triggers, associations and limb/trunk treatment Scalp psoriasis treatment
4.5	COPD	**Respiratory health** 'Common and important conditions – COPD' 'Local and national guidelines to manage … COPD' 'The importance of lifestyle changes, particularly smoking cessation and pulmonary rehabilitation'	From the GOLD guide: • Diagnosis, assessment of severity and management of COPD • Different types of inhalers

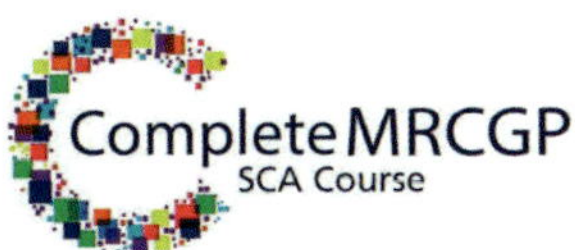

Links to the RCGP Curriculum

In this chapter, the cases are drawn from the following clinical topic guides:

- Neurodevelopmental conditions and neurodiversity
- Learning disability
- Metabolic problems and endocrinology
- Renal and urology
- Dermatology
- Respiratory health

And the following life stages topic guide:

- People with long-term conditions, including cancer

Scope of Conditions

Here are some examples of cases – this is not a complete list of all possibilities.

Conditions that may be present alone or as part of multi-morbidity include:

- Developmental coordination disorders (e.g. dyspraxia)
- Developmental disability (e.g. autism, autism spectrum disorder, ADHD, cerebral palsy)
- Learning disability (genetic and non-genetic causes)
- Hearing, speech, visual disorders and impairments
- Sleep disorders
- Physical health disorders across the systems
- Mental health disorders
- Cognitive disorders
- Cancers
- Chronic pain conditions
- Communicable diseases

Skills and Pitfalls

In addition to the information in Chapter 1 'Your Role as a GP' and 'How to Demonstrate Skills: The Marking Scheme Made Easy' consider the following challenges for this blueprint group:

- Physical, psychological and social conditions and challenges – how they interact and a holistic approach to care.
- The impact of the long-term health condition on a person's social wellbeing, integration, relationships, communication and self-care.
- The impact of the long-term health condition on a person's psychological wellbeing.
- The impact of the condition on carers and family.
- The recognition of coexisting depression or anxiety.
- The support network or lack of support network around the patient.
- The transition from paediatric to adult services.
- The opportunity to untangle the complexity of co-morbidities, communicate options and empower patients to care for their own health and wellbeing.
- The opportunity to coordinate and integrate care across services, teams and primary and secondary care.
- The recognition that third-sector providers may have a role in the patient's care.
- The importance of continuity of care.
- The opportunity to educate and work collaboratively with patients, family and carers to promote self-care.
- The identification of the patient's needs and priorities and working in partnership to develop shared plans.
- Managing comorbidity and long-term illness over time through discussing goals or future appointments.
- The opportunity for health promotion to prevent further disease.
- The opportunity and discussion required for education, surveillance and follow-up.
- The reoccurrence of disease and detection of new disease which long-term conditions could disguise.
- Where is the patient, within the natural history of their illness?
- The opportunity to reduce the burden of multi-morbidity on the patient.

Doctor's Notes

Patient	Matthew Dalton	24 years	M
PMH	Down syndrome		
	Closure ASD		
	Sensorineural deafness, hearing aids		
Medications	None		
Allergies	None		
Consultations	Out-of-hours appointment 4 days ago. Otitis externa. No wax. Drum seen – no perforation. Afebrile. Chest clear		
	Prescribed Otomize spray and advised to speak to GP if not improving		
Investigations	BMI 32 (2 months ago)		
Household	No household members registered		
Alert	Overdue annual review. Last review 3 years ago. No bloods done		

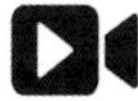

Example Consultation

Down Syndrome

Open ☐ How are you, Matthew? Thank you for speaking with me today.

ICE1 ☐ Please can you tell me more about why you think you need a new hearing aid?

ICE2 ☐ Is there anything that is particularly worrying you about your hearing or hearing aid, Matthew? Is your mum worried about anything?

Flags ☐ How is your ear now? Any discharge or yellow fluid coming from your ear? Is it painful? How is your hearing? Are you feeling well or poorly?

History ☐ What happened with your ear? How does the hearing aid feel? Can you remember what health problems you have had in the past? Can we go through the body to see if you have had any other problems? Let's start at the top – do you have any headaches? Can you see everything okay? When did you last have your eyes checked? Have you seen the dentist this year? How often do you feel out of breath? Do you have any other strange feelings in your chest? Does your back hurt? Do your arms and legs feel okay? How often do you go for a wee? Does it ever hurt? How often do you have a poo? Is the poo hard like stones, soft or runny? Does anywhere hurt? Who do you live with? What do you do during the day? You have a job: that's great! Do you enjoy it? Do you have friends who live nearby? Do you have a girlfriend or boyfriend? Is it going well? What do you enjoy doing on your own? It sounds like you are very independent. Are you happy or sad most of the time? Do you worry about anything? What is going well for you? What has been difficult this year?

Empathy ☐ I'm sorry to hear that. Do you miss her? Do you cry when you think of her?

Curious ☐ Why don't you like going to the doctor? What can you remember? That must have been horrible. I'm sorry you have had that experience.

ICE3 ☐ Apart from a new hearing aid, is there anything else I can help you with today?

SummarICE ☐ So it sounds as if you have had an upsetting time with losing your gran but Laura has made you feel happy. Your hearing aid is rubbing. You enjoy swimming but it makes your ear sore so you were thinking a new hearing aid may help. Was there anything else you were thinking?

Impression ☐ Your hearing aid may have contributed to your ear infection. I agree with you, Matthew, let's ask Audiology if they have a different hearing aid that may be more comfortable for you.

Empower ☐ Matthew, I'm now thinking about your general health. Your weight is a little high. How do you feel about me saying that? Do you do any exercise? What exercise would you most like to do? Who cooks your meals? Would you like to lose weight? What do you eat that is unhealthy? Do you think you could cut out some crisps, biscuits and cakes? How would you feel about me asking our dietician to see you to discuss your diet?

Future ☐ It would also be helpful to do your annual blood test and examine you for a check-up because we haven't seen you for a while. At that appointment I would like to examine your heart, blood pressure, tummy and check there are no lumps anywhere including the testicles. How would you feel about coming to see me next week for that? Oh dear, do you not like blood tests? It is important to monitor your blood to make sure you're healthy. If I ask the nurse to use a small needle would that help? I can give you some cream to make your skin numb so you won't feel it, if you like? It is a good idea to do exercise together with Laura. Would you like me to write down what we have decided to do next?

Specifics ☐ I will ask reception to make you an appointment for a blood test tomorrow then an appointment with me next week. You will receive a text message to remind you about the date. Can you please bring a urine sample to the appointment with the nurse tomorrow? I will write to Audiology and they will invite you for an appointment for your hearing aid. You should receive a letter in the next few weeks. If not please let me know. I will also ask the dietician to invite you to a consultation to talk about healthy food with you.

Safety net ☐ If your ear becomes sore, red or you have yellow discharge from it again please call a doctor. If you need help on an evening or at the weekend you can call 111 on the telephone to receive help.

Patient's Story

Down Syndrome

Doctor's notes Matthew Dalton, 24 years. PMH: Down syndrome, closure ASD, sensorineural deafness, hearing aids. Medications: none.

Consultations: out-of-hours appointment 4 days ago. Otitis externa. No wax. Drum intact, no perforation. Afebrile. Chest clear. Prescribed Otomize spray and advised to speak to GP if non-resolution.

Investigations: BMI 32 (2 months ago).

Alert: overdue annual review.

How to act Pleasant but quiet.

PC *'My mum said I need a new hearing aid. This one rubbing gave me an infection.'*

History *'I don't like talking to doctors.'* If asked why say: *'Because I had to go to the hospital and I didn't like it.'* If asked why, say: *'Operations hurt.'*

No other symptoms on systemic enquiry. You saw the dentist and optician a month ago. You are unsure of your medical history.

Social You live with your mum. You do not know your dad. You do not smoke or drink alcohol. You work in the hardware store. You have been saving money and hope to buy a house one day.

Your girlfriend's name is Laura. Laura has Down syndrome. You met at a party 3 months ago and you look pleased when you tell the doctor this. Your gran died earlier in the year. You cried a lot but not since you met Laura.

Your mum makes your meals but your diet is unhealthy and you do not exercise.

If encouraged to think about how you could be healthier, suggest going swimming with Laura and say you will tell your mum what the doctor said. You would be interested in losing weight.

ICE If the doctor mentions any new medical conditions, say you don't know. You have no understanding of any medical problems.

However, if the doctor says you need tests say: *'I don't want a blood test.'* If the doctor explains in simple language why you need tests, agree.

You are worried that your hearing aid is rubbing. You would like a new one. Your mum told you the doctor should see you for a check-up every year. She has been trying to convince you to come. If the doctor doesn't mention this you can prompt *'Mum said I have to have a check-up, is that true?'*

You don't know what the doctor will want to talk to you about. Your mum said the doctor will do a blood test. (Wrinkle your nose at this.)

Practices are encouraged to have a 'Learning Disability register'. This helps ensure that all patients with intellectual disabilities have an annual review. It is a good idea to send out a questionnaire before the appointment for the patient to complete with their carer. If your practice adopts this approach, make sure you ask to see the questionnaire at the appointment!

The annual health check should include:

- Health screening: observations, weight, height, urine dip, discussion about smoking, alcohol, drugs, diet and exercise, breast or testicular awareness, cervical screening, CVD screening (BMI, BP and blood tests).
- Social assessment: dependence and independence. Discussion regarding social skills.
- Vulnerability assessment: risk of abuse (neglect, physical, sexual, emotional).
- Advice regarding check-ups: vision (e.g. for cataracts), hearing (e.g. for SNHL) and dental.
- Systemic enquiry looking for undiagnosed problems (see below).
- Full physical examination: top-to-toe approach including ears, neck, chest, abdomen, genitalia, skin, nails, etc.
- Mental health assessment.

Discussion of potential issues specific to the condition and life stage[1,2]

Prenatal Heart disease, hypothyroidism, dislocation of the hip and cataracts.

Childhood Signs of developmental delay, duodenal atresia, pyloric stenosis, Hirschsprung's disease. Constipation and tracheo-oesophageal fistulae. Hearing and visual impairment. Symptoms of hypothyroidism (may be congenital or acquired). Ongoing cardiac conditions.

Atlantoaxial instability: have they had X-rays?

Once diagnosed – neurological assessments.

Ask about schooling.

Adolescence Growth and obesity. Dental care. Menstruation may be slightly delayed. Annual TFTs. Skin and hair.

Late adult Glaucoma and dementia screening.

Ongoing Recurrent URTIs – urine dip and MSU if signs of infection.

Create a **Health Action Plan** at the end of the annual review. This may be fairly simple, such as changes to diet/exercise, coming for blood tests or booking a dental review. It is a good idea to write this down for the patient and some may even have a Health Action Plan booklet which you can write this in. The RCGP provides an example of the questionnaires and action plans that can be used in its document *A Step-by-Step Guide for GP Practices: Annual Health Checks for People with a Learning Disability*.[3]

'Ageing and the problems of old age are particularly relevant to people with Down syndrome as some of these age-related problems develop earlier in life than would normally be the case.'[1]

'The astute GP will remember that the child with Down syndrome is susceptible to the same range of childhood problems as any other and that not all symptoms will be due to the syndrome.'[2]

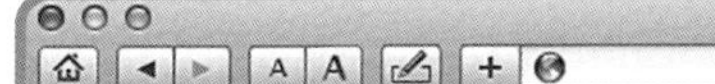

Doctor's Notes

Patient Fatima Sayed 47 years F

PMH Graves' disease (hyperthyroidism) 1 year ago

Medications Carbimazole 10 mg once daily

Propranalol 40 mg TDS PRN (not issued for 6 months)

Allergies No known drug allergies

Consultations 12 months ago – goitre palpable, confirmed on USS, no thyroid nodules. Diagnosis Graves' disease. Started carbimazole 30 mg once daily

10 months ago – T4 on the normal range. TSH remains low (expected). Decreased carbimazole to 20 mg daily

8 months ago – TSH normal range. Asymptomatic. Decreased carbimazole to 10 mg daily

1 month ago – request for repeat blood tests. Home observations supplied by patient. HR 70 bpm, BP 120/70

Investigations

	1 month ago	1 year ago	Normal range
TSH	2.2 mIU/L	2.2 mIU/L	(0.2–4.0 mIU/L)
T4	8.0 pmol/L	32 pmol/L	(10–20 pmol/L)
T3	2.0 nmol/L	3.4 nmol/L	(0.9–2.5 nmol/L)

TSH receptor antibodies positive

Household Aaqil Sayed 49 years M

Alert Overdue annual review

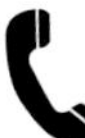

Example Consultation

Open ☐ Thank you for phoning. How are you? How are you getting on with the treatment?

Experience ☐ Would you mind taking me back to the start? I'm interested to know what it was like for you before you commenced treatment. What is your understanding of your condition? What is your understanding of the blood results?

ICE1 ☐ Have you had previous conversations with a GP about when to stop treatment? What are your thoughts about this?

ICE2 ☐ Has anything been worrying you about your thyroid or treatment?

History ☐ Have you noticed any new or troublesome symptoms? Tell me about your tablets; what dose are you taking of the carbimazole? How often are you taking the tablets? Have you any other medical history? Any medical problems that are in the family? Do you take other medicines or supplements? Any stressors at work? Or home? Do you drink? Or smoke?

Flags ☐ Is your weight stable? Did you ever have any problem with your vision? Any swelling of the eyes? Have you noticed any neck lumps?

Impact ☐ And what impact has the Graves' disease had on your life?

Sense ☐ I see you have not seen the GP for 8 months and I'm sensing there may be a reason why you decided to talk to me today about the treatment.

Curious ☐ Tell me more about your thoughts about the treatment. I'm wondering why at this stage you feel it would be beneficial to see a specialist?

ICE3 ☐ As well as discussing your carbimazole treatment and whether to stop or continue it, was there anything you were hoping we might do today?

SummarICE ☐ To summarise, you feel well, all your symptoms of Graves' disease have gone. You started reading about when to discontinue the carbimazole and this led you to forums that discussed the risk of the drug, which has alarmed you and led you to reassess the situation. You are wondering if the benefit of carbimazole no longer outweighs the risk and you would like to discuss stopping treatment with a specialist. Is that correct?

Impression ☐ It appears you have simple Graves' disease; high thyroid levels without signs of eye disease.

Explanation ☐ You are correct; there is a risk of agranulocytosis, 1 in 1000. With any treatment we need to weigh up the benefit of the treatment versus the risk.

Empathy ☐ I can appreciate that when you hear about the frightening risks associated with a tablet and, particularly now that you are well again, it is natural to revisit the decision as to whether the benefits of the tablet continue to outweigh the risks.

InCludE ☐ The scan was important at the beginning, in order to help make the diagnosis.

Options ☐ We usually treat Graves' disease for about 18 months. Your recent thyroid levels were in the normal range, therefore I would usually suggest 5 mg carbimazole for the next 6 months. Then, if the blood tests remain normal, aim to stop it after 18 months of treatment.

Recommend ☐ If you would like to stop it early that is your decision, but there is a risk of your symptoms returning and the disease not being completely treated. I suggest decreasing the carbimazole to 5 mg for 6 weeks, then we can reassess in 6 weeks with a blood test after you have had a chance to think about it. What are your thoughts?

Future ☐ If at any stage the TSH drops below the normal range, we need to increase the carbimazole. Once we have stopped the carbimazole I would like to continue to check your TSH level initially after 6 weeks then every 3 months for a year.

Empower ☐ If there were 100 people like you, after 18 months, 50 of them might need to continue carbimazole.[1] Smoking is a risk factor for this and if you would like to stop smoking I can help. Would you be interested in seeing our stop smoking advisor?

Safety net ☐ If you ever notice a sore throat, rash or infection then arrange a blood test straight away and withhold the medication until you know the blood test is normal.

Patient's Story

Hyperthyroidism

Doctor's notes Fatima Sayed, 47 years. PMH: hyperthyroidism – 1 year ago

Medication: carbimazole 10 mg once daily.

Consultations: 1 year ago – goitre palpable, confirmed on USS, no thyroid nodules. Started carbimazole 30 mg once daily.

How to act Pleasant.

PC *'Good morning, Doctor. I was hoping to discuss when I could stop my carbimazole please?'*

History Over a year ago you began to lose weight and feel generally unwell. You remember your bowels were loose and you felt quite jittery. Your doctor started carbimazole for high thyroid levels.

Since the treatment you have felt much better. You have always been healthy, take no other medicines and have no FH.

You have read about Graves' disease and have a good understanding of the terms TSH, T3 and T4. You called a month ago and the receptionist said the blood tests were normal.

Social Barrister, married with three children who have now all left home.

You drink no alcohol but smoke five cigarettes a day.

You are active and attend art classes.

ICE *'I should come off it as soon as I can.'*

A pragmatic suggestion you believe; however, if the doctor explores your thoughts behind this … You were reading about when to stop carbimazole and came across website forums which reminded you of the risk of the tablet. This led you down the path of reading frightening stories about agranulocytosis and you realised that now you feel well you should stop this tablet. You do not want this problem to happen to you. You wondered whether you should see the specialist again before you finished treatment so she could do a further scan to see if the treatment needs to continue. You presume she would rescan and you would like this. You follow the doctor's advice if they seem to know what they are doing. Otherwise, you push to see a specialist.

Learning Points

Hyperthyroidism[1,2]

History: Rapid-onset malaise, fever and pain in thyroid (suspect acute thyroiditis)
SOB, hoarseness, dysphagia, neck pressure
Exercise intolerance, fatigue, muscle weakness
$\uparrow$sweating, heat intolerance. $\uparrow$appetite $\uparrow$weight
Women: subfertility, oligo-/amenorhoea. Men: reduced libido, gynaecomastia
See NICE guidelines for full list

Examination: General: agitation, weight loss
Cardiovascular: sinus tachycardia, AF, heart failure, peripheral oedema
Thyroid: enlargement
Hands: fine tremor, palmar erythema
Skin: warm and moist, pruritus, urticaria, vitiligo, diffuse alopecia
MSK: muscle wasting, brisk reflexes
Eyes: exophthalmos, lid retraction, lid lag, chemosis, conjunctivitis, corneal ulceration, strabismus. See NICE guidelines for full list

Next tests: Repeat TSH, T4, T3. FBC (anaemia)
Calcium and LFTs may be raised
Thyroid receptor antibodies (85% positive in Graves')
If positive no need to do a thyroid scintigraphy scan
ESR (raised in Graves' or thyroiditis)
Thyroid scintigraphy scan if unsure on palpation of the thyroid
(GPs may be able to request if antibody negative)

Examine the thyroid

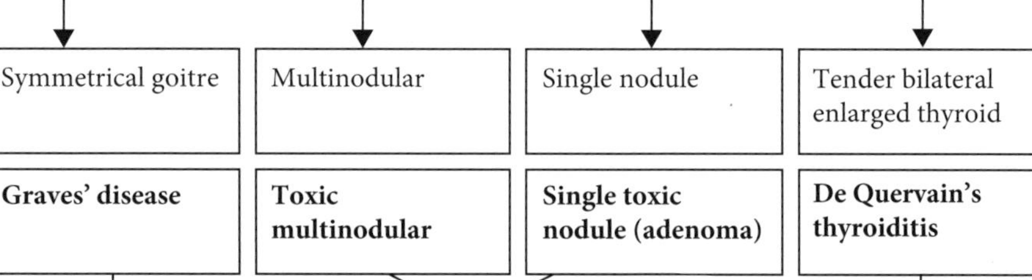

Radioactive iodine or surgery. Consider a 2WW referral for an unexplained thyroid lump

Beta-blockers and NSAIDs
Monitor TFTs

Emergency admission if thyrotoxic crisis
Refer urgently to endocrinology if pituitary or hypothalamic disorder suspected
For all others with new-onset hyperthyroidism: refer to, or discuss with, endocrinology for specialist Ix and management (urgency depends on clinical judgement). Whilst waiting:

- Consider prescribing beta-blocker (titrate dose to clinical response – palpitations/tremor/anxiety/tachycardia). Taper and stop once euthyroid
- If uncertainty about prescribing beta-blocker – seek specialist advice
- Seek specialist advice about starting carbimazole in primary care:
  - If symptoms troublesome despite beta-blocker
  - At risk of complication of hyperthyroidism
  - Taking amiodarone or lithium (liaison with specialist prescribing this drug may be needed)
- Give information leaflet[2]

Doctor's Notes

Patient	Arthur Smalling	49 years	M
PMH	Hypertension		
	Irritable bowel syndrome		
	Depression		
Medications	Amlodipine 5 mg OD		
	Mebeverine 135 mg TDS		
	Citalopram 20 mg OD		
Allergies	None		
Consultation	3 weeks ago: reporting urinary symptoms for 4 months. Request for PSA and counselled about test		
	Temperature 36.3°C. HR 68 bpm. BP 136/88		
	Abdomen soft and non-tender		
	Testicular examination normal		
	Slightly enlarged smooth prostate on rectal examination. Tender examination		
	Urine dipstick: leucocytes +		
Investigations	1 week ago: normal including PSA, MSU, HbA1c, FBC, U&E, CRP		
	E. coli UTI 1 year ago treated with trimethoprim		
Household	Patricia Smalling	42 years	F

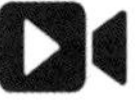

Example Consultation

Open ☐	Please don't be embarrassed. Please tell me about the problem. How is going to the toilet?
History ☐	Some specific questions about your symptoms … these are a little personal. Can you take me back to the start please? What sort of pain is it? Does anything bring it on or make it worse? How are your waterworks? Any pain passing urine? Going more often or in the night? Do you have to rush to the toilet? Does the urine flow start straight away or is there a pause? How is the stream? Does the flow stop and start? Any dribbling at the end when you think you have finished? Have you had any problems sexually? Any new sexual partners?
ICE1 ☐	Have you had any thoughts about what could be causing your symptoms?
ICE2 ☐	Are you worried about anything in particular in relation to these symptoms?
Flags ☐	Have you ever seen blood in your urine? Or blood in your semen? Have you had a fever? How are your bowels? Any changes, like blood or mucus? Or any weight loss?
Impact ☐	How have these symptoms affected you? And your relationship? How is your mental health?
Curious ☐	You mentioned being saddle sore. Have you been cycling a lot recently?
SummarICE ☐	You've had pain in your back passage and between your privates and bottom and discomfort passing urine. Your stream isn't as fast as before and there are some sexual issues and pain on ejaculation. You wondered if cycling caused these, but a month off didn't help. You've had no fever nor passed blood, and your bowels are fine. When your prostate was examined, it was not enlarged. Your blood and stool tests are normal. You had a urine infection a year ago.
ICE3 ☐	I have recommendations to share but were you hoping I would do anything specific today?
Impression ☐	I believe the cause of your symptoms is chronic prostatitis, which means inflammation of the prostate that has lasted for more than 3 months. There are no signs of a current urine infection. Your PSA level is reassuring so there is no sign of prostate cancer.
Experience ☐	Do you know much about the prostate?
InCludE ☐	You thought you might be saddle sore, but this may be an inflamed prostate.
Explanation ☐	The prostate is a gland found in every man and is located in the pelvis. In prostatitis, the gland becomes inflamed. Sometimes there is no obvious reason why. It is not a form of cancer and isn't usually caused by sexually transmitted infections. Any questions so far? Classic symptoms are pain in the region between your scrotum and anus, pain in the back passage and problems passing urine or with intercourse. Because the symptoms have been there for more than 3 months, we call the condition chronic. Unfortunately, it can be tricky to treat, but most men notice an improvement within 6 months. Taking regular paracetamol or ibuprofen may help. Ibuprofen may irritate the stomach lining so, if it does help, we can prescribe a tablet to protect the lining. What are your thoughts?
Future ☐	It would be helpful if you could complete a couple of questionnaires to identify how the symptoms have been affecting you. One is called the International Prostate Symptom Score and the other is the National Health Institute Chronic Prostatitis Symptom Index. I will email these to you and you can return them to me electronically. We can firstly treat prostatitis with a month of antibiotics. Do you have any allergies?
Specifics ☐	May I start you on doxycycline 100 mg twice daily for 1 month.* Antibiotics may have side effects, e.g. this tablet could cause nausea or diarrhoea. How would you feel about trying this treatment? Other potential treatments we could consider at our next appointment include a tablet to help urine flow, called tamsulosin. Perhaps a gentle stool softener called lactulose may help you to be more comfortable – shall I prescribe this today? If we are not making progress, we can ask a specialist to see you. (*Check local guidance.)
Safety net ☐	Should your symptoms worsen at any time or you develop a fever or pass blood, please let me know straight away. If the surgery is closed, call 111 for a doctor.

Patient's Story

Prostatitis

Doctor's notes Arthur Smalling, 49 years. PMH: HTN, IBS, depression. Medications: amlodipine 5 mg OD, mebeverine 135 mg TDS, citalopram 20 mg OD.

Consultation 3 weeks ago: reporting urinary symptoms for 4 months. Request for PSA and counselled about test. Temperature 36.3°C. HR 68 bpm. BP 136/88. Abdomen soft and non-tender. Testicular examination normal. Slightly enlarged smooth prostate on rectal examination. Tender examination. Urine dipstick: leucocytes +.

Investigations 1 week ago: normal including PSA, MSU, HbA1c, FBC, U&E, CRP. *E. coli* UTI 1 year ago treated with trimethoprim.

How to act Embarrassed.

PC *'Hello Doctor. I'm rather embarrassed; I've been getting a lot of pain in my bottom.'*

History You saw the GP a month ago to ask for a PSA test. They examined you and suggested some tests which you understand are all negative.

For the last 4 months you have been experiencing pain in your rectum. The pain can be sharp or a burning pain. You have been opening your bowels normally but sometimes passing a stool makes the pain worse. Your stools are formed but you are not constipated. No PR bleed or mucus. For the last 4 months, you have also had intermittent discomfort when passing urine but this hasn't increased recently. You feel tender in the region between your *'privates'* and anus. Your stream isn't as good as it used to be and you get up once or twice a night to pass urine. You have noticed occasional frequency or urgency in the daytime for the past 4 months. You have not seen blood in your urine. You don't suffer with hesitancy or terminal dribbling. You have had a couple of episodes of ED which you thought were due to your age (and possibly cycling), but you have also had pain during ejaculation which you thought was odd. No weight loss. No fever. You had a UTI a year ago and two others in the past. You have been married for 25 years and have not had any other partners. You have been very well with your mental health.

ICE You are a keen cyclist so initially thought cycling may be causing your symptoms. You have been training for a 100-mile bike ride for charity. You stopped cycling 4 weeks ago but unfortunately you haven't got any better so you thought you should get checked out.

'I thought I'd got a little saddle sore!'

Prostatitis

Acute prostatitis[1]

Symptoms A urinary tract infection. Perineal, penile or rectal pain. Acute urinary retention, obstructive voiding symptoms (difficulty voiding, hesitancy, straining to urinate, weak stream). Low back pain, pain on ejaculation.

Examination Gentle DRE – tender, enlarged or boggy prostate, leucocytes on urine dipstick.

Investigations MSU and STI screening. Blood cultures. FBC.

Acutely unwell If severely ill, unable to take oral antibiotics or acute urinary retention, admit to hospital.

Urgent referral Immunocompromised, diabetes, pre-existing urological condition or catheterised.

Oral antibiotics Two-week course of ciprofloxacin 500 mg BD or ofloxacin 200 mg BD or trimethoprim 200 mg BD.

Follow-up After 48 hours, or when cultures are back, review antibiotics, admit if not improving, refer to GUM if STI suspected.

Chronic prostatitis

'At least 3 months of urogenital pain, which may be perineal, suprapubic, inguinal, rectal, testicular, or penile and is often associated with lower urinary tract symptoms and sexual dysfunction.'[2]

Cause

1. Chronic prostatitis/chronic pelvic pain syndrome (CP/CPPS) – multifactorial? Infection or inflammation. Pain may be neuropathic.
2. Chronic bacterial prostatitis (CBP) – thought to be caused by recurrent UTIs, undertreated acute bacterial prostatitis, ascending urethral infection or lymphatic spread from the rectum.

Symptoms

Pain Perineum, inguinal, suprapubic, penis, scrotum, testes, rectum, lower back or abdomen.

LUTS Hesitancy, urgency, poor stream, terminal dribbling, frequency, nocturia or dysuria.

Sexual ED, painful ejaculation, premature ejaculation or decreased libido.

History needs to identify/exclude: a UTI, acute prostatitis, haematospermia (prostatitis, prostate cancer or STI), IBS (present in up to 30% of men with chronic prostatitis). Generally not systemically unwell.[2]

Assess symptom severity using the National Institute of Health Chronic Prostatitis Symptom Index (NIH-CPSI) or IPSS if UTI symptoms. Assess for **depression/anxiety** if cues to suggest this.

Examination Observations (rule out acute infection/sepsis), abdominal examination (tenderness, bladder distension or retention), external genitalia (urethral discharge, phimosis, meatal stenosis, penile cancer), costovertebral angle. DRE (prostate size, lumps? and tenderness).

Differential Acute prostatitis, prostatic abscess, UTI, urethritis, pyelonephritis, epididymitis, BPH, cancer of prostate/bladder/colon, urethral stricture, obstructive calculus in urinary tract or foreign body and pudendal neuralgia.

Investigations Urine dip and MSU (try sending MSU after DRE to increase microbiology yield).
Consider full STI screen (especially if <35 years or new partner).
Bloods: consider PSA testing and routine bloods, e.g. FBC, U&E and CRP.
NB: MSU may be negative in chronic bacterial prostatitis so look for old MSUs.

Management 4–6 week antibiotic (check local guidance). Trial alpha-blocker if LUTS present.
NICE – ciprofloxacin, ofloxacin or trimethoprim if quinolones not tolerated/allergy.
Paracetamol, NSAID, laxatives if constipation also present.

Refer If diagnosis in doubt, severe symptoms or if chronic bacterial prostatitis is suspected.

Doctor's Notes

Patient	Maureen Staples	70 years	F
PMH	Psoriasis		
	2 × normal vaginal deliveries		
	Hypertension		
	Never smoked		
Medications	Dermovate ointment, as directed		
	Cetraben cream PRN		
	Ketoconazole shampoo PRN		
	Amlodipine 5 mg once daily		
Allergies	No information		
Consultations	Recent private medical		
Investigations	1 week ago: private medical – 'Psoriasis moderate on trunk and mild on scalp. Height 164 cm, weight 72 kg, BMI 26.7. BP 138/80. Heart sounds normal. Hb1Ac 43 mmol/mol. Total cholesterol 5.6. Cholesterol/HDL ratio 4.2'		
	QRISK 13.2%		
Household	Brian Staples	72 years	M

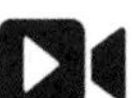

Example Consultation

Psoriasis

Open ☐ Thank you for calling. Please tell me about your medical history. And I see you had a recent medical. What did you learn from that? Yes, let's discuss your blood sugars.

ICE1 ☐ What thoughts have you had about your psoriasis and your sugars?

Impact ☐ What aspect of the psoriasis troubles you the most? In what way is it a nuisance?

ICE2 ☐ Is there anything you have been worried about or would like to talk about?

ICE3 ☐ Is there anything you thought or hoped we may decide today?

History ☐ Please tell me more about your psoriasis from the beginning. Where is it a problem at present? How bad is it now? What treatments have you tried? How often do you apply the Cetraben? What do you wash with? What shampoo do you use? How often do you apply the Dermovate? Does it help? How many days each month would you not apply it? When was the last time you had a longer break from it? Does the scalp shampoo work? How often do you use this? Tell me about a time when your psoriasis was problematic. Any other symptoms elsewhere in the body? Any nail changes? Are your eyes and joints okay? And your general health? I'm wondering about your mental wellbeing. How is your mood? Have you passed more urine recently? Or increased thirst?

ICE1 ☐ The clinician at the private medical thought that your psoriasis was moderate in severity and mild on your scalp. What do you think?

Curious ☐ What would you change or try to improve if you could?

SummarICE ☐ To summarise, the psoriasis is a nuisance, rubbing on and damaging clothes. You would like to improve this. Cetraben helps; you use it twice daily and in the shower.

Impression ☐ The psoriasis is troublesome and is affecting you every day. I'm sure we can, together, find ways to improve your symptoms and your general health.

Empathy ☐ You've lived with this all your life – it must have been wearing.

Experience ☐ What do you know about psoriasis? Has anyone explained the risks of steroid cream?

Explanation ☐ Psoriasis is caused by increased cell turnover. The Dermovate is a very strong steroid. You can use this daily for 8 weeks but then you should have a 4-week break as there are risks of too much steroid being absorbed into the body. For example, it can lead to changes in your hormones, a rise in blood pressure, diabetes and thinning of the bones.

Options ☐ Thinking about your general health, your high BP is currently under control. Your blood sugars have crept into the pre-diabetes range. Your cholesterol was 5.6 which is slightly raised. It's possible we could reduce your cholesterol and blood sugars with lifestyle changes such as exercise, dietary changes and reducing alcohol. What are your thoughts?

InCludE ☐ What do you know about pre-diabetes?

Future ☐ Because you are post-menopausal, we should consider your bones. I will use a calculator to determine your risk of frail bones so we can discuss this next time. How does this sound?

Recommend ☐ I recommend that you continue the Cetraben at least four times daily and please now stop the steroid cream for at least 4 weeks and use the Dovonex cream instead, which contains vitamin D, for the next 4 weeks, twice a day. How do you feel about this? For the scalp, because it looks mild you could try Cocois ointment at night and wash it off in the morning with Capasal shampoo. How do you feel about trying this regime?

Future ☐ If these don't work, we could try coal tar for the body and a steroid mousse for the scalp. We can repeat the blood sugars in 6 months. If we are not winning, we can ask the dermatologist to see you – you may be suitable for UV treatment. What are your thoughts about this?

Specifics ☐ I'll send your prescriptions to your pharmacy. Please can you arrange the follow-up appointment with me in a month to monitor progress?

Safety net ☐ If ever the skin looks red and is weeping, it may be an infection, so see a doctor.

Patient's Story

Psoriasis

Doctor's notes Maureen Staples, 70 years. PMH: psoriasis, pre-diabetes, 2 × NVD and hypertension.

Medications: Dermovate ointment, Cetraben cream, ketoconazole shampoo and amlodipine 5 mg daily.

Investigations: private medical 1 month ago. BMI 26.7, height 164 cm, weight 72 kg. Heart sounds normal. Hb1Ac 43 mmol/mol, BP 138/80. Psoriasis moderate on trunk and mild on scalp. QRISK 13.2%. Cholesterol/HDL ratio 4.2 units.

How to act Polite and playing down symptoms

PC *'I'd like my annual review please.'*

History You do not like to bother the doctor but the pharmacist told you that you are due for your medication review.

The psoriasis has been present all your life. You do not think about the impact it has on your life as you are used to it. But it does bother you: ***'It is a nuisance.'*** By this you mean it itches, rubs against clothes and the dry skin ruins your clothes.

You use the Dermovate most days so you are unsure if it makes a difference. Your last steroid break was 4 months ago. You apply this to your elbows and knees.

You like the Cetraben and use this in the shower and morning and night.

Your head irritates you the most. It is itchy. You use the shampoo twice a week and OTC anti-dandruff shampoo the rest of the week.

You were told that your blood sugar level from the recent blood tests was slightly high.

No family history.

Social You are an accountant. Your husband is well. With work you have not been exercising recently; however, if asked you could take up walking again and cycling.

You are a proud grandmother of seven grandchildren.

You enjoy a whisky with your husband every night. You have never smoked.

ICE Your psoriasis has been with you ever since you can remember. You were very interested in the psoriasis in your 20s and read all about it, but you have forgotten most of it now. You have no concerns. You expect the doctor will just give you the same creams. You are interested in any suggestions the doctor has.

Psoriasis in Adults

Remember 'associated morbidity; physical, e.g. CV disease; and psychological, e.g. depression.'[1]

Ask/Triggers Trauma, infection, pregnancy, sunlight, drugs, stress, alcohol, smoking and HIV.[2]

Aetiology Good evidence this is an autoimmune condition.[2]

Associations Psoriatic arthropathy 'in 30% of patients ... early intervention can reduce joint damage.'[2]

Cardiovascular disease, metabolic syndrome, venous thromboembolism.

Inflammatory bowel disease, coeliac disease. Anxiety and depression.

Examine Joints and nails, BP, BMI.

Investigate CVD: BP, lipids and HbA1c.

NICE suggests Offer topical Rx, consider if referral needed if lesions extensive, severe or unresponsive. Options:

Emollient – to reduce scale and help relieve itch.

Steroid + vitamin D – potent topical steroid + topical vitamin D, each applied once a day at different times. Explain risks of steroid Rx. Stop steroids when skin nearly clear.

Salicylic acid – consider if scale is a particular problem.

Review after 4 weeks – if good response, continue until skin is clear or nearly clear. Max. 8 weeks topical potent steroids, then 4-week break. Continue vitamin D throughout.

If poor initial response, first check compliance. If no explanation, continue steroid + vitamin D for a further 4 weeks. If no response after 8 weeks, stop steroid and continue topical vitamin D only. If poor response after 8–12 weeks with vitamin D alone, offer:

- Potent topical steroid BD for 4 weeks or coal tar preparation applied OD or BD.

If no response, consider combined corticosteroid + vitamin D once daily for 4 weeks.

If persistent, consider alternative diagnosis, dithranol or dermatology referral.

Scalp psoriasis

NICE CKS suggests:[3]

- First – commencing with a potent corticosteroid daily for up to 4 weeks, or vitamin D preparation or coal tar shampoo (do not use alone if severe scalp psoriasis).
- Second, at 4 weeks – if no improvement, change preparation (e.g. shampoo or mousse) or add scalp treatment such as salicylic acid, coconut oil or emollient to remove scale. Apply before the steroid.
- Third, at 8 weeks – combined Vit D preparation + potent corticosteroid or Vit D product alone.
- Fourth, at 16 weeks – diagnosis correct? Consider 2-weeks very potent steroid or coal tar or seek advice.

If mild – an example regime as advised by a dermatologist

Start with Ointment at night and wash off with a shampoo in the morning.

Ointment: Sebco™ scalp ointment (coal tar, salicylic acid, sulfur) or Cocois.

Shampoo: Capasal (coal tar 1%, coconut oil 1%, salicylic acid 0.5%), T gel or Polytar.

No improvement Above plus steroid and vitamin D preparation.

Steroid: betamethasone valerate (Bettamousse) 0.1% (potent).

Vitamin D: calcipotriol scalp solution.

When improved Stop the Sebco and continue shampoo and the Bettamousse.

When controlled Stop the steroid (Bettamousse) and continue antipsoriasis shampoo PRN.

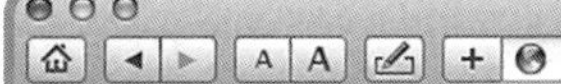

Doctor's Notes

Patient	Chao Lin 82 years M
PMH	COPD
	Current smoker
	Bowel cancer 9 years ago – bowel resection and chemotherapy
Medications	Salbutamol inhaler BD
	Tiotropium inhaler, once daily
Allergies	No information
Consultation	COPD review 1 year ago with the nurse. No changes made. Using salbutamol on hills. Tiotropium daily. Saturations 96%. MRC dyspnoea scale 2
	COPD review with specialist nurse 1 week ago: chest – air entry and wheeze throughout. No accessory muscle use. Saturations 94%. HS normal. HR 72 bpm regular. No leg oedema or raised JVP. Weight 72 kg. BP 130/70. Peak flow 20 L/min. No supraclavicular lymphadenopathy. No clubbing
Investigations	Last colonoscopy 1 year ago. FIT 2 months ago normal
	Weight 72 kg
	Spirometry 1 year ago
	FEV 48%, FVC 80%, FEV1/FVC 0.6
	FEV1 following salbutamol 50%
	Asked to make appointment with doctor
Household	No household contacts registered

Example Consultation

COPD

Open □ Thank you for calling Mr Lin. How are you? Please tell me about your health. Any changes? What is most difficult? Any recent changes with your bowels? Or elsewhere?

ICE1 □ Is there anything you wanted to talk to me about?

ICE2 □ Has anything been on your mind or worrying you? What is your biggest fear?

Sense □ I noticed when we were first speaking together your breathing was harder but seems to have eased now. Have you been struggling with your breathing whilst moving around?

Empathy □ After a cancer diagnosis life can feel different. How does it affect you?

Impact □ What are you not able to do? How long can you walk for? Do you have stairs in your home? Do you do your meals and shopping? Are you able to keep the home clean?

History □ Have you had any other previous health issues? Tell me more about your breathing. When do you take your inhalers? Do you use a spacer? Who is important to you? I'm sorry, that must still be very painful. How are you coping? How often do you see your son? And work?

Risk □ Did that involve exposure to asbestos? Are you still smoking? Growing up, were you exposed to much pollution or smoke? Did your family in China have any health problems?

Flags □ Do you cough up any phlegm or blood? Any chest pain? Breathlessness at night? How many pillows? Do your legs swell? Is your weight steady? When was your last chest infection?

Sense □ You seem concerned about infections.

Curious □ Why might that be? How is your mood? Do you feel isolated? Or depressed? Do you ever want to not wake up? Do you have a faith? With your faith is there anything important to you that I should know about now or in the future?

ICE □ Did you have any thoughts about what we may talk about today?

SummarICE □ For the past 6 months, you've struggled to walk as far as before without stopping. You worry about a chest infection and how your breathing may change over time. You fear dying and struggling to breathe. You have worried about asbestos and if this has damaged your lungs. Years ago you had bowel cancer and although all seems well, the fear remains.

Impression □ I'm afraid your airway disease does seem to have worsened.

Experience □ What do you know about the term COPD? Or chronic airways disease?

Explanation □ It is a long-term condition of the airways which have been damaged over time. Smoking is the usual cause, but you're right that asbestos can affect the lungs too.

Empathy □ I can imagine it is frightening to notice that your breathing does not allow you to do what you used to, and fear that soon you will not be able to reach the shops.

Recommend □ There are things we can try which should help. I would like to change your inhaler for a stronger one called Anoro Ellipta. It contains a medicine like your capsule inhaler but also a long-acting version of your blue inhaler. You may also find a spacer helps you take your blue inhaler. I will ask our pharmacist to demonstrate the new inhaler and spacer.

InCludE □ It's not easy to know if the asbestos has contributed, but let's do a CXR to look for signs.

Empower □ Stopping smoking is hard but may help slow the disease. I can refer you to our rehab service to help get your lungs working better. Would that be helpful? I can prescribe a COPD rescue pack containing antibiotics and steroids to start if you become unwell. You take prednisolone 30 mg daily (steroid) if your breathing gets worse, with amoxicillin (antibiotic) if more phlegm or it changes colour. Would you like to see our social support team? They may make suggestions, e.g. meals delivered to you. What are your thoughts?

Future □ Can we meet soon to discuss what might happen to your breathing over time? We could make a plan, talking through different scenarios and what you might like doctors to do.

Specifics □ I will ask our COPD nurse to see you in 6 weeks, and request a CXR. Please go to X-ray any time and just give your name. Please arrange your flu vaccine with reception.

Safety net □ Meanwhile, if you are more breathless, in pain or unsure, please speak to a doctor promptly. I'm pleased you came today and hope that the new inhalers will help your breathing.

Patient's Story

COPD

Doctor's notes Chao Lin, 82 years. PMH: COPD. Bowel cancer – 9 years ago – resection and chemotherapy. Last colonoscopy 1 year ago. FIT 2 months ago normal. Medications: salbutamol and tiotropium inhalers. Smoker.

Consultations: 1 year ago, COPD review with PN. Sats 96%. MRC 2. Letter to patient: COPD review now due.

How to act Breathing initially fast but this settles after a short while.

PC *'Hello, Doctor. I had a letter asking me to call for a check-up.'*

History You don't like to bother the doctor. Apart from your breathing you are well. You have noticed no recent bowel changes. You are compliant with your tiotropium and use the salbutamol twice daily. You have no allergies. You remember your grandparents were heavy breathers. You never knew your father and your mother died when you were small. You believe you are 82 years old but don't know exactly. Your breathing hasn't been very good for the past 6 months. You started to wheeze about 3 years ago. You wheeze when walking to the shop but you are okay in your home although occasionally wheeze after a shower. You have no orthopnoea and sleep on two thin pillows. You have no fluid collecting in the legs. You have no cardiac symptoms. Where you grew up, your grandparents used to light fires throughout the day to keep you warm. You had no siblings. You had three infections last winter and once you were in hospital overnight. This was a frightening experience as you had never been in hospital.

Social You moved to the UK when you were 36 years old and worked in the shipyards. You live alone and find life tiring. You walk to the local shop a couple of hundred yards away and stop for a rest midway. You use a shopping trolley to wheel your food back to the house but this is getting harder. You do not drive. Your son owns the local garage in the next village and he always offers to help you and you see him twice a week. He takes you wherever you need to go. You lost your wife to Alzheimer's 3 years ago. You feel quite lonely but feel you should not complain. Your mood is a little low but you have no thoughts of not wanting to be alive and generally you feel grateful for life. Your faith (Buddhism) is important to you.

You continue to smoke and would like to stop. The surgery is on the next street to your home so convenient if needed. You have no problems within your bungalow.

ICE You worry about an infection or whether you will one day struggle with your breathing. Your biggest fear is the cancer returning.

Is it likely you will die of not being able to breathe? You also worry about asbestos as you have heard about old colleagues who have been affected by this from working on ship repairs. You have no expectations from the consultation and would follow any advice that the doctor gives. However, a preference would be to avoid any risk of infection if possible. If the doctor can help reduce your worries about asbestos you would appreciate this.

Learning Points

The advice below is based upon the GOLD (Global Obstructive Lung Disease) Guidelines.[1] COPD is diagnosed using spirometry; post-bronchodilator FEV1/FVC <0.7. Exclude asthma/reversibility because it is dangerous to prescribe a LABA without a steroid in asthma.

Assessment of severity mMRC dyspnoea score + CAT (COPD assessment test) + number of exacerbations over last 12 months. Use to categorise as GOLD A, B or E group:

- GOLD A – mMRC 0–1, CAT <10, 0–1 exacerbations (not leading to admission).
- GOLD B – mMRC ≥2, CAT ≥10, 0–1 exacerbations (not leading to admission).
- GOLD E – mMRC ≥2, CAT ≥10, ≥2 exacerbations or ≥1 leading to admission.

Without exact scores to hand, A roughly equates to few symptoms and few exacerbations, B to few exacerbations but symptomatic and E to exacerbations but minimal interval symptoms or symptomatic and frequent exacerbations.

FEV1 indicates severity of airflow limitation but doesn't directly impact management.

Initial therapy Group A – PRN SABA or LABA.

Group B – LABA + LAMA.

Group E – LABA + LAMA + ICS if eosinophil count ≥300 cells/μL or if concomitant asthma.

Pulmonary rehab Offer if mMRC ≥3 or recent hospitalisation for acute exacerbation.[2]

Home oxygen Consider referral for LTOT if sats ≤92% on air, cyanosis, polycythaemia, peripheral oedema, raised JVP, severe or very severe airflow obstruction.[2]

Health promotion Smoking cessation. Flu and pneumococcal vaccine.

Carer support Involve the carer in the management plan.

Self-management plan For exacerbations – when to step up inhalers and take rescue medications.

Example inhalers (refer to own local formulary)

The patient should receive an explanation of how to use their inhaler. Following this, prescribe the same brand:

- SABA – salbutamol. Good practice to prescribe a spacer device as well.
- LAMA – Incruse Ellipta, Seebri Breezhaler.
- LAMA/LABA – Anoro Ellipta 2, Ultibro Breezhaler, Duaklir Genuair often first line after SABA.
- ICS/LAMA – Relvar Ellipta, Fostair 100/6.
- ICA/LABA/LAMA – Trelegy Ellipta, Trimbow (MDI – prescribe with spacer, good for those who struggle with poor inspiratory effort or difficulty using inhalers).

CHAPTER 5

OLDER ADULTS, INCLUDING FRAILTY AND PEOPLE AT THE END OF LIFE

	Cases in this chapter	RCGP 2025 curriculum	Learning points
5.1	Deafness and Tinnitus	**ENT, speech and hearing** 'Hearing problems including deafness and associated speech or language disorders' 'Ensure that a patient's hearing impairment or deafness does not negatively impact on the communication between the patient and doctor'	Deafness: • Red flags • When to refer and how urgently • Weber's and Rinne's tests Tinnitus: • When to refer and how urgently • Association with CV disease
5.2	AMD and Cataract	**Eyes and vision** 'Recognise how sight loss can interfere with mobility and lead to social isolation and difficulty in communication (such as use of telephones or computers) as well as the impact of poor eye health on loss of confidence, mental health, activities of daily living, independent living and ability to work'	AMD and cataract: presentation and management DVLA driving regulations
5.3	Angina	**Cardiovascular health** 'Risk factors for coronary heart disease and other thromboembolic diseases such as lipid disorders, diabetes and hypertension'	Angina: diagnosis and management Stable and unstable angina Syndrome X Managing complex cases in the exam
5.4	Lung Cancer/End of Life	**Respiratory health** 'Respiratory malignancies' 'Indications for chest X-rays, CT and MRI scans'	Causes of coin lesions Lung cancer: urgent suspected cancer referral criteria
5.5	Peripheral Neuropathy	**Neurology** 'Sensory and/or motor disturbances (peripheral nerve problems) including mono- and poly-neuropathies such as nerve compression and palsies'	Peripheral neuropathy: prevalence, causes, investigations, red flags and management

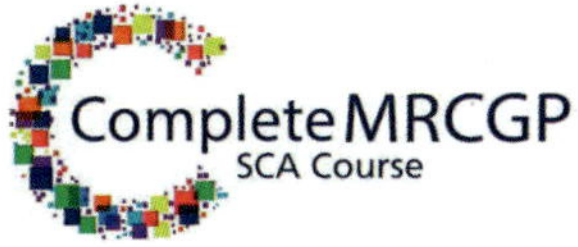

Links to the RCGP Curriculum

In this chapter, the cases are drawn from the following clinical topic guides:

- Ear, nose and throat, speech and hearing
- Eyes and vision
- Cardiovascular health
- Respiratory health
- Neurology

And the following life stages topic guides:

- Older adults
- People at the end of life

Scope of Conditions

Older adults may have health problems – acute and chronic – from many areas of the clinical curriculum. They may well also have psychosocial issues such as loneliness, isolation and depression. Many older adults may already be taking medication so it will be important to consider drug interactions and the risks of polypharmacy. The following are examples of cases in this clinical curriculum group:

- Dermatology – varicose eczema
- Ear, nose and throat, speech and hearing – deafness
- Eyes and vision – cataract, glaucoma
- Gastroenterology – malabsorption, GI tumours such as pancreatic cancer
- Haematology – anaemia, leukaemia, myeloma
- Mental health – depression
- Metabolic problems – diabetes
- Musculoskeletal – arthritis, joint replacements
- Neurology – Parkinson's disease, peripheral neuropathy
- Renal and urology – chronic renal failure, kidney cancer
- Respiratory health – COPD, lung cancer
- Urgent and unscheduled care – any of the above clinical scenarios may present acutely

Skills and Pitfalls

In addition to the information in Chapter 1 'How to Demonstrate Skills: The Marking Scheme Made Easy' consider the following challenges for this blueprint group:

- Full exploration of the presenting problem including psychological, social and physical features, including risk factors for disease in older people.
- Awareness that some illnesses are more prevalent in this age group than others.
- Recognise that there may be challenges when communicating with older people, for example due to hearing difficulty, cognitive impairment and the involvement of families and carers.
- Know your team – demonstrate that you can coordinate care with other health professionals such as social services, care homes and community nursing team.
- Recognise the different facets of clinical management – the acute problem, continuing care, self-care, chronic disease monitoring and awareness of the implications of polypharmacy.
- Legal and ethical issues – 'living wills', ReSPECT forms, DNACPR discussions, power of attorney for health and use of the Mental Capacity Act.

Doctor's Notes

Patient	Anthony Warren	72 years	M
PMH	Hypertension. Vasectomy		
Medications	Atorvastatin 20 mg daily		
	Enalapril 5 mg daily		
Allergies	None		
Consultations	Practice nurse 2 weeks ago. BP 132/80. U&E, LFT, HbA1c, FBC, cholesterol all normal. Mentioned hearing loss – advised to see high street provider to get this checked		
Investigations	All bloods normal, 2 weeks ago		
Household	Julie Warren	69 years	F

Note from high street provider dated yesterday:

'This 72-year-old man has sensorineural hearing loss and tinnitus. Both ear drums appeared normal and there was no wax. I have arranged hearing aids and advised him to see you to discuss treatment for tinnitus.

Yours sincerely,

Audiologist'

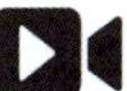

Example Consultation

Open ☐ Hello, Mr Warren – I'm sorry about your hearing and very happy to explain what the note means. Please tell me more about your hearing. Have your family noticed a problem?

History ☐ How did this start? When are you most affected? Any situations when it seems particularly bad? And the ringing in the ears? What is it like? When do you notice this?

ICE1 ☐ You said you didn't really want hearing aids – what thoughts do you have about them?

Flags ☐ Are both ears affected or just one? Any discharge or pain in the ears? Has your nose been blocked? Have you had any nose bleeds? Any episodes of dizziness or loss of balance? Any blurring of vision or weakness or numbness of arms and legs?

Impact ☐ Tell me how this is affecting you – in your home and social life.

ICE2 ☐ What worries you most about all this?

Risk ☐ Please tell me about your work over the years. Have you ever worked in a noisy environment? Do you have any hobbies that involve noise? Do you scuba dive? Do you take any medications? Anyone in the family with hearing problems?

Experience ☐ I'm interested to know more about your father.

Empathy ☐ I'm sorry to hear that – he must have felt very isolated.

Curious ☐ What do you know about deafness? Have any of your friends experienced this?

ICE3 ☐ Did you have anything in your mind you thought I might be able to do today to help?

Sense ☐ I sense you are embarrassed about this as well as frustrated at how it affects you.

SummarICE ☐ To summarise, for several years you have noticed a problem with your hearing, and the high street firm has confirmed this and arranged hearing aids. You are also troubled by noises and ringing in the ears.

Impression ☐ As well as the sensorineural hearing loss, you also have what we call tinnitus.

Explanation ☐ Sensorineural deafness means the tiny hairs in the ear or the nerves to the ear are not working well so that the nerve signals that carry sound are weaker, causing deafness. The ringing in your ears is called tinnitus and it is very common in this type of deafness. Sometimes it can be linked with heart problems, but I can see that your blood tests and BP are normal, so I don't think this applies to you. I suspect playing music in loud environments for many years has contributed to the problem.

Empathy ☐ It must be very upsetting – your home life and hobbies are affected, and you are worried you may go very deaf and become isolated like your father.

Recommend ☐ Hearing aids should really help, though they may feel strange at first.

Options ☐ For the tinnitus, I would like to give you a PIL from the British Tinnitus Association. There are lots of suggestions to try, such as having a little background noise at night, e.g. the radio at very low volume. You asked about a referral to ENT – I don't think we need to do this because there is nothing different that they could do.

InCludE ☐ How do you feel about this now? Hearing aids can take some getting used to but try to persist as they'll help. Modern hearing aids are also discrete so your band mates may not even notice.

Empower ☐ There are some things you can do to help. Please protect your hearing by always using good ear protection in a noisy environment, for example when playing at concerts.

Future ☐ Please arrange to talk to me again, or come and see me, in about 2 months – book the appointment through our website – and we can see how you are getting on with the hearing aids and help for tinnitus.

Safety net ☐ If you have a sudden change in hearing or develop severe earache, discharge, nosebleeds, dizziness or any weakness or numbness in your face or limbs, please see a doctor straight away.

Patient's Story

Deafness and Tinnitus

Doctor's notes Anthony Warren, 72 years. PMH: hypertension, vasectomy. Medications: atorvastatin 20 mg daily, enalapril 5 mg daily.

Note from high street provider: 'This 72-year-old man has sensorineural hearing loss and tinnitus. Both ear drums appeared normal and there was no wax. I have arranged hearing aids and advised him to see you to discuss treatment for tinnitus.'

How to act Concerned, embarrassed. If the doctor does not face you and speak clearly, you will struggle to hear what they say and will need to ask the doctor to repeat themselves.

PC *'I went to get my hearing checked – they sent a note for you – have you got it? And what is this sensorineural hearing loss?'*

'I never wanted hearing aids anyway – they're only for old people'

History For the last few years you have noticed increasing problems with your hearing. At home you have to have the TV louder than everyone else would like. Your wife remarks that you often don't hear her and are always saying '*Pardon?*' Your father went very deaf at a relatively young age and you remember how socially isolated he became, almost a recluse and cut off from the family. You also have bilateral tinnitus and notice this especially at night when it's quiet and you're trying to sleep. In fact, you wondered if it was the neighbour's burglar alarm, but your wife couldn't hear it at all.

Social Retired history teacher at local comprehensive school. You live with your wife and have two grown up children and four grandchildren. Your wife is a retired hairdresser. Social drinker, never smoked. Hobbies – play guitar with a local band – you are by far the oldest member. Gigs once a fortnight in pubs and clubs, often noisy.

ICE Ideas – *'I am going deaf like my father. It must be inherited. There's probably nothing that can be done to help.'*

Concerns – *'How am I going to continue playing the guitar? I don't really want to wear a hearing aid as the band members would tease me about this.'*

Expectations – possibly a referral to ENT.

Learning Points

Deafness[1]

Red flags
Unilateral.
Sudden onset.
Fluctuating hearing levels.
Facial droop (consider stroke).
Persistent tinnitus, especially if pulsatile or causing distress.

Immediate referral
NICE advises referral to be seen within 24 hours for:
- Sudden onset (3 days or less) severe or rapidly worsening sensorineural deafness.
- Hearing loss with facial droop – urgent admission ENT or stroke pathway if stroke suspected.
- Immunocompromised + deafness + otalgia + discharge with no response to 72 hours of treatment.

Urgent suspected cancer referral
To have diagnosis or cancer ruled out within 28 days for:
- Sudden onset (3 days or less) >30 days ago.
- Rapid worsening of hearing (over 4–90 days).
- Adults of Chinese or South East Asian heritage with hearing loss and middle ear effusion not associated with infection.

Examination
Ear drums and canals, palpate neck for lumps. Use Weber's/Rinne's to differentiate sensorineural from conductive hearing loss.

Vulnerable adults*
Consider audiology referral for assessment then every 2 years for hearing test.

Sensorineural hearing loss
Caused by damage to acoustic nerve, the cochlea or the hair cells.
Risk factors – age, noise exposure, atherosclerosis, smoking.

Conductive hearing loss
Caused by ear wax, perforated ear drum, problems with ossicles.

Weber's
Unilateral conductive loss – sound is louder in affected ear.
Unilateral sensorineural hearing loss – sound is louder in non-affected ear.
Heard equally in both – normal hearing or hearing loss is bilateral.

Rinne's
Air conduction better than bone conduction (AC > BC) – normal hearing or sensorineural deafness.
BC > AC – conductive deafness.

Treatment
Encourage early use of hearing aid. May need persistence.

Tinnitus[2]

Immediate referral
High suicidal risk; sudden-onset severe neurological symptoms or signs; acute uncontrolled vestibular symptoms; suspected stroke; sudden onset and pulsatile; head trauma.

Very urgent referral
Tinnitus that has developed suddenly – over 3 days or less – in last 30 days.

Urgent referral
Unilateral; pulsatile; associated with unilateral hearing loss; associated with persistent otalgia.

Cardiovascular risks
Association, not causation, but tinnitus and IHD may have similar risk factors so check CV risks if patient presents with tinnitus.[3]

Treatment
Reassure, treat cause if possible, check medications and review, discuss sound therapy, refer for counselling or CBT.

*People with dementia or suspected dementia, learning disability or cognitive impairment.

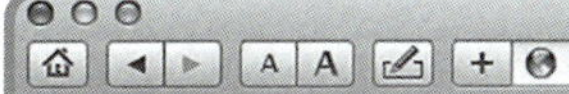

Doctor's Notes

Name	Fred Scott	81 years	M
PMH	Hypertension		
Medications	Atenolol 100 mg daily		
Consultations	BP check with nurse 1 week ago – 160/90. To come back in 1/12		
Investigations	U&E, cholesterol, HbA1c, LFT normal 1 week ago		
Household	Daisy Scott	84 years	F

Note from the optician, dated today:

'Dear Doctor

This patient attended for a routine eye check today. His vision is:

- Right eye – 6/60 (corrected to 6/18)
- Left eye – 6/60 (no improvement with correction)

This is below the legal limit for driving. I have advised him not to drive and to see you for referral to an ophthalmologist for treatment of his AMD and cataracts.

Yours sincerely,

High Street Opticians'

Example Consultation

AMD and Cataract

Open ☐ Hello, Mr Scott – yes of course – yes we received the note. Thank you. What do you think particularly worried the optician?

ICE1 ☐ And what thoughts have you had since you had your eyes tested?

History ☐ Tell me what problems you have noticed, for example with reading or distance vision.

Risk ☐ Are you currently driving? How about driving at night? Have you had any near misses?

Impact ☐ Please tell me more about your home situation. What do you use the car for? How far are you from the shops? Does anyone else drive? Any family nearby? Can you use the internet for grocery shopping?

ICE2 ☐ Tell me what else worries you particularly about your sight or not driving.

Flags ☐ May I ask if you smoke? And your diet? Do you eat fruit and veg?

Sense ☐ I sense that you have had some concerns yourself about your sight and whether it's safe to drive, even before you saw the optician.

Curious ☐ You mentioned your father went blind; I'm sorry to hear that. Please can you tell more?

ICE3 ☐ Was there anything you were hoping I might suggest today?

SummarICE ☐ After the near miss you were worried about your sight and your optician has confirmed your worst fears and told you not to drive, which is a real blow. You were hoping I would say that they were wrong and that it would be OK to drive short distances.

Empathy ☐ It must have been a shock for you – the car is a lifeline for you.

Impression ☐ The optician says you have two problems: one is that you are developing cataracts and the other is age-related macular degeneration or AMD.

Experience ☐ I know your father had eye problems; have you heard of either cataracts or AMD?

Explanation ☐ Cataracts are a cloudiness of the eye lens so the light can't pass through it so well. The other problem means that the most sensitive and the important area of the back of the eye is becoming worn and less sensitive, so your sight will not be as sharp as it used to be.

InCludE ☐ You mentioned vitamins. Eating a balanced diet is important and there is some evidence that supplements with vitamin C and antioxidants can slow AMD.

Options ☐ Controlling your BP well may also help and we should recheck that in a couple of weeks. It's good that you don't smoke. Surgery will cure the cataracts and I can refer you for this, if you like. There is no need to wait until the cataracts are worse. It will not help the AMD but your sight could be reassessed after the operation and it might mean you can drive for a while longer. Your vision may deteriorate with time, but this can be quite a slow change.

Empower ☐ How do you feel about this? Would you like me to refer you? Would you like me to send you a PIL about AMD? I can print it off in large print and post to you so it is easier to read. If your children can help you with the internet, you can also listen to the leaflet being read out loud.

Future ☐ May I book you in for a BP check in 2 weeks? We can do some blood tests to make sure everything else is okay, e.g. your blood sugar. You shouldn't drive for now – your insurance would not cover you if you had an accident. I'm really sorry but it isn't safe to drive even short distances. Could one of your children help with shopping for now? Could they shop on the internet for you and get groceries delivered to your home? Or perhaps take a taxi to the shops?

Safety net ☐ If your sight deteriorates further whilst waiting for the appointment, please call.

Patient's Story

Doctor's notes Fred Scott, 81 years. PMH: hypertension. Medication: atenolol 100 mg daily.

Consultations: BP check with nurse 1 week ago – 160/90. To come back in 1/12.

Investigations: U&E, cholesterol, HbA1c, LFT normal 1 week ago.

Optician's note: 'This patient attended for a routine eye check today. His vision is right eye – 6/60 (corrected to 6/18); left eye – 6/60 (no improvement with correction). This is below the legal limit for driving. I have advised him not to drive and to see you for referral to an ophthalmologist for treatment of his AMD and cataracts.'

How to act Polite, concerned about your eyesight.

PC *'I went to the optician this morning and she wrote a note for you – I handed it in this morning.'*

History You went for an eye check today and the optician told you that you are developing cataracts and AMD. She said your sight was just below the legal limit for being able to drive and suggested you stop. She told you to see your GP to discuss this. You had noticed that your sight seemed a bit worse than usual and troublesome 'haloes' around street lights had already made you give up night-time driving. You had a near miss last week when you did not see a car and pulled out of a junction. You have had to stop buying a newspaper as you cannot read the print anymore.

You have hypertension which is normally well controlled but the practice nurse said that your BP was up a bit when you last had an appointment a week ago. A re-check was booked for 1/12 after that appointment.

Social You are a retired accountant and live with your wife who is also retired. You live quite a way from the shops and rely on being able to drive to do the shopping and get out and about. The car is your 'lifeline'. Your wife has never driven; you have always been the family 'chauffeur'. There are no family members close by. Your father went blind in later life, when he was about 83. You remember how he struggled and became virtually housebound before he fell over at home, fractured his hip and died shortly afterwards. You have never smoked and eat a balanced diet. You are a basic computer user, not internet literate.

ICE You are now very worried about your sight.

Understanding You have never heard of AMD and will react badly to the use of this acronym that means nothing to you (unless described). You saw your father lose his independence once he started to lose his sight and are worried you are going the same way. You are sure you are still safe to drive to the shops – it's not far and you know the way.

Ask the doctor *'What is AMD? Is it okay to drive short distances?'*

'Am I going blind?'

'Will an operation help?'

'Why can't I have an operation now?'

Cataract[1]

Epidemiology Mainly >60. Women more at risk than men.

Aetiology Changes in proteins that make up lens.

Symptoms Cloudiness. Especially night vision with haloes around lights.

Risk factors FH, diabetes, eye surgery or injury, uveitis, prolonged or high-dose steroids. Other risk factors: smoking, hypertension, alcohol, poor diet, low socioeconomic status, sunlight, myotonic dystrophy, neurofibromatosis type 2 and atopic dermatitis (independent of possible risk factor from use of topical corticosteroids).

Treatment Surgery. No need to wait 'until cataract is ripe' anymore. Usually LA, go home same day. Lens removed and replaced with plastic one. May still need glasses for near vision. Clarity and colour vision should be improved.

Consider How the cataract affects vision and quality of life. What surgery involves, including risks and benefits. Whether the patient wants surgery, if they can cooperate with eye examinations, surgery and post-operative care. Pre-op assessment if systemic co-morbidities and consider individual care plan if social support at home, disabilities, reduced mental capacity or first language not English.

Age-related macular degeneration (AMD)[2]

Epidemiology More common in people of northern European ethnicity.

Symptoms Affects central but not peripheral vision. Reading and facial recognition more difficult. Size or colour of objects may appear different with each eye.

Risk factors FH, age (>50), smoking, obesity, alcohol, poor diet, sunlight, hypertension, history of CVD, lack of exercise.

Referral Urgently to be seen in 1 week, especially if symptom onset rapid. Advise go to Eye casualty if delay >1 week or symptoms deteriorate whilst waiting for appointment.

Dry (geographic atrophy) AMD Most common type, macula cells become damaged by build-up of drusen deposits. Visual loss is gradual, over many years. Treatment – limited options: diet rich in vitamins A, C, E may help. Consider antioxidants (AREDS2 combination).* Stop smoking, modify CV risk factors.

Wet (neovascular) AMD 4–12% people with dry AMD may develop wet AMD, which is much more serious.[3] Abnormal blood vessels develop beneath the macula and damage the cells.

Much more serious than dry AMD – vision can deteriorate in days.

Treatment: injections of anti-vascular endothelial growth factor (anti-VEGF). Laser treatment largely superseded but may be suitable for some.

Additional points Also consider referral to low vision services, group-based rehabilitation programme, eccentric vision training, support with depression and psychological problems.

*AREDS2 = vitamin C 500 mg, vitamin E 400 IU, lutein 10 mg, zeaxanthin 2 mg, zinc 80 mg and copper (cupric oxide) 2 mg.

DVLA driving requirements

Check current DVLA driving requirements at https://www.gov.uk/driving-eyesight-rules

Tip – when a patient has sight problems, think about how you can give them accessible patient information, e.g. auditory leaflet or large print. Don't make assumptions about an older person's internet skills, check.

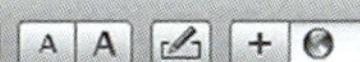

Doctor's Notes

Patient	Hibiki Hayashi 75 years M
PMH	Hypertension
Medications	Ramipril 5 mg once daily Bendroflumethazide 2.5 mg once daily Atorvastatin 20 mg daily
Allergies	NKDA
Consultations	3 days ago with advanced nurse practitioner: 'Getting chest pains. Pulse 69 regular. BP 132/78. Heart sounds normal. Check bloods and ECG'
Investigations	FBC, U&E, LFT, HbA1c, cholesterol and lipids – all normal. Resting 12-lead ECG normal
Household	No household members registered

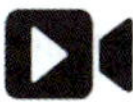

Example Consultation

Open ☐ Tell me about this pain, perhaps from when it first began.

ICE 1 ☐ When you get pain, what has gone through your mind? What do you think is causing it?

History ☐ Please tell me how often you experience this pain. Have you noticed anything that brings it on? What, if anything, takes it away? Any other symptoms with the pain? I was wondering about shortness of breath. Nausea or sweating?

Flags ☐ How long does the pain last? Have you ever had pain lasting more than 10 minutes? Any pain when you are sitting or lying down? Is this pain becoming more frequent?

Impact ☐ Has it stopped you from doing anything?

ICE2 ☐ Please tell me about any specific worries you had about this pain.

Risk ☐ Apart from high BP, any other medical problems? Has anyone in your family had heart problems or a stroke? Do you smoke? Any lower leg pain when walking?

Sense ☐ You seem really quiet - I'm wondering if you might perhaps be very worried?

Curious ☐ I'm sorry to hear you lost Maho and Hisae. That must have been devastating. You sound low just now. Sometimes when people feel so low, they don't want to be alive. I'm wondering if you have felt that? It's a very sensitive question, but may I ask if you have had thoughts about ending your life?

ICE3 ☐ Did you have thoughts about what we should do about this pain?

SummarICE ☐ So you have been feeling lonely and, since Maho died, you have had chest pains which you thought may be a heart attack. You thought I might say you need an operation, but you don't want this. Is that right? Is there anything else you would like to add?

Empathy ☐ The past 2 years have been life-changing for you.

Impression ☐ Mr Hayashi, I think this may be angina. I don't think it's a heart attack because the pain goes away when you stop moving. Your mood seems low; this is not uncommon, as angina can significantly affect a person's daily life.

Experience ☐ Have you come across angina? Do you know anyone with it?

Explanation ☐ Angina is where the blood flow to the heart is reduced due to furring of the vessels – like clogged drains. In a heart attack, the pipe becomes completely blocked.

Recommend ☐ I can make some recommendations to help your symptoms and protect your heart.

Options ☐ May I give you a spray to use, once under the tongue, if you have pain? It's quickly absorbed and widens your heart vessels. If pain is still there after 5 minutes, take a second spray. If you feel unwell or still have pain 5 minutes later, call 999. If you have a headache or feel dizzy, sit quietly for a few minutes. Please also use this spray before exercise. Are you happy to try it? We should consider aspirin to thin your blood to help blood flow through the vessels. Any tummy ulcers, because aspirin can make stomach problems worse? We should also start bisoprolol to slow the heart and prevent pain on walking. If it makes you feel tired or lightheaded, let me know. May I prescribe all three medications? May I send you to our chest pain clinic? You will be seen within a fortnight to confirm the diagnosis. Any concerns from what I've said? I will write it down, as there is a lot to remember.

InCLudE ☐ Yes, you can drive, unless pain occurs during driving, in which case stop driving until the angina is controlled.

Empower ☐ You've mentioned getting another dog to go for walks and for company. When your angina is under control, this would be an excellent idea to help both your mood and heart.

Future ☐ Have you ever wondered about stopping smoking? We can help you with this. Have a think about whether you might be interested in talking to someone about your loss and if information on community groups would be of interest.

Specifics ☐ I'll make you a double appointment with me in 2 weeks so we can talk more about your angina and your mood and I can answer any questions you may have. Is that okay?

Safety net ☐ If the pain becomes more frequent or occurs after a shorter distance let a GP know immediately. If pain occurs at rest or has been present for 10 minutes, call 999.

Patient's Story

Angina

Doctor's notes Hibiki Hayashi, 70 years, M. PMH: hypertension.

Medications: ramipril 5 mg daily, bendroflumethiazide 2.5 mg daily, atorvastatin 20 mg daily. NKDA. Last BP 132/78. Seen ANP last week: chest pains. Bloods and ECG normal.

How to act You are subdued.

PC *'Doctor, I keep getting these chest pains.'*

History It started 3 months ago when you were walking to get the paper. Since then, it has happened a few times a week, usually after about 500 m, particularly if you are in a hurry. The pain makes you stop. The pain is then gone after about 2 minutes.

You have not had pain before this distance and no rest pain. The pain is in the centre of your chest and feels very heavy. There is no radiation. There are no associated cardiac symptoms. You have not felt the pain after eating, only when walking.

No claudication pain.

You take two tablets for BP and a cholesterol tablet because your doctor said it was a good idea. You have no FH.

You saw the nurse practitioner 3 days ago who examined you, did an ECG and organised some blood tests and said you should see the GP.

Social You are a retired engineer and live in a bungalow having moved from Japan 40 years ago. Your wife, Hisae, died 2 years ago. Since then, your dog, Maho, kept you going and you used to walk her 2 miles a day but she died 4 months ago. Perhaps you will get another dog, but you aren't sure. These days, you feel very lonely and low and have stopped going to get the paper. Indeed you hardly go out at all anymore and don't see anybody. Your only son lives 2 hours' drive away. You have not had pain when at home. You smoke 20/day. You do not drink alcohol.

ICE You are not worried about the pain and think you have probably had a heart attack. You don't want to die and have had no thoughts about ending your life, but you do sometimes think it would be nice to be with Hisae and Maho. You expect the doctor will tell you that you need an operation, but you don't want this and would refuse it. You believe angina is a small heart attack.

Ask the doctor *'Am I allowed to drive?'*

Learning Points

Angina[1–4]

Refer to full NICE Guideline CG126[1] and NICE CKS guideline *Angina*.[3]

Prevalence 3.05% men and 1.79% women experience angina. Increased age = increased incidence.

Demographics of risk: South Asian > European > Afro-Caribbean origin.

Investigations ECG. Abnormal ECG makes diagnosis of coronary artery disease more likely but does not confirm that chest pain is stable angina.

FBC for anaemia. U&E, fasting blood glucose (if no diagnosis of diabetes), LFT, TFT.[3]

Referral To confirm diagnosis – refer to specialist chest pain service. Re-refer if symptomatic despite medical therapy.

Classification **Stable angina** –may be **typical** (all of the following features) or **atypical** (two of the following features) of:

- Constricting pain.
- Precipitated by exertion.
- Relieved by rest or GTN.

Unstable angina – deterioration or angina at rest. Requires immediate admission.[3]

Medications in angina GTN before exercise and during angina (unless taken Viagra).
Beta-blocker or CCB. If cannot tolerate one, switch to the other.

If both are contraindicated or not tolerated, consider monotherapy with:

- Long-acting nitrate (e.g. ISMN).
- Nicorandil.
- Ivabradine.
- Ranolazine.

Secondary prevention drugs Aspirin 75 mg OD. Continue clopidogrel if on this for another reason.
Statin.

ACEI if DM or other conditions, in line with NICE.[4]

Cardiac syndrome X Consider in ongoing symptoms and normal angiography. Continue anti-anginal if effective. No evidence of benefit with secondary prevention treatment.

Tip – you may be faced with a complex case in a simulated surgery, as well as in real life, when you may need to manage multiple problems. In this example we suggest completing a risk assessment for depression, then focusing on the chest pain and finally signposting the need to manage the low mood/depression at a later date. You are not expected to be able to fully manage multiple problems within the 12-minute consultation, but you must show that you can prioritise correctly and deal with the most pressing problems, with a clear plan about how and when to manage the others.

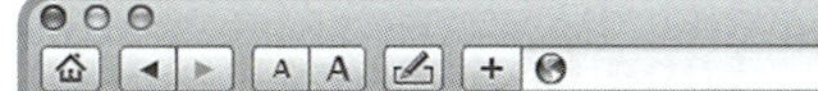

Doctor's Notes

Patient	Doris Ripley	76 years	F
PMH	Infective exacerbation of COPD		
Medications	Anoro Ellipta inhaler OD		
	Salbutamol inhaler PRN		
Allergies	No information		
Consultations	2 weeks ago – chronic cough, sputum, sometimes containing streaks of blood. Feeling more SOB. Diagnosis: infective exacerbation of COPD. Management: antibiotics + steroids, will arrange CXR due to haemoptysis		
	1 week ago – still coughing with haemoptysis. Temperature 37.0°C. Sats 94%. HR 84 bpm, RR 16, BMI 18. Chest – examination clear. Abdo soft, non-tender, no mass		
Investigations	Chest X-ray result received today		
	'Coin lesion right upper lobe, suggestive of malignancy. Forwarded to lung MDT.'		
Household	Peter Ripley	78 years	M

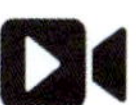

Example Consultation

Lung Cancer/End of Life

Open ☐ How can I help? That must be worrying; I'm sure together we can find the answers.

ICE1 ☐ What has been going through your mind?

Explanation ☐ Unfortunately the CXR has shown something unexpected. There is a shadow on your right lung. It is possible this is a patch of pneumonia but it could be something more serious. To better understand the CXR, it would be helpful to know a little more about you and the symptoms you have been having.

History ☐ Could tell me what led to the CXR being suggested? Can you tell me anything more about the cough? Have you had any chest pain? Any fever or sweats? Do you feel short of breath? Have you brought anything off your chest?

ICE2 ☐ What is your biggest fear?

Flags ☐ Have you coughed up any blood? Have you noticed any weight loss?

Impact ☐ How has the cough been affecting you? Has it stopped you from doing anything?

Risk ☐ Do you smoke or have you been a smoker in the past? Is there any family history of lung problems? What did you used to do for a living?

Experience ☐ Have you known anyone with similar chest problems? Or an abnormal CXR?

Curious ☐ That must have been a difficult time; how is Peter now?

ICE3 ☐ There are clearly questions which need answering, but were you hoping for anything specific today?

SummarICE ☐ So you have had a cough for about 12 weeks. You initially thought it was your COPD playing up but when you coughed up blood you were more worried. You are concerned that the usual antibiotics and steroids haven't worked this time. You've noticed yourself being more breathless and have experienced some weight loss. You've had a CXR and been told by the hospital you need to see a specialist. You'd like to know what this all means and what the next steps are. Is there anything else?

Impression ☐ Unfortunately, you have some worrying symptoms that suggest the shadow on your lung could be lung cancer. (Pause about 10 seconds.)

Empathy ☐ I'm sorry, this must be a shock; what's going through your mind?

Options ☐ Would you like to talk about what happens next? It's good news that you have an appointment with the lung specialist so soon. The sooner these things are investigated the better the chance of successful treatment. When you see the specialist, they will likely arrange a detailed scan of your body to get a better idea of the cause of the shadow. They may offer you a test to put a small flexible camera into your lung so a sample of any lump there can be taken. If it did turn out to be lung cancer, possible treatment options are surgery, radiotherapy or chemotherapy. What are your thoughts? I would like to arrange some blood tests to help the lung specialist decide which scans and possible treatments would be best. Is this okay?

Empower ☐ To help yourself, try to keep your strength up by eating regularly. There will be support groups and information you could access should it turn out to be bad news.

Future ☐ I would really like to talk to you again after your hospital appointment next week. May I book you an appointment here?

Specifics ☐ Please make an appointment for blood tests at reception. I will see you again on Tuesday, after your appointment with the lung specialist. If you have any more questions or problems please give me a call.

Safety net ☐ If you're unable to make your appointment, start feeling more poorly, particularly with fever or breathlessness, please call us straight away.

Patient's Story

Lung Cancer/End of Life

Doctor's notes Doris Ripley, 76 years. PMH: infective exacerbation of COPD. Medications: Anoro Ellipta inhaler OD, salbutamol PRN.

Consultations: 2 weeks ago – chronic cough, sputum, sometimes containing streaks of blood. Feeling more SOB. Diagnosis: infective exacerbation of COPD. Management: antibiotics + steroids, will arrange CXR due to haemoptysis.

1 week ago – still coughing with haemoptysis. Temperature 37.0°C. Sats 94%. HR 84 bpm, RR 16, BMI 18. Chest – examination clear. Abdo soft, non-tender, no mass.

Recent CXR results: 'coin lesion right upper lobe, suggestive of malignancy. Forwarded to lung MDT.'

How to act Upset. Push the doctor for the X-ray result. Be shocked if cancer is mentioned.

PC *'I've had a phone call from the hospital saying I need to see a specialist next week. What is going on?'*

History You visited the doctor 2 weeks ago with a cough which had been going on for 12 weeks. Initially you thought it was just your COPD, so you ignored it. However, when you started to notice blood in your spit you went to the doctor. The doctor was nice and said it was probably a chest infection, so you were given antibiotics and steroids, but wanted a CXR to be 'on the safe side'. You saw the doctor again last week and they examined you and said your temperature and oxygen levels were OK. They listened to your lungs and examined your abdomen and said both were fine. Yesterday you received a phone call from the hospital stating your CXR was abnormal and you had been booked into an urgent suspected cancer appointment next week. You don't know what this means and are worried. You don't feel much better after the antibiotics and steroids. You are still short of breath and occasionally see blood when you cough. You have had some right-sided chest pain, sharp in nature. You have noticed a 2-stone weight loss over the last few months but put this down to lack of appetite. No fevers or night sweats. No foreign travel. The cough has been keeping you awake at night and the breathlessness has made your weekly shop more difficult. You are able to get yourself dressed without being too breathless but have to walk slower than you used to due to shortness of breath.

Social You live with your husband. He is reasonably fit and well. You have two children but they are grown up and live in a different part of the country – 200 miles away. You are an ex-smoker – you gave up 6 years ago, previously smoking 20 a day since you were 15. You don't drink alcohol. You are a retired seamstress.

ICE You presume the CXR was looking for pneumonia so are worried why there is a fuss. You were given antibiotics anyway.

'Is it pneumonia? Should the antibiotics have cleared it?'

Your husband Peter had pneumonia a few years back and was quite poorly. You expect the doctor to explain the CXR results. You would like the doctor to explain why you have been referred to the hospital and what is likely to happen when you get there.

'A coin lesion refers to a round or oval, well-circumscribed solitary pulmonary lesion. It is usually 1–5 cm in diameter and calcification may or may not be present. Typically but not always the patient is asymptomatic.'[1]

Causes of coin lesions[1]

- Malignancy: primary lung tumour or metastases.
- Infections: pneumonia, TB, abscess, hydatid cyst.
- Benign disease: granuloma (e.g. sarcoidosis), rheumatoid nodule, AV malformation.

Lung cancer: Urgent suspected cancer referral criteria[2,3]

Refer people using a suspected cancer pathway referral for lung cancer if they:

- Have CXR findings that suggest lung cancer. Or
- Are aged >40 with unexplained haemoptysis.

Offer an urgent CXR (to be performed within 2 weeks)[3] to assess for lung cancer in people aged 40 and over if they have two or more of the following unexplained symptoms, or if they have ever smoked and have one or more of the following unexplained symptoms:

- Cough.
- Fatigue.
- Shortness of breath.
- Chest pain.
- Weight loss.
- Appetite loss.

Consider an urgent CXR (to be performed within 2 weeks)[3] to assess for lung cancer in people aged 40 and over with any of the following:

- Persistent or recurrent chest infection.
- Finger clubbing.
- Supraclavicular lymphadenopathy or persistent cervical lymphadenopathy.
- Chest signs consistent with lung cancer.
- Thrombocytosis.

'Unexplained' is defined as symptoms or signs that have not led to a diagnosis being made by the healthcare professional in primary care after initial assessment (including history, examination and any primary care investigations).

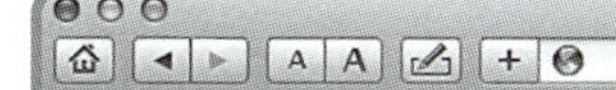

Doctor's Notes

Patient	Maggie Freestone 72 years F
PMH	Bereavement. Death of husband 2 years ago
	2 × NVD
	Gastritis
	Miscarriage
Medications	No current medications
Allergies	No information
Consultations	Saw consultant neurologist last week. Letter reads:

'Dear Doctor,

Thank you for referring this 72-year-old lady with symptoms of numbness in both feet, present for about 12 months. She has no relevant past medical history, family history or drug history. Full clinical and neurological examination revealed sensory loss in both feet and ankles, normal motor function.

Her blood results – FBC, U&E, LFT, B12, folate, TFT, cholesterol, vasculitis screen, antibody test, infection screen, immunoglobulins – were all normal. MRI head and spine normal. Nerve conduction studies confirm peripheral neuropathy. In the absence of any identifiable underlying cause I have given her a diagnosis of idiopathic peripheral neuropathy and have advised her to see you for further advice. I have discharged her from my clinic.

Signed,

Consultant Neurologist'

Investigations	As above. Urine dipstick normal
Household	No household members registered

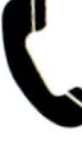

Example Consultation

Peripheral Neuropathy

Open ☐ Yes of course, I'm sure I can help with that. But first please can you tell me about this problem from the beginning. Then what did you notice? Anything else that isn't right?

Curious ☐ When you say you don't trust your feet, what do you mean?

Sense ☐ I can see you are a positive person, but I'm worried how this is affecting you.

Impact ☐ Has this changed how you live or your behaviour? Or your mood?

ICE1 ☐ What do you think has caused this? What has been on your mind?

History ☐ What does it feel like? Any other symptoms? I'm sorry that I am not aware, but what caused your husband's death? How are you getting on without him? Who else is in your life?

Flags ☐ How are you on the stairs or rising from a chair? Any weight loss? Is it painful?

ICE2 ☐ Please tell me what worries you most about this.

Risk ☐ Have you fallen at all? How confident do you feel going out? Do you drive?

Experience ☐ Have you known anyone who has had a similar problem?

ICE3 ☐ Other than explaining this diagnosis, was there anything else you thought we might do today?

SummarICE ☐ To summarise, your feet have been gradually becoming more numb over the last year. This has stopped you cycling and you have fallen. You have worried about what may have caused this and so has your son. You sometimes have pain in your feet too. The hospital doctor said you had peripheral neuropathy but didn't explain this. Have I understood?

Empathy ☐ I imagine it knocks your confidence when you can't trust your feet, especially after a fall.

Impression ☐ Let's discuss idiopathic peripheral neuropathy and the problems it can cause.

Explanation ☐ Peripheral means the parts of us furthest from the heart, and neuropathy means a problem with the nerve. When working well, our peripheral nerves transmit instructions from our brain to our muscles, skin and everywhere else, and then back again. So peripheral neuropathy means that there is a problem with this communication between the nerves and brain. Unfortunately, this describes the problem but doesn't tell us the cause. We know that it is more common in older people and is linked with some illnesses like a recent infection, diabetes, lack of vitamins and alcohol use, but you don't have any of these risks. Sometimes no cause is found, we term this idiopathic. Not knowing the cause can be difficult. Peripheral neuropathy doesn't always get worse with time, and most patients can adjust to manage with it. But you should take care; make sure you always wear something on your feet to prevent injury because you can't properly feel them.

InCludE ☐ You told me you've been worrying about this; hopefully understanding what is happening will help you feel less worried and more in control.

Recommend ☐ I'd like to arrange for our falls team to see you to help rebuild your confidence.

Options ☐ We can try different pain relief – would you like to hear about the options?

Empower ☐ What do you think would give you more confidence on your feet? Perhaps something to give you some support when walking? I could ask our health coaches to help you find a type of exercise you feel you can manage as you've had to stop cycling. Would you like to read more about peripheral neuropathy? I can give you a patient information leaflet that explains more about what it is, if that would be helpful. Would you be able to see a podiatrist/chiropodist now and then to help keep your feet healthy?

Future ☐ Perhaps we could catch up again after you've seen the falls team and exercise team? Please book a review in 6 weeks and bring any questions to that appointment.

Safety net ☐ If ever you notice weakness or new symptoms, or you fall, please contact a doctor promptly, as you would need to be examined again. I don't expect this, but, in particular, if you notice a change in your bladder or bowel control or new back pain or difficulty breathing, please let a doctor know straight away so we can make sure it is nothing serious.

Patient's Story

Peripheral Neuropathy

Doctor's notes Maggie Freestone, 72 years. PMH: bereavement. Death of husband 2 years ago. 2 × NVD. Miscarriage. Gastritis. Medications: none. Urine dipstick normal.

Saw consultant neurologist last week. Letter reads: 'Thank you for referring this 72-year-old lady with symptoms of numbness in both feet, present for about 12 months. She has no relevant past medical history, family history or drug history. Full clinical and neurological examination revealed sensory loss in both feet and ankles, normal motor function.

Her blood results – FBC, U&E, LFT, B12, folate, TFT, cholesterol, vasculitis screen, antibody test, infection screen, immunoglobulins were all normal. MRI head and spine normal. Nerve conduction studies confirm peripheral neuropathy. In the absence of any identifiable underlying cause I have given her a diagnosis of idiopathic peripheral neuropathy and have advised her to see you for further advice. I have discharged her from my clinic.'

How to act Chirpy and chatty.

PC *'Hello, Doctor. Well, the hospital doctor said I had peripheral neuropathy. Can you tell me what that means?'*

History You have always been very healthy with no other symptoms apart from your feet. About a year ago you started to notice your left foot felt a bit odd at times and then the right started about 6 months ago. Now both feet don't really feel normal most of the time, so you watch your feet as you walk. You have no symptoms of diabetes and don't drink alcohol or smoke. No medication. Your memory is good and you have never had a head injury. You have no back pain or bladder/bowel dysfunction. Your strength is good apart from when you can't feel what you are doing. You have no problems in the proximal muscles. How does it feel? Not like pins and needles but *'peculiar … like my feet have become sponge'*. You can still feel warm/hot water. No FH.

Last week you went to the hospital where they were very thorough and did lots of tests and told you that you had 'peripheral neuropathy' which they didn't explain. They said there was no cause and nothing they could do for you and discharged you. They sent you a letter after your appointment but you don't really understand what it means.

Social You miss Des, but you get on with life and love seeing people. Des died of prostate cancer which had spread to his bones and caused his kidneys to fail. You remain very active for the church, often raising money. Overall, you are very proud of how good you are for your age. Until last year, you were still riding your bike but then it became a problem. You miss exercising. You don't drive; there are good local buses and taxis you use if it's too far to walk.

'Now, I don't trust my feet.' Say this with laugh.

You live on your own. Your son visits frequently.

ICE You try to laugh this off; however, you have been lying awake wondering what this is. But you like to stay positive and you shrug it off when your children mention it. Your son is worried since you fell and banged your shoulder. He bought you a pendant alarm just in case you ever fall and you do wear this. The shoulder recovered but it did knock your confidence. Only if the doctor specifically asks you, you mention the burning pain the problem causes but you do not want any medicine for this.

Learning Points

Peripheral Neuropathy[1]

As well as sensory and motor symptoms, ask about features of autonomic dysfunction, which may include a change to the bowels, sweating, sphincter disturbance and postural hypotension.

Prevalence About 1 in 50 people have some form of peripheral neuropathy.[1]

Causes Diabetes or diabetic amyotrophy (most common cause in Europe).
Alcohol.
B12/folate deficiency.
Chronic kidney disease.
HIV.
Shingles.
Rheumatoid arthritis.
Lyme disease.
Sjögren's syndrome.
Amyloidosis.
Uraemia.
Guillain–Barré syndrome/chronic inflammatory demyelinating polyneuropathy (CIDP).
Porphyria.
Charcot–Marie–Tooth disease.
Malignancy or paraneoplastic syndrome.
Vasculitic neuropathy.
Side effects of chemotherapy including drugs used to treat HIV and more.

Ensure you are aware of how the rare conditions above may present.

Remember the Complete MRCGP motto: '**Common things are common … but what mustn't I miss?**'

Blood tests FBC, U&E, LFT, GGT, TFTs, CRP, ESR, ANA, B12, folate, serum and urine electrophoresis.
Urine dipstick for protein and glucose.

Other tests CXR – sarcoidosis, malignancy.
Consider – Lyme or HIV serology, urinary porphyrins and an autoimmune screen.
Nerve conduction studies will often support the diagnosis.
MRI scan may be needed to rule out other causes, e.g. spinal cord issues.

Red flags Always look out for cauda equina syndrome.

Management tends to focus on treating the underlying cause. However, you also need to consider the impact (e.g. falls) and the risk of tissue damage from reduced sensation. Foot ulcers and serious infections are more common in the presence of peripheral neuropathy. Drivers must inform the DVLA if they have a diagnosis of peripheral neuropathy.

CHAPTER 6

MENTAL HEALTH, INCLUDING ADDICTION, SMOKING, ALCOHOL AND SUBSTANCE MISUSE

	Cases in this chapter	RCGP 2025 curriculum	Learning points
6.1	Anxiety	**Mental health** 'Anxiety including generalised anxiety and panic disorders, phobias and situational anxiety'	Managing anxiety The 'Stepped care' model Diagram of CBT model
6.2	Depression Review	**Mental health** 'Mood (affective) problems such as depression, including features of a major depression such as psychotic and biological symptoms; cyclothymia and bipolar disorder. Self-harm, including putting themselves in dangerous situations as well as self-poisoning and cutting; suicidal ideation and behaviou'	Self-management NICE guidance on first-line treatment options Medication – how long to treat
6.3	Personality Disorder	**Mental health** 'Personality disorders including borderline, antisocial, narcissistic'	Personality disorder: • Identification • Management • Classification – different types
6.4	Postnatal Psychosis	**Mental health** **Maternity and reproductive health** 'Pregnancy-associated disorders such as antenatal, perinatal and postnatal anxiety and depression, puerperal psychosis'	Postnatal mental health: • Identification and diagnosis of depression and anxiety • Management of postnatal psychosis
6.5	Harmful Drinking	**Smoking, alcohol and substance misuse** 'Identify and offer interventions, including effective advice and treatment, to people who smoke or misuse alcohol or substances'	Harmful drinking: identification and management When to refer to the detox team DVLA considerations

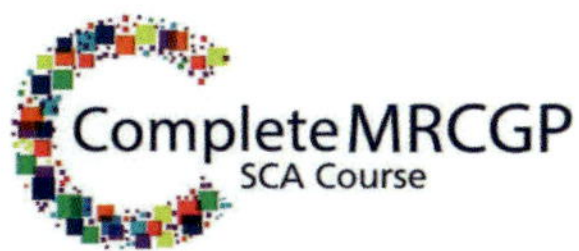

Links to the RCGP Curriculum

In this chapter, the cases are drawn from the following clinical topic guides:

- Mental health
- Maternity and reproductive health
- Smoking, alcohol and substance misuse

Life stages topic guides: all life stages

Scope of Conditions

Consider these examples of acute and chronic mental health conditions:

- Alcohol and substance misuse
- Psychoses or delusions
- Mood disorders, anxiety, phobias and obsessive compulsions
- Somatic disorders, stress, trauma or neurosis
- Behaviour or emotional disorders
- Learning difficulties
- Bereavement reactions
- Eating disorders
- Organic causes, e.g.
    - Delirium secondary to infection or medication
    - Secondary to other conditions such as Parkinson's or thyroid disorders
- Pregnancy and postpartum

Skills and Pitfalls

In addition to the information in Chapter 1 'How to Demonstrate Skills: The Marking Scheme Made Easy' consider the following challenges for this blueprint group:

- Full exploration, e.g. psychological, social and physical features, red flags and risk factors.
- Assessment of risk with a management plan that reflects the assessment and is safe.
- Show that you can diagnose and manage a mental health condition.
- Recognition and sensitive communication of the complexities of how the physical/psychological and social problems are connected or impact on the patient.
- Awareness of the health needs of the patient in full, avoiding diagnostic overshadowing (this means unintentionally neglecting the physical and other health problems of a patient with mental health issues, e.g. cardiovascular disease and diabetes risk), with a plan to address all in time.
- Communication with the patient to enable informed decision making where possible.
- Coordination of care with the wider team (e.g. CMHT) with an explanation of next steps.
- Continuity of care with general practice and a discussion of future plans.
- Demonstration of an adequate safety net with clear communication.
- If required, knowledge of the Mental Health Act and mental capacity.

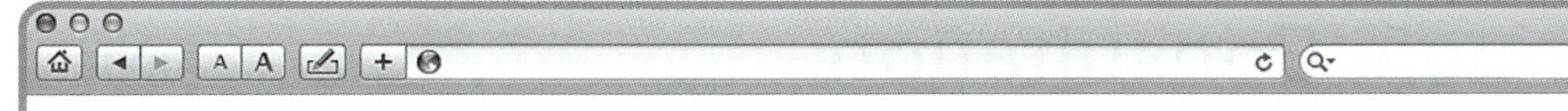

Doctor's Notes

Patient	Stephen Harper	42 years	M
PMH	Irritable bowel syndrome		
Medications	No current medications. Previous medications include mebeverine		
Allergies	No information		
Consultations	2 days ago: GP consultation		
	Intermittent bloating. No red flags. Abdomen examined – NAD, PR normal. 70 kg weight (no change). Impression IBS. Check bloods		
	2 weeks ago: A&E attendance with chest pain		
	Bloods and ECG all normal – reassured and discharged		
Investigations	FBC, U&E, LFT, TFTs, GGT, CRP, HbA1c, ESR and coeliac screen – all normal 2 days ago		
Household	Judith Harper	43 years	F
	Bridget Harper	15 years	F
	Aidan Harper	14 years	M

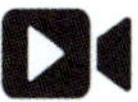

Example Consultation

Open ☐ Tell me more about your bowels? Anything else you've noticed? How do you feel?

ICE1 ☐ What do you think is wrong? Has any other diagnosis crossed your mind?

ICE2 ☐ When you think about your symptoms, what is your biggest fear?

Curious ☐ I'm interested to know what you mean by *'turning 40 … a mid-life crisis'*. Where has this has come from? Has a terminal illness happened to anyone you know?

Impact ☐ What triggers these thoughts? Does it make you feel unwell? Then what do you do?

History ☐ Any other problems in the past? Have you taken any medication? Did it work? As it's the first time we've spoken, please tell me more about you. How are things at home? Who is important in your life? Tell me about your work. How is it going? How do you relax?

Flags ☐ Any change in your bowels? Any bleeding? Any weight loss? Any pain? How do you sleep? Your appetite? Are you able to enjoy activities? How do you see the future?

Sense ☐ You seem quiet today; is there anything else on your mind?

Risk ☐ Any thoughts of hurting yourself or suicide? And alcohol? Any other drugs?

ICE3 ☐ What did you think we may decide today? Any other thoughts about this?

SummarICE ☐ You are worrying about your health, in particular the risk of bowel cancer and the possibility of dying from this or from a heart attack.

Impression ☐ I would like to reassure you that you have no worrying symptoms of bowel cancer. There is no weight loss, bleeding or change in your bowels and your blood tests were reassuring. I am a cautious doctor but am confident that you don't need a colonoscopy. I think anxiety is driving your symptoms and fears, causing panic attacks.

Experience ☐ Has anyone else you know suffered with anxiety? Do you know of ways to help?

Explanation ☐ Everyone has negative thoughts, but when these start to affect your life we need to recognise and address the triggers. Panic attacks occur when normal hormones in the body get released inappropriately. These reactions are normal when we are in danger but, when you have anxiety, they can occur when there isn't any danger.

InCludE ☐ Your symptoms of loose bowels, heart racing and breathlessness are physical responses to anxiety and panic, rather than a physical cause. There are some things that you can do to help; other things I can help with, and we may seek input from other health professionals too. Relaxation exercises may help. You could contact MIND about local support groups. I can help with suggestions, monitoring and prescribing if needed, but talking therapies can be just as powerful or more so. For example, a therapy called CBT teaches you tools to use when you feel anxious. Family, friends or therapists may also help. There are useful resources, including websites such as FearFighter.com and, on the Mindfulness website, a '3-minute breathing space' exercise. What do you feel might help you best?

Empathy ☐ Anxiety can have a huge impact on one's life. Let me show you a diagram that helps explain the therapy called CBT.* Let's take the example of someone who thinks they have a terminal illness. We would expect *emotional* and *physical* responses. These are natural. The *behaviour* response and initial *thought* is where the CBT can help, over time, gradually giving tools to step out of the circle. *See later in this section.

Empower ☐ Do any of these suggestions sound like they might work for you? Who else could help?

Future ☐ Recognising that your symptoms are due to anxiety can be helpful but if you feel you might benefit from counselling, I can give you the contact details.

Specifics ☐ You can self-refer by phone or online. Shall we catch up next month? You can prebook an appointment online. Phone me earlier if you need to.

Safety net ☐ If you feel your mood drops or you have new symptoms, for example your bowels change, you lose weight or you see blood in the stool, please tell a doctor.

Patient's Story

Doctor's notes Stephen Harper, 42 years. PMH: irritable bowel syndrome. Medications: no current medication; past medication: mebeverine.

GP consultation 2 days ago: intermittent bloating. No red flags. Abdomen examined – NAD, PR normal. Impression IBS. Check bloods.

A&E attendance 2 weeks ago with chest pain – discharge letter, tests all normal and reassured.

FBC, U&E, LFT, TFTs, GGT, CRP, HbA1c, ESR and coeliac screen all normal 2 days ago.

How to act Hesitant and quiet.

PC *'It's my bowels again, Doctor.'*

History You go to the toilet three times every morning. Your bowels are loose (not watery) but then they settle down. No other GI symptoms. No red flags – no weight loss, no bleeding and no change in bowels. You have seen previous doctors and *'they said it is irritable bowel'*.

You have been struggling with financial pressures.

Your children want to go to university.

You have no thoughts of hurting yourself or anyone else.

You have no features of depression, only worry. You eat and sleep okay.

Social You work at an electronics store. At work, your concentration is good. You exercise to keep healthy. Your parents are elderly, which upsets you. Your relationship with your wife is good. She knows you worry. Children aged 15 and 14. You do not drink much alcohol. No drugs.

ICE Deep down you think this must be due to stress.

You often have anxious thoughts when alone and especially on waking. Thoughts include financial worry and waiting to be told you have a life-limiting illness. Lots of things remind you of this: adverts and articles. You think about death a lot and it frightens you. It can make you cry.

Your chest can become tight, you feel sweaty and can feel breathless. You recently had an episode of chest pain which frightened you, so you went to A&E and were told it was muscular. You had a mild pain in your lower chest which had no features of cardiac, gastric or respiratory disease. You accepted this but you fear you have bowel cancer, perhaps near the top of the tummy because of the recent chest pain.

If the doctor senses you are quiet say: *'Well, you get to 40.'*

If asked what you meant, you say: *'A mid-life crisis.'* If asked about it further, tell the doctor *'You hear of people going to the doctor and 6 weeks later they are dead.'*

No one you know has had this happen.

You don't know what to do but wondered if you should have a colonoscopy.

You do not want medication at this time. You expect the doctor will restart your mebeverine but you know it doesn't help. You would follow any guidance from the doctor.

Open questions help the real problem to surface. Red flags steer diagnosis. Risk assessments guide management. **'Has anything else crossed your mind?'** was useful here to avoid missing his multiple ICE. There were no red flags for lower GI symptoms, but this fear needed to be acknowledged and resolved.

NICE guidance – the stepped care model for the management of generalised anxiety[1]

Step 1 'Identification and assessment; education about GAD and treatment options; active monitoring.'[1]

Step 2 'Low-intensity psychological interventions: individual non-facilitated self-help, individual guided self-help and psychoeducational groups.'[1]

Step 3 'High-intensity psychological intervention (CBT/applied relaxation) or a drug treatment.'[1]

SSRIs. Side effects: upset stomach and may increase anxiety initially.

Propranolol may be required in addition. Consider contraindications, e.g. asthma.

Alternative drug treatments: SNRI and pregabalin.

Benzodiazepines may be used for crisis management only.

Step 4 'Highly specialist treatment, such as complex drug and/or psychological treatment regimens; input from multi-agency teams, crisis services, day hospitals or inpatient care.'[1]

A simplified version of the CBT model adapted from Williams[2] and Williams and Garland[3] can be used in whole or in part even in a normal length consultation after excluding red flags for the physical causes. This model helps patients to visualise why their physical symptoms are linked to their anxiety and not a sign of something sinister. It is also a great way of summarising and demonstrating you have listened.

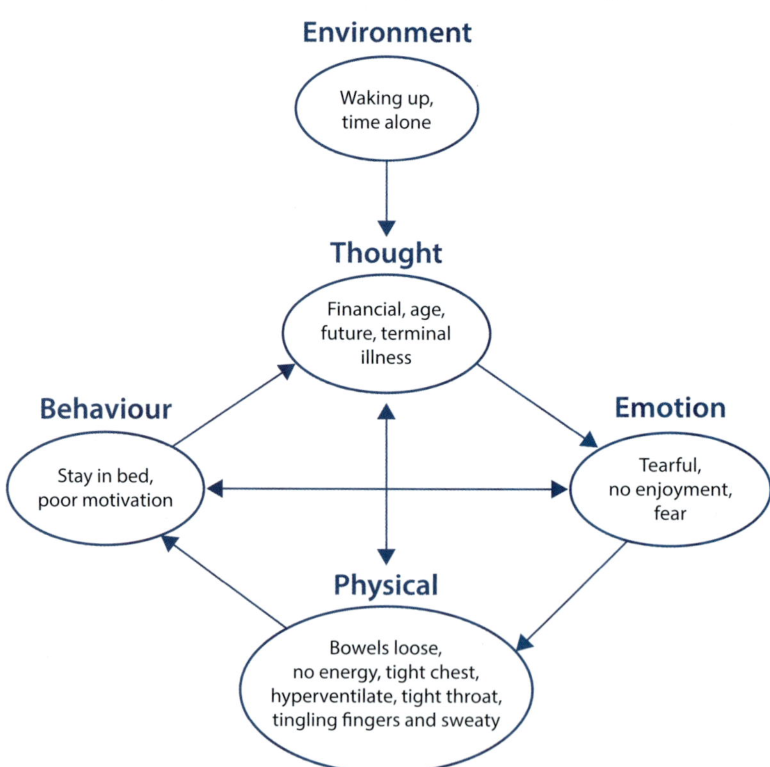

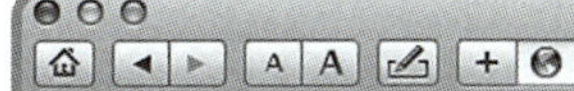

Doctor's Notes

Patient Jessica Miller 24 years F

PMH Depression diagnosed 3 months ago

Medications Sertraline 50 mg daily

Allergies No information

Consultations No recent consultations

Investigations No recent investigation

Household No household members registered

Example Consultation

Depression Review

Open ☐ Thank you for phoning. How have you been since starting the sertraline?

Sense ☐ You seem very quiet today.

ICE1 ☐ What has been going through your mind?

History ☐ Please take me back to the beginning. When do you think you started to feel this way? What was happening in your life at the time? How is the job going? I'm sorry to hear that. Please tell me about your family. Are you close to them? Can you confide in anyone? Do you live with anyone? Have you felt this way before? Tell me what happened then. What helped? Have you been able to take the sertraline regularly, each day? Any side effects?

Curious ☐ What does your mum think? What have you told her? What haven't you told her? Are people at work aware? Do you have any difficult thoughts? Or thoughts you cannot explain?

ICE2 ☐ What worries you about this?

Flags ☐ How do you sleep? Do you use an alarm? Do you enjoy activities? How is your concentration? How do you picture the future? Are you eating? Any thoughts of not wanting to be alive? Have you ever hurt yourself or someone else? Do you think you might? Who would you tell if these thoughts became stronger? How much alcohol do you drink? Do you take any drugs?

Impact ☐ How do you spend your days? And what about when you are not at work?

SummarICE ☐ So to summarise, you have been feeling this way for 6 months now, impacting on your energy levels. You have had upsetting thoughts of how you could end your life but have made no plans to do this as you do not want to upset your mum. You started sertraline 3 months ago and don't feel any different at all. You are wondering if they are working and whether we should change them. Work has been tough lately.

ICE3 ☐ I already have a number of thoughts about what we could do, but is there anything particular you were hoping I might suggest or do today?

Impression ☐ I wonder if we should increase the dose of tablets? Sertraline is an effective drug for depression but takes time to work and often a higher dose than 50 mg is needed.

Experience ☐ Do you know anything about the causes of depression?

Explanation ☐ These include new life challenges or a chemical imbalance in the brain. Sertraline helps but it takes time and you need to keep taking them: 50 mg is a good starting dose but I recommend that we now increase that to 100 mg daily. How do you feel about that?

Empathy ☐ It is very hard to move away from those you love for both you and your mum.

Options ☐ Depression makes it harder to look after yourself and perform well at work. It sounds as if your mum would like you to go home; have you considered this? That sounds sensible to me but what do you think? Going home may provide time to decide what to do longer term. For depression there are things that I can help with, for example increasing medication and a work note for 4 weeks. Others – your parents or counsellors – can provide support. How do you feel about talking to a counsellor? Whilst off work, some things that may help your wellbeing are getting more exercise and eating well; how might you spend this time?

Empower ☐ What sort of exercise appeals? Could anyone else help – perhaps an exercise buddy?

Future ☐ Can we catch up in a couple of weeks? Would you like me to talk with your mum? We need to make sure you are safe and so if your mum is aware of what thoughts you have had she can help you … would it be okay if I explained to her what you have told me?

Specifics ☐ If you decide to stay with your mum, can you book another telephone appointment to let me know so we can discuss the ongoing plan? Avoid alcohol as it lowers mood.

Safety net ☐ If you feel your mood is dropping or you have thoughts of hurting yourself, call a GP, me if available or the on-call GP. Out of hours, phone 111 or the Samaritans. You could even go to A&E. I'll send you the contact numbers by text so you have them to hand.

Patient's Story

Depression Review

Doctor's notes	Jessica Miller, 24 years. PMH: depression diagnosed 3 months ago. Medications: sertraline 50 mg daily.
How to act	Quite short sentences. Your depression makes it hard work for the doctor to retrieve information from you. Often initially answering, *'I don't know.'*
PC	After a pause … *'I don't know what's wrong with me. The tablets aren't working.'*
History	You started to feel this way when you moved for your job about 6 months ago. No physical symptoms but you have no energy. No psychotic features. You experience anhedonia and hopelessness. You felt like this in the past, whilst doing your GCSEs, and were seen by the school counsellor – you found this helpful. You saw the GP 3 months ago and were started on sertraline. You have been taking the tablets regularly and not missed any. No side effects from the tablets. You are struggling at work and making mistakes. You have no features of psychosis.
Risk	You have had occasional thoughts of not wanting to be alive. You sometimes think it would be good if you didn't wake up in the morning. You drink some alcohol – if asked, up to 7 units per week: a small glass of wine each day. You take no drugs. No thoughts of hurting others. Never self-harmed. You have never made a plan to harm yourself, though you have had thoughts of self-harm including jumping off a bridge or taking an overdose. If the doctor asks whether you intend to do this say, *'I don't believe I would'* and if they ask if you would tell someone say, *'Yes but I won't do that'.*
Protective factor	You are very close to your mum and you would hate to upset her by committing suicide.
Social	You work in marketing. You have been late for work as you struggle to get out of bed, despite being awake since 4–5 a.m. Your boss is nice and told you to talk to the GP. You have fallen out with your flatmates over bills. You moved here for work 6 months ago. You are eating less and can't even think about cooking. You spend your days in your room watching TV and don't see your friends. You have no hobbies. You do not exercise. Your parents live 4 hours away and you confide in your mum on the phone every night – she is worried about you.
ICE	You are not sure why you feel like this. You are not worried about anything. You don't know what to expect today. You accept a work note and a prescription for an increased dose of antidepressants. You will go on walks with your mum. You will also see your local vicar. If offered, accept a referral to counselling services. You give consent for the GP to speak with your mum if the GP offers this.

Recommend a few suggestions tailored to their needs and capacity. Provide a list of the suggestions and contact numbers for organisations. You may have a collection of books you can recommend. Structure your management plan: you can do (self-help), I, the GP can do, what others can do and other resources. For example:

> *'What you can do: a healthy sleep and meal regime to give you energy, avoiding alcohol which lowers mood, and exercising every day should help to make you feel better. I can help with providing suggestions, monitoring and prescribing medication if needed. Other people who can help may include family, friends or professionals. You could contact MIND who will advise on local support groups. I suggest arranging counselling if you feel there are emotions or experiences you want to talk about. There are other useful resources: websites such as MoodGym or Mindfulness. There are helpful books also, such as* Living in the Moment *by Anna Black, which includes very useful mindfulness meditations.[1] I have a list of all of these suggestions and here are the contact numbers.'*

NICE guidelines on discussing first-line treatments for less severe depression[2]

- Discuss options and match treatment to clinical need and preferences.
- Consider the least intrusive and least resource-intensive treatment first.
- If the person has a clear preference based on previous treatment, support their choice if possible.
- Don't routinely offer antidepressants first, unless this is the person's choice.

NICE suggestions in order of recommended use, based on cost, clinical and cost effectiveness, and implementation factors

- Guided self-help.
- Group CBT.
- Group behavioural activation.
- Individual CBT.
- Individual behavioural activation.
- Group exercise.
- Group mindfulness and meditation.
- Interpersonal psychotherapy.
- SSRI antidepressants.
- Counselling.
- Short-term psychodynamic psychotherapy.

Duration of treatment of medication therapy

First episode of depression: continue for 6 months after the depression has improved.

Second episode: continue for at least 2 years.[2]

Combining drug medication in the patient resistant to first-line therapy needs careful consideration and 'should only normally be started in primary care in consultation with a consultant psychiatrist'.[2]

Be aware of:

Serotonin syndrome – see https://patient.info/doctor/serotonin-syndrome.

Malignant neuroleptic syndrome – see https://patient.info/doctor/neuroleptic-malignant-syndrome.

Doctor's Notes

Patient Andrea Lockwood 36 years F

PMH

15 years old – under Child and Adolescent Mental Health Services for depression

17–20 years old – under secondary care for major depression and self-harm. Discharged by mental health services for repeated failure to attend

Mid-20s – managed by GP for moderate depression and superficial wrist cutting

Overdose of paracetamol aged 27 years, seen by crisis team and discharged

Termination of pregnancy 29 years old, referred to counselling team. Disclosed a history of sexual abuse as a child (by stepfather), declined to inform police

Further episode of severe depression in early 30s, suicidal ideation but not attempts, wrist cutting, referred to secondary care but repeatedly failed to attend appointment. Discharged back to primary care

Medications Sertraline 50 mg daily

Several courses of antidepressants in the past including fluoxetine, sertraline, mirtazapine

Allergies No information

Consultations GP appointment 4 weeks ago:

'Becoming depressed again, feeling low. Not sleeping or eating well. Got into trouble at work. Only had the job for 4 weeks when got into an argument with a colleague, resulting in her quitting the job on the spur of the moment. Feels colleague was out to get her. Worried about money. Lives alone, no local family. Finds it hard to keep friends, says no close friends. Has a nice neighbour who looks in on her occasionally. Having fleeting thoughts of suicide, no plans or attempts. Has been cutting wrists again, superficial wrist wounds seen'

Plan: restart sertraline, TCI 3–4 weeks for review. Crisis team number given to patient and worsening advice given

Investigations No information

Household No household contacts

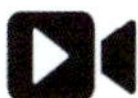

Example Consultation

Open ☐ I'm sorry to hear that. Can you tell me a bit more about how you feel? Can you explain what upsets you? Can you share more about your mental health over the years? That sounds really tough (pause). What other thoughts have you had?

Impact ☐ Has the way you are feeling caused you any difficulties in life recently?

ICE1 ☐ Do you have any thoughts about what could be causing all these problems for you?

History ☐ I'm sorry you are feeling so low. How do you sleep? And eat? Do you get out and enjoy yourself? I can see you've previously had mood problems. Tell me what contact you've had with health professionals. Does your mood affect your relationships? Who is in your life? How do you get on? Has anyone in the family had mood problems? Have you ever been in trouble with the police? Do you drink alcohol? Or smoke? Have you ever taken illegal drugs? Do you ever act impulsively? Has this had any bad consequences for you? Do you ever feel paranoid, as if people are watching you or out to get you? Do you ever hear or see things which other people cannot?

ICE2 ☐ Are you worried about anything specific?

Flags ☐ Last time, you said you had been harming yourself; is this still the case? How often? Can you tell me what drives you to cut yourself? Does it make you feel better afterwards? Have you ever felt so bad that you have wanted to end your life? Have you made plans to end your life? What would stop you from ending your life? Do you know where you can get help if you do feel suicidal?

Sense ☐ I sense that life can be very complex for you at times; would you agree?

ICE3 ☐ Was there anything specific you wanted today, or hoped we would achieve?

SummarICE ☐ You've had mood problems since you were a teenager, perhaps due to the abuse you experienced as a child. You've seen lots of different doctors, without much success. It's difficult to maintain relationships and you sometimes act on impulse without thinking of the consequences. Cutting yourself releases tension and makes you feel better. You sometimes think it would be better if you weren't around but haven't recently made plans to end your life. You would like help and for a medical team to stick with you. Anything I've missed or you would like to add?

Explanation ☐ You're clearly experiencing depression, Andrea, but I wonder if the problem runs a little deeper and if there may be another explanation as to why you have had such complex issues in your life. I wonder if you may have a personality disorder. Have you heard of this? Personality means a set of qualities that control how we think, feel and behave. Our personalities develop partly due to our genes but also due to our experiences and upbringing. In some people, personality develops in such a way that it causes them great difficulties in life. These difficulties can be mood, relationships or behaviour, such as committing crimes. Do you think this could be the case for you?

Recommend ☐ May I refer you to our complex needs team to assess you to see if you may have a personality disorder? If so, they can help by providing a community mental health nurse to visit. They may also offer a support worker and can help you access talking therapies. Sometimes medication, such as sertraline, can also help but I would like to be guided by their expertise. Is that okay?

Empathy ☐ I realise this is a lot to take in and may be a bit scary; how do you feel about it?

Future ☐ Let's continue the sertraline for now as it's helping and I will do the referral.

Specifics ☐ Can I talk to you again in 3 weeks? Please book online or by phoning reception.

Safety net ☐ If you are worsening in the meantime, please let me know. If you feel suicidal you can phone the Samaritans, but if you feel in danger call the crisis team. Thanks for talking to me today.

Patient's Story

Personality Disorder

Doctor's notes Andrea Lockwood, 36 years.

PMH: 15 years old – under Child and Adolescent Mental Health Services for depression. 17–20 years old – under secondary care for major depression and self-harm; discharged by mental health services for repeated failure to attend. Mid-20s – managed by GP for moderate depression and superficial wrist cutting. Overdose of paracetamol aged 27 years, seen by crisis team and discharged. Termination of pregnancy 29 years old, referred to counselling team. Disclosed a history of sexual abuse as a child (by stepfather), declined to inform police. Further episode of severe depression in early 30s, suicidal ideation but not attempts, wrist cutting, referred to secondary care but repeatedly failed to attend appointment. Discharged back to primary care.

Medications: sertraline 50 mg daily. Past medication: fluoxetine, sertraline, mirtazapine.

GP appointment 4 weeks ago: 'Becoming depressed again, feeling low. Not sleeping or eating well. Got into trouble at work. Only had job for 4 weeks when got into an argument with a colleague, resulting in her quitting the job on the spur of the moment. Feels colleague was out to get her. Worried about money. Lives alone, no local family. Finds it hard to keep friends, says no close friends. Has a nice neighbour who looks in on her occasionally. Having fleeting thoughts of suicide, no plans or attempts. Has been cutting wrists again, superficial wrist wounds seen.'

Plan: restart sertraline, TCI 3–4 weeks for review. Crisis team number given to patient and worsening advice given.

How to act Low.

PC *'So, things aren't much better, Doctor.'*

History You had a tough start in life as your natural father was an alcoholic so home life was chaotic. He died following an alcohol-related accident. Your mother was devastated but over time came to terms with this. She experienced anxiety and depression and was once hospitalised. She met a new partner whom you disliked. You told a counsellor that your stepfather abused you when you were 13 years old but you do not want to go to the police about this now. He and your mother are now separated and you no longer see him. Your relationship with your mother is variable. It's good at the moment. Over the years you have seen many health professionals about low mood. They never help you. You have repeatedly self-harmed and on one occasion took a paracetamol overdose, although you didn't really intend to die.

You easily make friends but often the friendships fail due to arguments; you feel that your friends don't really care about you. You have had different jobs but none for more than a few months. You will spend money that you don't have and react to situations without thinking of the consequences. You can be impulsive. You were arrested for shoplifting but let off with a caution. At present, you feel low and worthless. Cutting your wrists gives you a sense of relief. You have had thoughts that it would be better if you weren't alive but have no plans to end your life. The sertraline has helped a little. You have no symptoms of psychosis. You want your life to get better and feel you need help from people who *'won't let me down'*. Doctors always give you a tablet, then pass you on to someone else. You would like continuity of care. You call the Samaritans regularly. This helps to release anger if you don't want to cut yourself.

Social Currently unemployed, given a 'Med 3 fit note' at last GP appointment. Occasional alcohol. Smoke 15 cigarettes/day. No illicit drug use. Live alone, rented flat.

ICE You think you are depressed. You would like to continue sertraline. You are open to the idea of seeing a specialist if the doctor suggests this.

Personality Disorder

Personality disorders can be quite difficult to identify but be suspicious in patients with repeating patterns of behaviour, such as self-harm, emotional instability, criminal activity and problems maintaining relationships or difficulties functioning in day-to-day life (unable to keeps jobs, etc.). Personality disorders are thought to develop due to a combination of genetic factors and 'nurture' factors (early life experiences, abuse). Our personalities have normally formed between our mid-teens and early 20s. Although our personalities cannot be changed (hence personality disorders are often labelled untreatable), intervention can help patients cope with their difficulties and enable them to function better and have a more stable and fulfilling life. NICE recommends a structured approach to assessment and management. Psychotherapy can be effective and drug therapy may help in some cases (e.g. antidepressants to treat depressive symptoms). Antipsychotics or sedatives can be used for short-term crisis management but are not advised long term.[1–3]

In 2022, the guidelines for diagnosing personality disorder changed and UK doctors are now more likely to talk about categories and traits, but some may still use the different categories of personality disorder and their typical features summarised below (*source:* https://www.mind.org.uk/information-support/types-of-mental-health-problems/personality-disorders/types-of-personality-disorder/).

Paranoid	Find it hard to confide and difficult to trust others. See threats and dangers that others do not.
Schizoid	Emotionally cold, prefer being alone. Little interest in sex or intimacy.
Schizotypal	Eccentric behaviour, distorted thoughts, may feel anxious or paranoid. Hard to make and maintain relationships.
Antisocial	Lack of empathy, easily frustrated, easily bored and impulsive, aggressive, criminal activity or conduct disorder often <15 years old.
Borderline (emotionally unstable personality disorder)	Impulsive, hard to control emotions, features of depression/low mood/low self-worth, self-harm, difficulty maintaining relationships, may feel paranoid, can have auditory hallucinations.[3]
Histrionic	Over-dramatic, self-centred, suggestible, worry about appearance, look for excitement and new things, and can be seductive.
Narcissistic	Strong sense of self-importance; desire success, power and intellectual greatness; crave attention but don't reciprocate; take advantage of others and don't return favours.
Avoidant	Avoid work/activities that mean being with others. Anxious/tense, insecure, feel inferior, extremely sensitive to criticism.
Dependent	Low self-confidence, feel needy or weak, can't make decisions, submissive, difficulty coping with daily tasks, feel hopeless and abandoned.
Obsessive-compulsive	Worry, doubt, perfectionist, rigid routines, cautious and preoccupied with detail, difficulty adapting, judgemental, sensitive to criticism, obsessional thoughts.

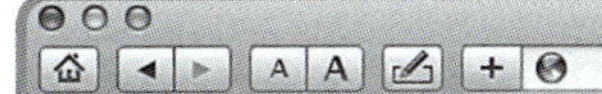

Doctor's Notes

Patient	Chloe Livingstone-Smith	28 years	F
PMH	Failed forceps delivery and emergency lower segment caesarean section 2 weeks ago		
Medications	None		
Allergies	None		
Consultations	Midwife visit at home yesterday: 'Baby doing well, no jaundice, yellow stool nappies. Regained birth weight. Forceps mark fading. Breastfeeding. Up 2-hourly in the night. Mum tired. Not been out, says worried baby will pick up an infection, made an odd comment about the government, seems a little tearful, suggested talks to GP, asked husband to make her an appointment tomorrow'		
Investigations	No information		
Household	Damian Smith	32 years	M
	James Smith	2 weeks	M

Example Consultation

Postnatal Psychosis

Open ☐ I see you had a baby 2 weeks ago, congratulations! Is James your baby's name? How has it been going? How are you? How is James? What has been the biggest challenge?

History ☐ How was your delivery? Is this your first child? How are you getting on with feeding? Is James sleeping well? Have you managed to get any rest? Who's at home? What support are you getting?

Sense ☐ You said that you couldn't talk for long; what is making you feel the need to rush?

ICE1 ☐ What do you think is happening to you?

Flags ☐ Have you felt sad or worried since James was born? Why do you think he may be getting an infection? What makes you think the government wants to take him away? Is the government speaking to you or sending you messages? Do you ever hear or see things which other people cannot? Have you ever had thoughts about harming James or yourself?

ICE2 ☐ Do you worry that the government can hear your thoughts or interfere with your thoughts?

Risk ☐ Any mood problems before? In the family, has any mum had mood problems after childbirth?

ICE3 ☐ Have you any thoughts about what you would like to happen? You are clearly worried that James may become ill and that the government may take him away; would you like my help with this?

Experience ☐ Have you known anyone who has become unwell with their mood after childbirth?

Curious ☐ What does your husband think? Is he worried about you or James?

SummarICE ☐ So you had your baby, James, 2 weeks ago. You had a tough time but recovered well. But now you feel unable to take James out of the house in case he becomes unwell and fear the government will remove him as it believes you are a bad mother. You have avoided other people and kept James clean by bathing him three times a day and changing his nappy hourly. You've unplugged the TV to stop the government spying on you and sending messages. You want to protect yourself and James but aren't sure whom you can trust. Is there anything else you would like to tell me?

Explanation ☐ It seems to me, Chloe, that you may be suffering from a condition that can develop after having a baby and causes the mother to have severe mood problems. The condition is called postpartum psychosis. It sounds like your grandmother may have had the same problem.

InCludE ☐ Your feelings of being scared and anxious are very real but they are because you are unwell, not because anyone wants to take James away from you.

Recommend ☐ I would really like to get you some help with this today. To get the best help, I would like to speak to our specialist colleagues at the hospital and ask them to see you today.

Empathy ☐ I understand this is a scary prospect and it must seem that we are ganging up on you but I would really like to get you some help.

Future ☐ There is a special mother and baby ward at the hospital where you and James can go until you are feeling better. You will both be safe there and you will be able to rest and recover. You may need some medication to help settle how you are feeling and the hospital team will prescribe this. James will stay with you, no-one will take him away, but there will be specially trained nurses to help you look after him, if you need any extra support or are tired. Many people start to feel much better after 2 weeks or so, but it may take longer and you will have all the help you need to make a full recovery so that you and James can come home when you feel well and confident. How does that sound? I think your husband is in the house. Can he take you to the hospital?

Safety net ☐ If you feel worried or change your mind about seeing the hospital doctor, let us know and we can talk it through again.

Specifics ☐ If I phone your husband, may I explain to him what you have told me? When you are discharged, please let me know and I will come and visit you and James at home.

Patient's Story

Postnatal Psychosis

Doctor's notes Chloe Livingstone-Smith, 28 years. PMH: failed forceps delivery and ELSCS 2 weeks ago. Medications: none.

Midwife visit yesterday:

'Baby doing well, no jaundice, yellow stool nappies. Regained birth weight. Forceps mark fading. Breastfeeding. Up 2-hourly in the night. Mum tired. Not been out, says worried baby will pick up an infection, made an odd comment about the government, seems a little tearful, suggested talks to GP, asked husband to make her an appointment tomorrow.'

How to act Agitated. You want to reassure the doctor that all is well; however, you open up to the doctor when they explore your thoughts.

PC *'Can we make this quick, Doctor. I can't talk for long.'*

History You had your first baby, James, 2 weeks ago. You were induced due to being overdue and had a torrid time in hospital. The induction took a long time and resulted in a failed forceps delivery followed by an emergency caesarean section as James had become distressed in the womb. You were in hospital a couple of days recovering. James needed to be monitored as he had inhaled some meconium and the doctors were worried about infection. Since being discharged, you have become extremely anxious about James becoming unwell, especially that he will get an infection. You change his nappy hourly to keep him clean and bath him three times a day. You worry that the government is trying to take him away from you. You think that it sends messages through the television to you, telling you to give him up as you can't look after him properly and keep him safe and clean. You have unplugged the television and won't allow your husband to watch it. James is at home in another room and you have agreed to a phone consultation as you didn't want the government to snatch him if you went out. Your husband has told you that you need a telephone consultation check-up to see how you are getting on after the caesarean. He booked the appointment for you. You remember your mother telling you that her mother went into an 'asylum' after giving birth to her. A friend is with you now, holding James whilst you phone the doctor. You have no thoughts of harming yourself or anyone else. You want to keep the baby safe. You trust your husband and friend.

Social You are a designer for a large fashion company; previously you have travelled the world through your work. You married a photographer, whom you met whilst working on a fashion show. Your husband was keen to have children as he is a little older than you. You weren't sure at first as you didn't want to take a lot of time off work but were happy when you fell pregnant. Your parents live in Miami, so you don't see them often. You are an only child. Your in-laws live fairly locally and have been helping out.

ICE You believe that your baby will be taken from you by the government as it thinks you are an unfit mother. You love your baby and have been doing everything you can to protect him, especially from infection. You do not want to go back to hospital. You think the doctor may be on the government's side but, if they explain kindly and empathetically, you agree to their plan. You are happy for the doctor to speak to your husband on the phone.

Postnatal Psychosis

Mood changes after delivery are common but we must all be on the look-out for women who may be struggling with a mental illness.

'Baby blues' – Very common (>50%). Low mood, irritability, anxiety and tearfulness are common symptoms. Usually occurs day 3–4 postnatally and has usually resolved by day 10. Be suspicious if symptoms persist beyond 2 weeks.

Postnatal depression[1] – Occurs in 10–15% of women. Typically begins within the first 8 weeks but can occur several months later. Often there is a history of depression during pregnancy, although this isn't always picked up. More severe and longer lasting than 'baby blues'. Same symptoms as with non-pregnancy-related depression, i.e. low mood, tearful, changes in sleep, changes in appetite, anxiety and anhedonia. May be some more specific symptoms related to having a new baby, e.g. difficulty bonding with the baby, lack of emotional connection to the baby, feeling guilty for not loving the baby enough, resenting the baby for the way they feel, thoughts of harming the baby. As with all patients with depression, it is essential to assess any risk posed by the patients to themselves or others. In postnatal depression, be especially alert to risk to the baby or other children in the household.

Screening questions – **NICE recommends the following screening questions to help identify PND:**

'During the past month, have you often been bothered by feeling down, depressed or hopeless?

During the past month, have you often been bothered by having little interest or pleasure in doing things?'

Any positive response should lead to further assessment, possibly using a tool such as the Edinburgh Postnatal Depression Scale.

NICE also recommends screening for anxiety with the following two questions (GAD-2):

'Over the last 2 weeks, how often have you been bothered by feeling nervous, anxious or on edge?

Over the last 2 weeks, how often have you been bothered by not being able to stop or control worrying?'[2]

Depending on the severity of the symptoms, the mother may be able to care for herself and her baby without much extra support, but in severe cases the mother may struggle to complete simple tasks. In milder cases, health visitors, community mental health teams, etc., can be called upon to help treat the patient in the community setting, with support from the family, partner or carer. In more severe cases, involvement of the perinatal psychiatry team or even admission to a specialist mother and baby unit may be required. Where possible, the mother and baby should be kept together.

Postpartum psychosis (puerperal psychosis)[3] – Much rarer, occurring in 0.1%. Typically begins suddenly within the first 2 weeks following delivery. Symptoms vary but include severe depression, mania, hallucinations and delusions. It may occur in a woman with no history of mental illness, but the risk is increased if there is a personal or family history of mental illness (particularly of postpartum psychosis). There are frequently delusions about the baby: e.g. 'the baby is evil'. The patient may demonstrate typical features of psychotic illness, e.g. pressure of speech, knight's move thinking, delusions (e.g. paranoia, grandiose thoughts or ideas of persecution) or auditory/visual hallucinations. Postpartum psychosis is a psychiatric emergency and NICE recommends referral for immediate assessment (within 4 hours) and, where possible, the mother should be treated in a specialist mother and baby unit. Thankfully the prognosis is good with the worst symptoms usually improving around 12 weeks and the majority of cases resolving between 6 and 12 months. However, there is a 50% chance of recurrence in future pregnancies.

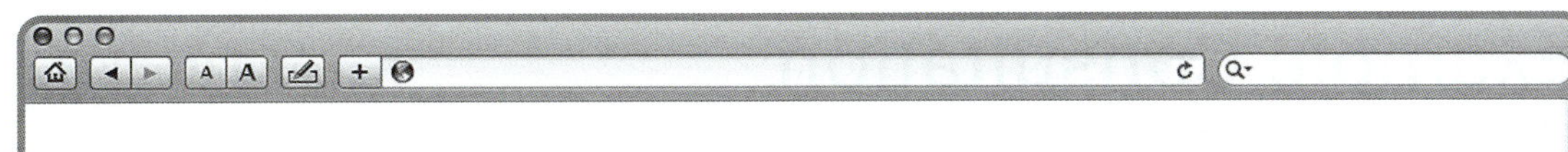

Doctor's Notes

Patient	Katherine Knight	68 years	F
PMH	None		
Medications	None		
Allergies	None		
Consultations	Appointment with GP 1 week ago – 'Concerned about alcohol intake. Examination – BP 130/80. No stigmata of liver disease. No tremor. Abdo examination normal – no liver edge. Check bloods and review 1 week'		
Investigations	FBC, MCV, clotting screen, U&E, GGT, LFT, amylase all normal		
Household	Barry Knight	63 years	M

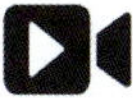

Example Consultation

Open ☐ Yes – I do have your blood results but first I would like to get to know you a bit. What prompted last week's appointment? Tell me about your drinking pattern. How do you feel about it?

ICE1 ☐ What do you think has led to this? What else have you been wondering? Have you known anyone else who struggled with alcohol?

Impact ☐ How has this affected your life? Or relationships? Or hobbies?

History ☐ Do you drink in the morning? Alone? Are you in good health? Any medicines? Any physical symptoms? Tremors? Stomach changes? Sleep problems? What do you do each day? Tell me about home life. Have you ever not done something expected of you due to drinking? Have you ever started drinking and felt you couldn't stop?

ICE2 ☐ What worries, if any, do you have about your health?

Sense ☐ You seem very sad. I'm interested to know why. Are there people you are close to?

Risk ☐ Do you feel isolated? Any mental health problems/depression? Do you take any drugs?

Flags ☐ Are there any dangers you can see associated with drinking? Any injuries? Are you down? Any thoughts of life not worth living? Have you acted on them? Do you have plans to end your life? Are either of you violent or unkind? Have you had thoughts of hurting another person? Do you eat well and look after yourself? Do you drive?

Curious ☐ What does your husband think about the alcohol? And the relationship? Any impact on him?

Empathy ☐ You've taken a big step, contacting us. It must seem like a difficult journey ahead.

ICE3 ☐ What did you think we may decide today?

Empower ☐ We can help. How would life be different without alcohol? Do you think you can stop? What steps could you take? Why might it be difficult? Who could help? What is your aim? When would you like to achieve that by?

SummarICE ☐ To summarise, you've been drinking more alcohol for 6 months. You feel low, due to being alone and bored. You hope to cut down and spend more time with your husband.

Impression ☐ Thankfully, all your blood tests have come back normal so there is no damage to your body, but it sounds like you have alcohol dependence and depression.

Experience ☐ What do you know about why alcohol is dangerous?

Explanation ☐ Alcohol affects most parts of the body. As well as damage to the liver it can cause problems with the nerves and the functioning in the brain. Sometimes people can suffer with a dementia-like illness because of alcohol. Alcohol keeps you awake at night. Alcohol is a false friend; it makes you more depressed.

Options ☐ There are things that you can do. It is actually dangerous to stop drinking straight away. We should either cut down gradually or provide support through a detox programme. What are your thoughts about these options?

Recommend ☐ Reducing your alcohol intake by 2–3 units (a large glass of wine) per day is a good starting point. Others can help with your recovery. Your husband, the alcohol team or Turning Point can support you through the process and afterwards. Would you like to see these teams? I can give you some vitamin tablets – thiamine – to prevent you becoming confused and unwell. The dose is one 100 mg tablet daily. How does this sound?

Future ☐ Can I talk to you again in 4 weeks? You could attend AA for ongoing support. There is also Relate which offers relationship counselling – you may find this helpful. What are your thoughts? I can send you these contact details by text message.

Safety net ☐ If you ever feel you are muddled, or start vomiting or feel shaky or generally unwell, or have thoughts of wanting to hurt yourself or anyone else, please see a doctor straight away.

Patient's Story

Harmful Drinking

Doctor's notes Katherine Knight, 68 years. PMH/medications/allergies: none.

Appointment with GP 1 week ago – 'Concerned about alcohol intake. Examination – BP 130/80. No stigmata of liver disease. No tremor. Abdo examination normal – no liver edge. Check bloods and review 1 week'.

Investigations: FBC, MCV, clotting screen, U&E, GGT, LFT, amylase all normal.

How to act Speak quietly. Do not be forthcoming with information.

PC *'Do you have my blood results, Doctor?'*

History Your husband made you come to the doctor last week as he was worried about your drinking. You started to drink one bottle of wine every night about 6 months ago. You just enjoyed it and the amount gradually increased. You are bored and don't have anything else to do! As well as the wine, you sometimes also have a brandy or two, usually starting to drink at lunchtime. If you don't drink, you feel shaky and you drink every day. You take no drugs. Your health has always been good and you take no medicines. You have no physical symptoms that you know of and your bowels are fine but your appetite is reduced. You often wake through the night. When others mention the alcohol, you feel upset. You drink alone and your husband has stopped drinking, *'To make me feel guilty.'*

Social You spend the day watching TV or you may wander to the supermarket. You eat quick meals these days and don't feel like cooking. You have never driven a car. Your husband is still working as a caretaker. *'He is too busy to notice.'*

You have lost touch with friends. You missed a catch-up with a friend as you'd been drinking and fell asleep on the sofa.

ICE Your husband told you to speak to your GP. Your relationship is not good. He is becoming upset. He is polite and kind to you but you feel very alone. You regret not having children.

You wanted to make sure your blood tests are normal and talk to the GP today but are unsure what you want from the meeting. You are worried that you rely on the alcohol and you don't know how to cut down. Although you would like to cut down, boredom may prevent it. However, overall, you believe you can and know your husband will help you.

You think you are depressed but want no medication.

You have occasional thoughts that life is not worth living but no plans and you would not attempt suicide.

You would like to get out of the house more. You would like to do more things together.

You agree with the doctor's advice about your relationship and self-help measures. You understand that alcohol is bad for the liver.

Learning Points

Harmful Drinking[1]

Perform a risk assessment	Self (neglect, harm, suicide, injury).
	Others (the public, children/vulnerable adults).
Assess psychological and social problems	E.g. mental health problems, work issues, housing issues, driving, criminal activity, relationship problems.
Investigations	U&E, LFT, GGT, FBC and clotting.
Questionnaires	AUDIT, SADQ and APQ.

Divide who can help into self, GP and others (friends, professionals or support groups: AA or SMART recovery). Involve families and carers in the recovery process with the patient's consent.

Consider the addition of acamprosate[2] or naltrexone to psychological therapy if this therapy alone has not been successful in mild alcohol dependence.[1] In practice, for most GPs, this will require a referral to the local drug and alcohol team.

When to offer community detox programmes

For those who 'drink over 15 units of alcohol per day and/or who score 20 or more on the AUDIT, consider offering: an assessment for and delivery of a community-based assisted withdrawal, or assessment and management in specialist alcohol services if there are safety concerns …'[1]

When to consider inpatient or residential assisted withdrawal[1]

- 15–30 units/day and 'significant psychiatric or physical co-morbidities … **or** a significant learning disability or cognitive impairment.'[1]
- SADQ score >30.
- History of: Epilepsy
  Withdrawal-related seizures
  Delirium tremens
  Consuming alcohol and benzodiazepines.

'Consider a lower threshold for inpatient or residential assisted withdrawal in vulnerable groups, for example homeless and older people.'[1]

'After a successful withdrawal for people with moderate and severe alcohol dependence consider offering acamprosate or oral naltrexone in combination with an individual psychological intervention **or** (third line) disulfiram after explaining the risks.'[1]

Advise patients wanting to cut down that this should be done slowly to prevent withdrawal symptoms and explain the importance of this to patients.

Remember driving – the law requires all dependent drinkers to inform the DVLA.

CHAPTER 7
URGENT AND UNSCHEDULED CARE

	Cases in this chapter	RCGP 2025 curriculum	Learning points
7.1	Chest Pain of Recent Onset	**Cardiovascular health** 'Risk factors for coronary heart disease' 'Manage cardiovascular emergencies in primary care'	Chest pain: differential diagnosis and management
7.2	Abdominal Pain	**Renal and urology** 'Abdominal pain including differential diagnoses' 'Acute abdominal conditions'	Differential diagnosis of abdominal pain
7.3	Hyperglycaemia	**Metabolic problems and endocrinology** 'Recognise and manage metabolic and endocrine emergencies' 'Systems of care for people with metabolic/endocrine conditions'	Tackling potential medication compliance issues Continuity of care and follow-up after the acute treatment of hyperglycaemia Ketones, HONK and lactic acidosis
7.4	Knee Pain	**Musculoskeletal health** 'Intervene urgently when patients present with emergencies or red flag symptoms...' 'Sprains, strains and other significant soft-tissue trauma' 'Coordinate care with other health professionals leading to effective and appropriate acute and chronic management'	Knee pain: assessing, investigating and managing Osteoarthritis: holistic assessment ACL injuries
7.5	Acute Asthma	**Respiratory health** 'Common and important conditions – asthma: acute and chronic' 'Specific procedures such as PEFR'	Acute asthma management Acute COPD management

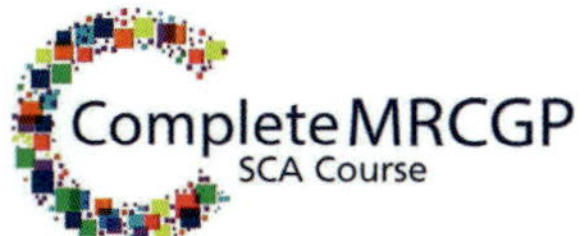

Links to the RCGP Curriculum

In this chapter, the cases are drawn from the following clinical topic guides:

- Cardiovascular health
- Renal and urology
- Metabolic problems and endocrinology
- Musculoskeletal health
- Respiratory health

Life stages topic guides: all life stages

Scope of Conditions

Here are some examples of cases – this is not a complete list of all possibilities.

Examples of conditions requiring immediate care include:

- Respiratory: acute COPD, asthma, pulmonary embolism
- Cardiovascular: aneurysms, heart failure, ACS, arrhythmias, limb ischaemia
- Gastrointestinal: appendicitis, intestinal obstruction or perforation
- Urological: urinary retention, renal colic
- Neurological: stroke-like conditions
- Infection
- Pregnancy related: ectopic, pre-eclampsia
- Complications of cancer: e.g. hypercalcaemia, neutropenic sepsis, spinal cord compression, superior vena cava obstruction
- Mental health: acute psychosis/mania

Skills and Pitfalls

In addition to the information in Chapter 1 'How to Demonstrate Skills: The Marking Scheme Made Easy' consider the following challenges for this blueprint group:

- Risk assessment of the condition.
- Recognition of when urgent or immediate assessment and care is required.
- Familiarity with appropriate referral pathways.
- Appropriate safety netting and explanation of how to seek urgent care.
- Appropriate, clear and sensitive discussion around the challenges and impact on the patient needing urgent care.
- Appropriate plan for review and monitoring.
- Recognition of and make plans for health beyond directing patient to an alternative or secondary service.
- Make the patient's safety a priority.

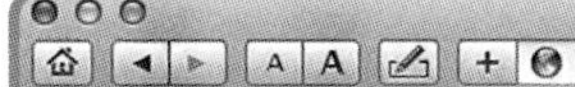

Doctor's Notes

Patient Mary Jones 45 years F

PMH New patient questionnaire: current smoker, BMI 40.2, three children

Medications None

Allergies None

Consultations None

Investigations None

Household No household members registered

Example Consultation **Chest Pain of Recent Onset**

Open ☐ Please tell me more about the pain, from when you first noticed it until now. How did it start? Please describe the pain to me. And tell me about any other symptoms.

Flags ☐ What are you typically doing when the pain comes on? Do you feel sick, sweaty or short of breath? Have you injured your neck? Any headache? Any weakness or tingling in the arms?

Risk ☐ Do you suffer with raised BP or cholesterol? Has a family member under the age of 65 had a problem with their heart? Do you smoke?

History ☐ Do you have any other medical conditions? Or take any medications?

ICE1 ☐ What do you think might be going on?

ICE2 ☐ What has been on your mind about this pain? Any other worries about your health?

Impact ☐ Has this pain stopped you from doing anything?

Summary ☐ So you've had this pain a few times, initially when quite active, but this time it came on whilst you were resting. It has now been present for 30 minutes in your chest and neck and you feel nauseous and sweaty.

ICE3 ☐ I'll be explaining my thoughts and recommendations today but apart from prescribing co-codamol, was there anything else that you were hoping I would do today?

Impression ☐ I am concerned that this pain is from your heart (pause); this could be a heart attack.

Explanation ☐ A heart attack is where a vessel to the heart becomes blocked and the lack of blood flow causes the pain.

InCludE ☐ I see why you thought it was a neck problem. However, pain from your heart is commonly felt in the neck.

Empathy ☐ I appreciate this is very frightening and completely unexpected.

Recommend ☐ To keep you safe and have an urgent assessment, you need to go to hospital as that is the only place where the right tests can be done to confirm or rule out a heart attack.

Empower ☐ I appreciate you need to go to your son. However, I must tell you what is at risk here. You need to go to the hospital now otherwise your life could be in danger.

Options ☐ I'm sorry. I am going to ask our receptionist to call an ambulance for you. Meanwhile can you call your husband and tell him to come straight home?

Future ☐ At the hospital I expect they will do an ECG which is where they put stickers on your chest to get an electrical tracing of your heart, and a blood test. They may take you to have a procedure which looks at the vessels to the heart. I'm so sorry this is a shock. Do you have any questions?

Specifics ☐ When you are discharged from the hospital, please make an appointment to see me so that we can discuss what has happened, make sure your medication is up to date and answer any questions you might have. Also, I know that sometimes when people are new to an area they can feel isolated. I'd really like to catch up with you soon and discuss your general health. There's lots we can do to improve this.

Patient's Story

Chest Pain of Recent Onset

Doctor's notes Mary Jones, 45 years. New patient. BMI 40.2. Smoker. Three children.

How to act You want to reassure the doctor it's just a pulled neck.

PC *'Doctor, I've got a pain in my neck.'*

History You have just returned from walking the dog. Your husband has now just left home for the afternoon shift at work so you are alone with your two younger children. You are going to the school soon to watch your older son perform in a play.

The pain in the upper left chest and neck has now been present for 30 minutes. It feels like something is pressing. You feel nauseous, sweaty and slightly SOB. You can't think of anything that takes it away. It just comes and goes but you think movement makes it worse because whenever you are doing something it comes on.

You also had the same pain 2 days ago when you were in the garden, but it went away after 5–10 minutes when you rested. You have had this pain a few times in the past 2 weeks, for example when running upstairs or watching television.

Your old GP gave you co-codamol for back pain so you would like this for your neck.

Your father died when you were a child due to his heart.

Social Mother of three. You have recently moved here as your husband has been relocated; he works in the building supplies industry. You used to work in a local tea room but have not yet found a job here. You smoke 10 cigarettes a day and rarely drink alcohol.

ICE You believe you have pulled your neck. You have not made any connection with the heart.

You would like a prescription for co-codamol and you will return another time if the doctor suggests anything else.

You can't go to hospital now. You have to go and watch your son in a school play.

You would just like the prescription. However, when the doctor explains the seriousness of the problem, you become upset and agree.

Initially, determine the cause of the chest pain by:

- Taking a detailed history.
- Examining the person.
- Organising appropriate investigations, **unless** immediate hospital admission is needed.

Do they need to go to hospital today?

Yes, if the clinical history suggests a serious cause for the chest pain. For example, suspected ACS with:

- Current chest pain.
- Complications such as pulmonary oedema.
- Pain free but chest pain within last 12 hours **and** abnormal ECG/no ECG available.

Consider admission if pain is resolved but there are signs of complications (e.g. pulmonary oedema).

Also consider admission if:

- Respiratory rate >30 breaths per minute or tachycardia >130 per minute
- Systolic BP <90 or diastolic BP <60 (unless normal for the person)
- Oxygen Sats <92% or central cyanosis if no history of chronic hypoxia
- Fever or altered level of consciousness
- Recent history of ACS[1] or if the patient shows signs of acute decompensation or other complications, or if clinical judgement concludes a troponin level is required.

Otherwise refer to RACPC.

Do I need to call for an ambulance?

Yes, if current chest pain, and consider in all cases if potentially ACS. Always refer to full guidance.

Differential diagnosis

ACS	Pain >10 minutes or increasing frequency or onset with less activity or at rest.
Stable angina	Precipitated by exertion, constricting discomfort. Relieved by GTN within ~5 minutes.
Dissection	Sudden tearing pain radiating to the back between the scapulas.
Pericarditis	Sharp, relieved by sitting forward ± radiation, fever, cough and arthralgia.
Acute heart failure	Orthopnoea and breathlessness.
Arrhythmias	Associated with palpitations and syncope.
PE	SOB, tachycardia, hypoxia ± haemoptysis ± leg swelling ± risk factors for VTE.
Pneumothorax	Risk factors include injury, tall male and COPD.
Pneumonia	SOB, fever, purulent sputum, cough ± pleuritic pain. Check the CRB-65 score.
Pancreatitis	Epigastric pain, severe, continuous and boring in nature.
GORD/PUD	Belching, reflux and sharp/burning pain ± melaena.
MSK causes	From Tietze's, costochondritis or rib fracture. Recent activity, tender to touch.
Anxiety	Tight chest, tingling in fingers, feeling of needing to breathe.
Referred pain	Back pain with possible back pain red flags.

Other treatment

Give O_2 if Sats <94% and not at risk of hypercapnic respiratory failure (aim for 94–98%). If at risk, use 28% Venturi mask with 4 L/min flow (aim for 88–92%). Consider GTN and 300 mg aspirin unless clear allergy.

Doctor's Notes

Patient	Rosie Carpenter 40 years F
PMH	Irritable bowel syndrome
	Renal colic 2 years ago
	BMI 31
Medications	Desogestrel 75 mcg daily
	Trimethoprim 200 mg BD – started yesterday
Consultations	Contraception check 1/12 ago and no problems with progesterone-only pill
	Seen by nurse yesterday for ?UTI and prescribed trimethoprim
	Urine dipstick: leucocytes positive, nitrites positive. HR 72 bpm, 37.2°C
	Abdomen – suprapubic discomfort. MSU pending

Example Consultation

Open ☐ I'm sorry to hear that. What have you noticed? I appreciate you explained to my colleague, but please can you go back to when you noticed something wasn't right? Anything else that you have noticed? Can you describe the pain? How is passing urine?

Flags ☐ Have you had a high temperature? Have you vomited? How much are you drinking? Any blood in your urine? When was your last period? Have you had any unusual discharge from the vagina? A personal question now – are you sexually active? Any pain during sex or bleeding afterwards?

ICE1 ☐ What are your thoughts about what's caused your symptoms?

Risk ☐ I see that years ago you had kidney stones. Can you describe that experience to me please? How is this different or the same in comparison? Before 2 days ago, had you noticed any symptoms that might suggest kidney stones returning? Including blood in the urine? Or discomfort in the back or passing urine?

ICE2 ☐ What concerns you most about what it might be?

History ☐ What other medical problems have you had in the past? Do you take any medicines? Are you allergic to anything? Do you have regular periods on the desogestrel? Have you tried anything for the pain? As we haven't met before please tell me more about yourself. Do you work? How is home life?

ICE3 ☐ I will be making my recommendations but was there anything specific you were hoping we would arrange today?

SummarICE ☐ To summarise, you feel the antibiotics given for a urine infection are not effective and you are hoping we can prescribe new ones today.

InCludE ☐ I agree with you. The urine infection, which was detected on your urine dipstick, seems to have progressed upwards and different antibiotics are needed.

Impression ☐ I think this may be an infection of the kidney, called pyelonephritis. Pyelonephritis can be treated with stronger antibiotics for longer.

Experience ☐ I'm concerned that you have had kidney stones in the past. You seem to feel this is different?

Explanation ☐ If you are very unwell, with a fever or in severe pain, you may need to be treated in hospital with antibiotics through your veins. Also, if kidney stones are present, hospital is required.

Empathy ☐ It sounds like you have been knocked sideways from this infection making you feel unwell.

Recommend ☐ I've been asking questions to assess whether you need treatment in hospital or at home. You haven't had symptoms of your kidney stones returning, and no fever. Your pain sounds very uncomfortable, but perhaps not severe enough to need hospital. I suggest we try antibiotics at home, with a low threshold for admission if anything gets worse or you are no better in the next 24 hours. But what are your thoughts?

Future ☐ Ok, so I will prescribe you 10 days of a different antibiotic, cefalexin. May I just check that you are not allergic to this? Like all antibiotics there may be side effects, in this case dizziness or diarrhoea, and many others could be possible. Any thoughts or questions about this? If you feel you are improving, then continue the antibiotics. If not improving by this time tomorrow, please call the surgery and I will arrange admission.

Specifics ☐ I will look out for the urine result to confirm this antibiotic is a good match for the infection. I will put you on my callback list to discuss this in 2 days.

Safety net ☐ If you develop a fever, feel more unwell, have more pain or worsening symptoms, please seek medical help immediately. If we are open, call us as we can sometimes arrange hospital assessment without going through A&E. Out of hours, 111 doctors may also be able to offer this. But, if you are worried and your symptoms have become severe, please go directly to A&E. Any questions?

Patient's Story

Doctor's notes Rosie Carpenter, 40 years. PMH: irritable bowel syndrome. Renal colic 2 years ago. BMI 31. Medication: desogestrel 75 mcg daily.

Contraception checked 1/12 ago and no problems with progesterone-only pill.

Seen by nurse yesterday for ?UTI and prescribed trimethoprim 200 mg BD.

Urine dipstick: leucocytes positive, nitrites positive. HR 72 bpm, 37.2°C.

Abdomen – suprapubic discomfort. MSU sent (no result yet).

How to act In discomfort. Not able to sit still. Worried.

PC ***'I don't think the antibiotics are working for my urine infection, Doctor.'***

History Two days ago you started going to the toilet to pass urine frequently which is uncomfortable and stinging when passing. Initially only a little urine was coming out at a time but you are continuing to drink well so you are still passing good amounts. You have not seen any blood. The pain is now in your right lower back and lower abdomen. 5/10 severity. You don't feel well in yourself. Your temperature at home is 37.4°C and HR is 88 bpm. You feel nauseous.

Two years ago you had a different pain where you felt you couldn't keep still because of pain in your left side and you had blood in your urine. It was very different. You have not had this since.

LMP was normal 2 weeks ago. Your periods are regular and you have no gynaecological symptoms.

Social You work in publishing. You live with your husband and two children.

You don't drink alcohol or smoke.

ICE You feel you have a urine infection which needs different antibiotics. You are hoping from this phone call that the doctor will prescribe and you explain you cannot attend the GP surgery again today. You feel it is safe to try a different antibiotic at home and accept the GP's advice about what to do for worsening symptoms.

Differential diagnosis of abdominal pain[1]

Acute pancreatitis	Tender, distention, fever and tachycardic. Causes include gallstones, alcohol and raised cholesterol.
Peptic ulcer	Reflux symptoms (belching, heartburn, nausea) ± melaena.
Cholecystitis	Murphy's sign (RUQ pain) or mass + fever or raised CRP/WCC ± vomiting, radiation to back, distention. Usually from gallstones.
	RFs = raised BMI/women/diabetes. Can be more severe in men.
Acute intestinal ischaemia/infarction or vasculitis	Possible vascular history. Sudden onset. Systemically unwell. May appear SOB or vomit.
Acute appendicitis	Initial generalised pain before localising to RLQ + peritonitic.
Intestinal obstruction	Vomiting + constipation + distended + not passing flatus. Peritonitic if perforated.
Renal colic	Severe loin to groin pain ± haematuria (macroscopic or microscopic).
Pyelonephritis	Urinary symptoms + loin pain + febrile + positive dipstick ± rigors.
Ectopic pregnancy	Lower abdominal pain (may radiate to shoulder) + β-hCG positive ± systemically unwell.
Ovarian cyst torsion	Severe pain radiating to iliac fossa or flank usually with nausea and vomiting.
Ovarian cyst rupture	May be peritonitic or haemodynamically unstable.
PID	Adnexal tenderness or cervical excitation + negative β-hCG ± history of STI. May be systemically unwell.
AAA rupture	Pain (abdominal or back) + haemodynamically unstable.
MI	Crushing central chest pain may radiate to arm or jaw (may present as abdominal pain) with SOB, nausea or vomiting and sweating. May be haemodynamically unstable.

See patient.info acute abdomen[1] for full information and a very useful diagram showing the possible causes of the pain, according to the location in the abdomen.

Could the patient be pregnant?

Perform a β-hCG in any female (of reproductive age) despite recent LMP or contraception.

History can be 'taken in good faith' with good reason (e.g. not had sexual intercourse for a year).

Most of the differential diagnoses listed require admission. 'If you are concerned enough to be ordering blood tests or imaging, the patient should be referred to secondary care.'[1]

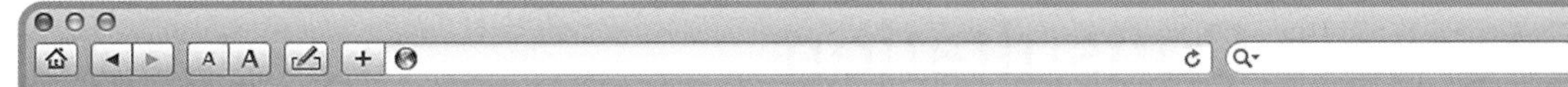

Doctor's Notes

Patient	Mary Owen 35 years F
PMH	Type 1 diabetes
	Diabetic ketoacidosis 1 year ago
	Anxiety
	Irritable bowel syndrome
Medications	Insulin glargine
	NovoRapid insulin
	Citalopram 20 mg once daily
	Buscopan 10 mg TDS PRN
Allergies	No information
Consultations	DNA letter from hospital diabetes clinic
Household	No household members registered

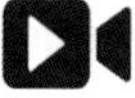

Example Consultation

Open ☐ Oh dear. In what way unwell? When did you last feel your normal self? Okay, take it from that day and tell me what symptoms you noticed in sequence if you can. How is your general health usually?

Flags ☐ How are your blood sugars at the moment? Do you have a ketone meter? Yes please – what numbers has your machine given? Thank you that's helpful. Are they higher than what you have had before?

Risk ☐ Any symptoms that may suggest infection, for example a cough, sore throat, diarrhoea, changes passing urine or tummy pain or abnormal vaginal discharge? Is it painful to pass urine? Are you racing to the toilet? Or passing a small or large amount each time? Any blood? Any rash, stiffness of the neck or discomfort looking at the light?

ICE1 ☐ What do you think may have caused this?

History ☐ Is the insulin regime appropriate for your lifestyle? Has everything been okay with taking your insulin recently? What was your past experience of DKA? Do you have any other medical problems? How is your anxiety? How are your bowels at present? Do you work? Tell me more about work. Is anyone at home? Are you in a relationship? 'Not really'? I'm wondering if there is a chance of pregnancy?

ICE2 ☐ What worries you about your symptoms?

Curious ☐ You say you have been forgetting to take the insulin. Why might this be? Why are you missing meals? You say you haven't got time to worry about work: is everything okay? I'm sorry your mother is not well.

Impact ☐ Have you been struggling with your normal day? Are you feeling low?

ICE3 ☐ What did you think I might suggest today?

SummarICE ☐ To summarise, you have felt unwell for 2 days. You believe you have a urine infection, are frightened by your blood sugars being so high and thought I would suggest how to bring them down.

Empathy ☐ It sounds like you are under stress physically and emotionally with a busy career, whilst taking care of your mother with whom you are very close.

Impression ☐ Mary, I believe the raised blood sugar has led to DKA again, likely due to a combination of stress and missing insulin doses.

InCludE ☐ And, I agree, a urine infection may have contributed to this. Urine infections are more likely after having sex and with raised sugars.

Experience ☐ What did the doctor explain about DKA?

Explanation ☐ Because you do not have a good supply of insulin to move all that sugar into your muscles, your body breaks down fat to make ketones.

Options ☐ You need to go to hospital for treatment through the veins otherwise you will be extremely unwell. I'm sorry. What are you thinking?

InCludE ☐ Unfortunately, although I know this is not what you hoped, we cannot give this care at home. Is your mother a patient with us? What does she need? I can call your mother and suggest arranging emergency care through the single point of contact team whilst you are in hospital. I will phone the medical team at the hospital to let them know you need to come in. I will arrange for an ambulance to take you to hospital.

Future ☐ At the hospital, I expect you will be given fluids, insulin and antibiotics. I will arrange a review for your mum; it sounds like she may be eligible for free long-term care.

Empower ☐ When you are better, please return to see me to discuss your general health, support we could offer and changes to your insulin regime to suit your lifestyle better. I also recommend going to the toilet after sex to prevent water infections as this helps flush out the bacteria that may be pushed up into the bladder during sex. Does this make sense?

Safety net ☐ If you feel unwell again, please don't hesitate to speak to a doctor.

Patient's Story

Hyperglycaemia

Doctor's notes Mary Owen, 35 years. PMH: type 1 diabetes, DKA 1 year ago, anxiety and IBS.

Medications: insulin glargine, NovoRapid insulin, citalopram 20 mg once daily, Buscopan 10 mg TDS PRN.

Consultations: DNA letter from hospital diabetes clinic.

How to act Slightly breathless and lacking in full concentration.

PC *'I keep being sick. I feel really unwell.'*

History Two days ago you started feeling unwell and tired and started to develop stomach pain. This morning you started vomiting with abdominal pain and a headache. You feel dehydrated. You have no rash and no fever. You have no neck stiffness and no neurological symptoms.

If the doctor asks you about your breathing, you do feel more breathless but have no other respiratory symptoms. Your blood sugar is 24 and your ketones are 2.8 mmol/L. Your blood pressure machine states 115/70 and a heart rate of 115.

'I have been forgetting to take the insulin.' This is usually because you are '***always on the go***' and you have missed meals.

You have no fever, but you have been passing urine more frequently over the past week. At first you thought you needed to go but then nothing came out and now you are passing much more urine, you have seen some blood and it is painful.

Your bowels are currently normal. Your anxiety has been controlled recently.

You have no other systemic symptoms. Last year you had DKA. You had abdominal pain, felt unwell and were vomiting.

Social You live alone. You are '***not really***' in a relationship. By this you mean you caught up with an old boyfriend and had sex 10 days ago. You used condoms.

You work in advertising and have been successful in your career which can be stressful and you have suffered with the stress of meeting deadlines and presentations to clients in the past but ***'I don't have time to worry about this now.'***

You only drink minimal alcohol socially. You do not smoke.

Your mother was diagnosed with leukaemia 3 months ago and she is currently having chemotherapy. You have been driving to see her after work and at the weekends, sometimes staying up with her through the night if she feels unwell. She isn't well at present but she made you contact the GP. You are very worried about your mum and will go back to see her after the consultation with the GP.

You need to return to be with your mother. She has no one else. However, if the doctor explains why you need to go to hospital you will go. Your mother is a patient at the same GP practice. Can the doctors help? She needs someone to check in on her and make sure she has fluid and food tonight. She is very weak and in bed.

ICE You are worried about your health and you are frightened because your blood sugars are so high. You believe you have a water infection after having sex.

If the doctor mentions DKA, you have heard of it. You expect the doctor will tell you what to do with your insulin today to bring your sugars down.

The consultation

When asking if a patient has been compliant with medication, avoid sounding confrontational, for example instead of *'Are you taking your medicines correctly?'* ask: *'I see you are prescribed … How are you getting on with …? When do you take it?'* This is a much softer question and more likely to yield a truthful answer. This case challenges your skills at managing an emergency, practising holistically and negotiation. Without a thorough social history and consideration of the patient's concerns, it is unlikely that the key information about the patient's mother will be uncovered. It is essential to address this concern and offer a solution to allow your patient to accept potentially life-saving treatment.

Most areas have a rapid access team who can put emergency care in place (either at home or within a care home) for short-term care issues. It is very important to invite the patient back to discuss ways in which she can access help with her mother (both practically and financially) or at the very least signpost her to local carers' support groups. It is likely she will need long-term support to prevent her own health suffering.

Ketones[1]	**<0.6 mmol/L**	A normal blood ketone value.
	0.6–1.5 mmol/L	Indicates that more ketones are being produced than normal. Test again in 2 hours.
	1.6–3.0 mmol/L	A high level of ketones, and could present a risk of ketoacidosis. It is advisable to contact your diabetes team or GP for advice as soon as possible.
	>3.0 mmol/L	A very high risk of DKA which will require immediate medical care.[1]
HONK	In type 2 diabetes: hyperglycaemic hyperosmolar non-ketotic coma. This may present with extreme thirst, frequency, confusion and nausea and may progress to coma if not treated promptly.	
Lactic acidosis	Diabetic patients may become acidotic especially if they are taking metformin.	

Doctor's Notes

Patient	Robert Hayes	32 years	M
PMH	None		
Medications	None		
Allergies	None		
Consultations	Physiotherapy this morning: the left knee is swollen with an effusion. The knee is not hot or red. There is tenderness along the medial side. There is limitation of movement. Lachman's test and the anterior drawer test are positive. The rest of the examination is normal. Doctor's assessment required		
Investigations	None		
Household	None		

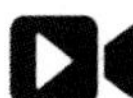

Example Consultation **Knee Pain**

Open ☐	I'm sorry to hear that. Can you tell me what happened? Talk me through the injury in slow motion if you can please. Then what did you notice? Can you describe the pain please?
ICE1 ☐	What do you think may have happened inside the knee?
Flags ☐	Did the knee swell straight away? Could you walk on it? Does the knee lock into a certain position stopping you from straightening or bending it? Has it given way?
Risk ☐	Have you injured your knee before? Any other injury?
Impact ☐	And the past couple of days, has it stopped you from doing anything? Do you work? How would a knee injury affect your work, hobbies or home life?
ICE2 ☐	Has anything else gone through your mind?
Curious ☐	Anything else you fear about this injury? Is there a reason you'd like to avoid the orthopaedic doctors?
ICE3 ☐	Is there anything you thought I might say we should arrange? Is there anything else you were hoping we could do? Are there any other thoughts you had about what may be helpful?
SummarICE ☐	To summarise, you believe you may have torn a ligament and fear needing an operation after your experience with your right ankle. You are hoping that I will organise an MRI scan to guide physiotherapy but would like to get better quickly because you don't want to be sat out for the rest of the season. Is that correct?
Impression ☐	It sounds as if it could be a torn ligament, and I'm wondering specifically if it is the anterior cruciate ligament injury. This can be very painful, as you have described.
Sense ☐	You sound disappointed and upset.
Experience ☐	Have you heard of this injury?
Explanation ☐	This ligament in the knee prevents your knee from overstretching, but unfortunately if you have had an injury which causes the leg to overstretch, it can tear.
Empathy ☐	It sounds as if you have been relatively isolated socially, so I appreciate that not being able to play football with friends in an evening is a huge disappointment.
Options ☐	To get you on the mend as soon as possible, we should consider referring you to the trauma clinic today.
InCludE ☐	You mentioned you were keen for physio; I think that sounds a good idea but wonder if we should get the orthopaedic opinion first.
Recommend ☐	I suggest that I give the trauma registrar a call, if that's okay with you.
Future ☐	If surgery is needed, keyhole surgery may be an option. I can also prescribe some codeine for additional pain relief if you need it. It can cause a few side effects such as nausea, constipation or drowsiness and please do not take more than the prescribed dose of two tablets every 6 hours. Perhaps once the injury has settled a little you could still go to matches to support your team and see your friends?
Specifics ☐	I expect the trauma team will call you in the next day or so. If you have not heard from them by Friday please let a doctor know.
Empower ☐	In the meantime, please keep it elevated with some ice on it to reduce the swelling. Whilst waiting to see the trauma team, I'd recommend paracetamol and an anti-inflammatory like ibuprofen but can prescribe something a little stronger if you need it.

Patient's Story

Knee Pain

Doctor's notes Robert Hayes, 32 years. PMH/medications: none.

Physiotherapy this morning: the left knee is swollen with an effusion. The knee is not hot or red. There is tenderness along the medial side. There is limitation of movement. Lachman's test and the anterior drawer test are positive. The rest of the examination is normal. Doctor's assessment required.

How to act Pleasant but concerned.

PC ***'I've injured my knee playing football.'***

History Two days ago, you were playing football. You felt something pop as you were changing direction – your studs seemed to stick in the mud. There was no contact with another player at the time. It was extremely painful, and you could not continue the game. You applied ice to your swollen knee, but the swelling is still present. The knee doesn't lock but has given way. You have had no previous knee injury. You have not been able to drive since the injury despite taking paracetamol and ibuprofen. You also find it painful walking and weight bearing. You have seen the team's physiotherapist this morning and they advised you to consult a doctor. They said it was a ligament injury.

You cannot get to the surgery now because you are looking after small children at home; you feel unable and unsafe to drive and there is no one available to give you a lift.

Social You work as a project manager and enjoy running, badminton and football. You live with your partner and two children. If the doctor asks you about what impact this injury may have, you have responsibility for most of the childcare because your partner has a high-pressure city job but you can work from home so do all the nursery and school pick-ups. You do not have family nearby and have felt lonely. Because your partner can be around in the evenings, when the football season started, you began to spend more time with your friends and felt less isolated.

ICE You believe you may have torn a ligament. You are worried that you will be ***'out for the season'***.

You also fear you may need an operation. You fractured your ankle falling out of a tree as a child and remember a lot of pain after the operation. For this reason, you would rather see an NHS physio than be referred to Orthopaedics; however, you will follow the doctor's advice. You would like an MRI of your knee – if asked why, you think this would help a physiotherapist. If the doctor asks you about your understanding of the diagnosis, you remember that Michael Owen couldn't play in the 2006 World Cup due to a cruciate ligament injury. The doctor is giving you terrible news as you fear you will now be isolated from your friends this season.

Osteoarthritis – New diagnosis

Suspect arthritis if:[1]

- Age ≥45 years.
- Clinical features are suggestive.
- Alternative conditions have been excluded.

Differential diagnosis: this includes gout/pseudogout, septic arthritis, inflammatory arthritis, malignancy, trauma, patellofemoral pain, pre-patella bursitis, greater trochanteric pain syndrome, iliotibial band syndrome, meniscal tear and anterior cruciate ligament tear. Don't forget referred pain from the hip.[1]

NICE CKS advise a holistic assessment of a person with OA: consider social situation and impact, health beliefs, mood, quality of sleep, support network, other MSK pain, attitudes to exercise, influence of co-morbidity and a full pain assessment including history of the pain, symptoms of joint instability, risk factors and atypical features.

GP management options: these include advice on sources of information and support such as www.versusarthritis.org, topical NSAIDs, muscle-strengthening exercises, advice about aerobic fitness and footwear, physiotherapy and steroid injections. Consider the additional need for TENS or aids and psychosocial support.

Possible referral routes:[1]

- Physiotherapy/MSK – strengthening exercises, manipulation, joint supports, joint injections.
- Occupational therapy – advice on helpful devices for ADL to reduce strain on different joints.
- Podiatrist – biomechanical assessment, orthotics device.
- Orthopaedic surgeon (irrespective of patient's age, BMI or co-morbidities) and **before** severe functional limitations and/or pain if:
    - Symptoms (stiffness, joint pain, functional impairment) are not improving with primary care management after 3 months, or if this is inappropriate.
    - QOL significantly affected.
    - Diagnosis is unclear or symptoms are atypical.
    - Symptoms suddenly get worse.
- Pain clinic if:
    - Pain uncontrolled despite optimised medical and/or surgical management.
    - Suspect chronic pain syndrome.
- Psychological services if co-morbid depression or anxiety despite primary care management.

ACL injury

Mechanism	Most commonly associated with a non-contact mechanism – 'knee in and toe out'.[2]
	The risk is greater in females.[2]
Injury triad	Anterior cruciate ligament + medial collateral ligament + medial meniscus.

Acute injuries

Refer acute injuries to Orthopaedics for assessment, imaging and management options.

NB: Immediate effusions following trauma/injury are often due to haemarthrosis which is associated with more significant joint injuries. Have a low threshold for referral of such cases (possibly same day or urgently to trauma/fracture clinic). If presenting as a chronic injury, you may be able to refer for direct access MRI to guide diagnosis and management – check local protocols.

Doctor's Notes

Patient	Daisy Fitton	24 years	F
PMH	Asthma		
Medications	Clenil 100 inhaler 2 puffs BD Salbutamol inhaler PRN		
Allergies	No information		
Consultations	9 months ago asthma review with nurse. Peak flow 450 L/min Asthma nurse appointment this morning. Peak flow 210 L/min. RR 24, Sats 95%, HR 104 bpm. Temperature 36.9°C. Speaking in full sentences. Good air entry, R = L. Vesicular breaths and wheeze throughout, expiration > inspiration 10 puffs given of salbutamol. No wheeze after 10 puffs and good air entry throughout. PEFR 300 L/min after treatment. Became upset when discussed the asthma deteriorating. Patient left stating she will call the doctor		
Investigations	No information		
Household	No household members registered		

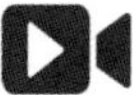

Example Consultation

Acute Asthma

Open ☐ Hello, Daisy. I understand you would like to speak to a doctor. I'm Dr X. I see your breathing is a problem, I'm sorry to hear that. Can you tell me about it please? What does your chest feel like? And your breathing?

Flags ☐ How often have you been using your blue inhaler? With a spacer? How often do you usually use the blue one? What about the brown one?

ICE1 ☐ What do you think has caused this?

Risk ☐ Have you ever been admitted with your asthma? Have you ever been in intensive care? Do you smoke? Has your asthma ever been as bad as this? Do you have a personalised asthma action plan?

History ☐ Do you have any other medical problems? Your brown inhaler – how have you been getting on with that? How often do you take it? What about the blue one? Do you take any other medicines? Is there anyone at home with you? What do you do in the day?

ICE2 ☐ What, if anything, worries you about your asthma?

Sense ☐ It sounds like you were upset this morning? What was going through your mind when you felt that way? When you think about hospital, what is it that you find frightening? Have you had any past experiences?

ICE3 ☐ From your experience of your asthma, what do you believe is necessary?

SummarICE ☐ To summarise, you have had a cold and sore throat and now you are struggling with your asthma despite regular use of your blue inhaler. You think this may have been caused by the weather and that you may need antibiotics and steroids. You feel upset with the thought of your lungs struggling for air and the thought of hospital frightens you.

Impression ☐ Your peak flow blowing test and your breathing and heart rate suggest this is a severe asthma attack.

Explanation ☐ Your oxygen levels have fallen slightly, your heart rate is raised and your peak flow has fallen. However, you have responded well to the treatment our nurse gave.

InCludE ☐ I think this has been caused by a viral infection. You are not coughing green phlegm and your sore throat and cold are typical of a virus so, although I agree that steroids will help, I don't think that antibiotics will be of any use.

Empathy ☐ Normally, you have been able to manage the asthma at home so it is frightening when your asthma is so much worse than usual.

Recommend ☐ I will also arrange for a prescription for 40 mg of prednisolone, a steroid. Can your boyfriend collect it for you from the chemist, now? I would want you to be able to manage at least an hour without the inhaler, and then 4-hourly at home. Hopefully, you will respond to treatment and will be able to stay at home.

Specifics ☐ The nurse gave you 10 puffs at 10 a.m. I would want you to go 4 hours without needing another inhaler. Can we see you at 1.30 p.m. again today to see how you are? Come in earlier if you need the inhaler before that. How do you feel about this plan?

Future ☐ When you are feeling better, I'd like to meet up again to optimise your inhalers. Guidance now suggests we manage asthma with a single inhaler where possible which would mean a change in inhaler for you. We would advise using it for both maintenance and to relieve symptoms. We can write all this down for you in your own asthma plan.

Safety net ☐ If you feel your breathing is getting worse, please return to the surgery. I don't expect this to happen, but if your breathing is feeling very bad, and you're close to using 10 puffs of your inhaler, this is when you must call 999 for an ambulance.

Patient's Story

Acute Asthma

Doctor's notes Daisy Fitton, 24 years. PMH: asthma. Medications: Clenil 100 inhaler two puffs BD, salbutamol inhaler PRN.

Nine months ago asthma review with nurse. Peak flow 450 L/min.

Asthma nurse appointment this morning. Peak flow 210 L/min. RR 24, Sats 95%, HR 104 bpm. Temperature 36.9°C. Speaking in full sentences. Good air entry, R = L. Vesicular breaths and wheeze throughout, expiration > inspiration.

10 puffs given of salbutamol. No wheeze after 10 puffs and good air entry throughout. PEFR 300 L/min after treatment. Became upset when discussed the asthma deteriorating. Patient left stating she will call the doctor.

How to act A little distracted by your breathing.

PC ***'My asthma isn't very good.'***

History You've had a cold and sore throat and for the past 2 days you've become wheezy. You are not coughing any phlegm and have no pain but feel tight in the chest. No fever. Your chest always feels like this at this time of year.

When you were a child, you were admitted to hospital once but no ITU admissions. You remember the nurses putting a mask over your face and you screaming and this was very upsetting. You generally cope with your asthma but it upsets you when your lungs are worse, making you feel scared and vulnerable. If the doctor says so, you would go to hospital, but this scares you because of your previous experience.

You use the Clenil BD and usually your salbutamol six times a week, especially after hockey.

You saw the practice nurse this morning. You have a peak flow meter but don't use it very often.

You last took four puffs of salbutamol 1 hour ago.

Social You are a solicitor. You live with your boyfriend. You have never smoked. All is well at home, at work and in your relationship.

ICE You believe the weather has caused this exacerbation. You are not too concerned.

You expect the doctor will give you steroids and antibiotics – if the doctor suggests you don't need antibiotics, question them about why – you usually get given them.

You will follow the doctor's advice regarding admission, stating: ***'You are the doctor.'***

Learning Points — Acute Asthma and Acute COPD

Life-threatening asthma

Peak flow <33% or asthma with any of the following features: Sats <92%, silent chest, cyanosis, poor respiratory effort, arrhythmia, hypotension, confusion or altered consciousness or exhaustion.[1]

Acute severe asthma

Peak flow 33–50% or RR >25 or HR >110 bpm in people >12 years or not able to complete sentences in one breath, or accessory muscle use, with O_2 Sats ≥92%, **and** no features of life-threatening asthma.[1]

Moderate asthma

Peak flow >50% best or predicted, normal speech and no signs of acute severe/life-threatening asthma.[1]

Management of acute asthma – adults

All: administer oxygen to keep the saturations between 94% and 98%.[1]

Give prednisolone 40–50 mg stat then daily to complete minimum of 5 days.[1]

Monitor PEFR (if person can comply) and O_2 Sats to assess response to treatment.

Follow up patients at home within 2 working days.

Life-threatening asthma Admit the patient *immediately*. Call 999. Give nebulised salbutamol 5 mg, preferably by O_2 driven nebuliser. May repeat salbutamol after 20–30 minutes if required whilst waiting for the ambulance. Consider adding nebulised ipratropium bromide – 500 mcg for adults, 250 mcg for children age 2–12. Do not repeat within 4 hours.

Severe asthma Consider admission if symptoms persist after initial treatment. Give 5 mg salbutamol via nebuliser, preferably O_2 driven, or spacer if nebuliser not available. If no response or still has features of acute severe asthma, admit.[1]

Moderate asthma Give salbutamol (100 mcg) via pMDI large vol spacer, one puff every 60 secs, up to 10, according to response. One puff at a time, inhaled separately using tidal breathing. If no response, give nebulised salbutamol and consider admission. If good response, continue or increase usual treatment and continue prednisolone for minimum of 5 days.[1]

On discharge Follow up within 2 days: F2F or telephone. Consider stepping up by increasing ICS. Advise how to recognise poor control. Ensure patient has a personalised asthma plan.

Asthma long-term management Move towards single maintenance and reliever therapy (MART) rather than separate SABA and ICS ± LABA due to over-reliance on SABA being associated with increased risk of death. For MART, the LABA must be formoterol which is both fast and long acting. See Global Initiative for Asthma (GINA) guidance for more information.[2]

Acute COPD[3]

Consider admission if severe breathlessness, inability to cope at home/lives alone, poor or deteriorating general condition, rapid onset, acute confusion/impaired consciousness, cyanosis, Sats <90%, worsening peripheral oedema, new arrhythmia, already on LTOT, failure to respond to initial treatment, or changes on CXR. Give supplemental O_2 whilst awaiting emergency transfer – aim for Sats 88–92%.[3] Provide O_2 via Venturi 24% mask at 2–3 L/min or Venturi 28% mask at 4 L/min or via nasal cannula at 1–2 L/min if no Venturi mask.

Where admission not required, advise the person to increase the doses or frequency of short-acting bronchodilators (not exceeding the maximum dose). Treat increased cough and/or breathlessness with 30 mg prednisolone, once daily for 5 days. Discuss adverse effects of long-term treatment and consider osteoporosis prophylaxis if more than three or four courses of steroids per year. Treat change in colour or increased volume of sputum with antibiotics (e.g. amoxicillin, doxycycline or clarithromycin).

CHAPTER 8

HEALTH DISADVANTAGE AND VULNERABILITIES*

	Cases in this chapter	RCGP 2025 curriculum	Learning points
8.1	Domestic Violence	**Smoking, alcohol and substance misuse** 'Social consequences of substance misuse, e.g. contact with the criminal justice system (including incarceration), domestic violence, homelessness, poor attendance or functioning at school or work, relationship issues, safeguarding concerns, unemployment'	Domestic violence Child protection Coercive controlling behaviour
8.2	Mental Health and Learning Disability	**Mental health** 'Communicate effectively, professionally and sensitively with patients, relatives and carers, recognising potential difficulties in communicating with people with mental health conditions' **Neurodevelopmental conditions and neurodiversity** 'Tailored physical and mental state assessments in neurodivergent patients, recognising that they may be unable to verbalise or describe symptoms typically' **Learning disability** 'Recognise the risk of diagnostic overshadowing and potentially atypical presentations, especially when unwell'	Diagnostic overshadowing in people with learning disability Questions to carers
8.3	Suspected DVT	**Haematology** 'Symptoms and signs of haematological disorders … DVT or PE' 'Anticoagulants: indications, initiation, management and reversal/withdrawal including heparin, warfarin, direct oral anticoagulants such as dabigatran, drug interactions and contraindications' **Urgent and uscheduled care** '... always needing urgent action if suspected'	Diagnosis and treatment of DVT Wells score Capacity to make a decision
8.4	Alcohol and Safeguarding	**Smoking, alcohol and substance misuse** 'Recognise and manage medical consequences of smoking, alcohol and substance misuse' 'Be aware of wider social issues, including the need to protect children and family members from the potential impact of smoking, alcohol or substance misuse, and respond to any safeguarding concerns'	Harmful drinking Hazardous drinking Alcohol dependence Safeguarding
8.5	LARC and Sterilisation	**Sexual health** 'Other important content: LARC; sterilisation.' **Mental health** 'The needs of and services for veterans, including the psychological effects of trauma and war (such as PTSD)'	Implant – IUS/IUD Injection Services for veterans

* INCLUDING VETERANS, MENTAL CAPACITY, SAFEGUARDING AND COMMUNICATION DIFFICULTIES.

Links to the RCGP Curriculum

In this chapter, the cases are drawn from the following clinical topic guides:

- Smoking, alcohol and substance misuse
- Mental health
- Neurodevelopmental conditions and neurodiversity
- Learning disability
- Haematology
- Urgent and unscheduled care
- Sexual health

Life stages topic guides: all life stages

Scope of Conditions

Here are some examples of cases – this is not a complete list of all possibilities.

Examples of vulnerable patients:

- Young adults and those who have just left home
- Patients transitioning to adult services
- Mental health conditions
- Patients new to the country
- Elderly people
- Pregnant women or new parents
- Patients with a disability
- Patients at risk of abuse from others
- Patients with communication difficulties
- Veterans
- Patients without employment

Skills and Pitfalls

In addition to the information in Chapter 1 'How to Demonstrate Skills: The Marking Scheme Made Easy' consider the following challenges for this blueprint group:

- Recognise patients who are vulnerable.
- Risk assess considering physical, psychological and social challenges and risks.
- Communicate appropriately and sensitively.
- When required, assess the mental capacity of patients.
- Find opportunities to empower patients.
- Optimise the patient's general health.
- Consider management options for physical, mental and social health challenges.
- Consider the wider team and services who may be able to support health challenges and inequalities.

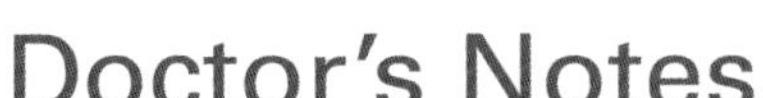

Doctor's Notes

Patient	Isabel Forster	33 years	F
PMH	Fracture of thumb 1 year ago		
Medications	None		
Allergies	None		
Consultations	None		
Investigations	None		
Household	No household members registered		

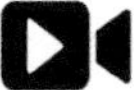

Example Consultation

Open ☐ Okay, what are your thoughts about this?

Sense ☐ You're mentioning David. I sense David is more concerned than you. Is that right?

Curious ☐ What do you mean by *'Not the right time anyway'*?

ICE1 ☐ What do you think may be contributing to you not getting pregnant?

ICE2 ☐ With everything that is going on, what is worrying you most today? Any specific worries about your health?

History ☐ Please tell me about you. Tell me about work. Do you take any medicines? Some personal questions: your periods – are they regular? How often do you have sex? Have you ever had an STI? When were you last checked? What made you have an STI check? How is your relationship now? What else do you argue about? Do you ever feel unsafe at home? Are you able to tell me more about that? Do you have any support from family/friends? Can you confide in them? Do you feel isolated? Do you drink alcohol? Or take drugs? Do you own your house? Do you have your own access to money? What do you enjoy doing? Would you like to investigate your fertility? Thank you for sharing this with me.

Flags ☐ Questions about David … Does he work? Abuse can be physical but also emotional. In what ways does he upset you? Does he hit you? Has he used objects to hurt you? Does he force himself on you sexually? Is anyone else aware? Does he spend time with children? What is he capable of? Do you feel that your life is at risk? Has he ever been arrested? Has he threatened to kill you or someone else? Does he have any mental health problems? How much alcohol does he drink? What about drugs? Thank you for telling me. I appreciate it must be upsetting to talk about. Is the abuse getting worse? Do you feel he is controlling you? How is your mood? Have you ever hurt yourself? Do you ever have thoughts that life is not worth living? Have you ever made plans or tried to end your life? Do you have any other injuries? Has he harmed himself? Have you tried to leave before?

Impact ☐ How do the violence and unkind words you receive affect you?

ICE3 ☐ Have you had any thoughts about how I can particularly help you today?

SummarICE ☐ To summarise, David is keen for a family but because of the violence in the relationship you are taking the Depo injection to give you time to think about your options.

Impression ☐ It sounds like you do not feel safe in your home and David's behaviour could be described as coercive and controlling.

Explanation ☐ Violence in the home is just as illegal as violence in the streets.

Empathy ☐ This must be very difficult for you to talk about. It can also be frightening telling someone.

ICE3 ☐ What are your thoughts about your options? What would you like to happen? Are you starting to think about planning to leave? What frightens you? What do you need? Have you thought about telling the police?

Experience ☐ Have you heard of any support groups? Are there family/friends who may be able to help?

Recommend ☐ If you are thinking of leaving, be careful who you tell, so David does not know. But there is help: the freephone National Domestic Abuse Helpline, available 24/7, offers confidential information and support without judging. Women's Aid responds to emails within 5 days and offers a survivor's handbook. There is also the Freedom Programme, Recovery Toolkit and Sanctuary Scheme. I can send you details electronically. Does David monitor your messages? If so, could you use a trusted friend's number instead? If you ever feel your life or health are at risk, phone 999 straightaway.

Empower ☐ We need to try and give you back control in your life. Which, if any, of these steps would you like to take? What would you do first? When could you take that first step?
I can post a sticker to you in a plain envelope. It looks like a barcode but with a crisis number on it – put it on something like a lipstick. What will you tell David about our consultation?

Safety net ☐ If you ever feel you need help you could call this number, us, 111 or the police.

Patient's Story

Domestic Violence

Doctor's notes Isabel Forster, 33 years. PMH: fracture of thumb 1 year ago. Medications: none.

How to act Very quiet. You have a concern that you have not shared with anyone else.

PC *'Doctor, we've been trying for a baby for over a year now.'*

History You are well. Fracture of the thumb after you tripped 1 year ago. You have regular periods. No STIs and smears are up to date.

You have had no other sexual relationships since this relationship with David.

'David thought I should call. He is at work.'

'He thinks something must be wrong.'

Social You met David 4 years ago. You work in the kitchen of the local primary school. David is a building manager for large corporation sites. He has no children. You drink no alcohol and take no drugs. David drinks *'too much'* alcohol.

ICE You tell the doctor it is likely that you haven't fallen pregnant because David is often at work or you have been busy around the time of ovulation.

'I'm not worried. I know it takes time. I'm not sure now is the right time anyway.'

'We argue about it.' If asked why, say you feel you should wait until you have bought a house.

'I thought maybe have some blood tests; that is what David would like.'

When the doctor asks about David or, if they don't, as soon as you can bring it into the consultation.

'David sometimes hurts me.' You have been receiving the contraceptive injection every 3 months at family planning since your coil was removed 1 year ago. You would like to leave the relationship but you are waiting for the right time. You have no concerns about your health. You had a GUM check 6 months ago because you were concerned David may have had an affair. It was normal. David drinks large amounts of alcohol after work.

He says hurtful things, e.g. that you are fat and ugly. He has never used a weapon and has never hurt another person or animal. He sometimes apologises and can be very loving. He takes no drugs and has no access to children. He has never been involved with the police and doesn't drink and drive. You do not feel he would kill anyone including yourself. You want to start thinking about ending the relationship. You tried before and he got very angry, then very remorseful and loving. You were scared and you stayed. He is controlling, but does not read your phone messages.

He pushes himself on you for sex but you do not resist. You need time to think about how and when to leave.

One year ago, you broke your thumb after he pushed you into a radiator. You have lived with his aggression for years but your mood is OK. You have never had suicidal thoughts. You have a best friend whom you may now tell. You have no money. You don't know where you would go or how you would pay for rent if you lost your job.

Discussing domestic violence

Asking about relationships is part of any social history. The doctor should always be prepared to sensitively ask about DV if there are any concerns or it crosses the doctor's mind. There are many opportunities to ask about DV: injury, pregnancy, contraception, pain (e.g. abdominal) and repeated minor illness.

Raising DV

'Tell me more about your relationship. Do you often argue?' 'Do they ever say or do anything that upsets you?'

'Do you ever feel threatened by anyone at home?' 'Is there any violence at home?'

Be aware of your local support groups for DV.

Child protection

Establish whether there is a child protection concern:

'Do they have any contact with children?' 'Do any children witness the violence?'

'Has a child been hurt?' 'How are the children getting on?' 'How are they getting on at school?'

'Is there any pet abuse?'

Ensure immediate reporting to the local safeguarding team if another adult or child is at risk. When children are in the home, even if the parent/guardian feels the children are not affected by the violence, they almost always are in some way and so reporting to the local safeguarding team should be discussed.

How to approach a consultation if the perpetrator, not the victim, presents

'You have honestly explained when you feel angry you …' 'And recognise this is serious.'

'It sounds as if you would like to receive help for this?' 'What thoughts have you had?'

'We have local teams … e.g. Give Respect – here is their number.'

'May I ask you to see me again and follow this up …?'

'Could you bring your husband/wife with you next time?'

Do not collude or offer relationship counselling.

Coercive controlling behaviour (CCB)[1]

As well as asking about DV, the doctor should be aware of the possibility of CCB – which is emotional abuse that is damaging to the mental health of the victim and is illegal in the UK. In the example consultation, there is evidence of CCB as well as DV. David says hurtful things, he is controlling, he became angry when Isabel wanted to leave and he forces sex. Some features of CCB include:

- Controlling aspects of another's life – where they go, who they can meet. Repeated 'put-downs' – *'You're fat and ugly'*.
- Controlling finances or access to money. Humiliating or degrading behaviour.
- 'Gaslighting', e.g. hiding things, denying something that's been said, telling lies so that the victim starts to question their own reality and even thinks they are losing their mind.

> **'The victim becomes captive in an unreal world created by the abuser, entrapped in a world of confusion, contradiction and fear.'**
>
> Professor Evan Stark[2]

Doctor's Notes

Patient	Janine Paton	33 years	F
PMH	Cerebral palsy		
	Severe learning disability		
	Constipation		
	Urinary tract infections		
	Epilepsy – no seizure for 2 years		
Medications	Laxido sachets 1 daily		
	Sodium valproate 1 g daily		
	Carbamazepine 400 mg BD		
Allergies	None		
Consultations	Nurse in minor illness clinic 2 days ago – seems tired and staff have noticed she looks pale. Eats reasonably well, bowels regular, no black stools. No symptoms of infection. No weight loss. Has heavy periods with clots – last 7 days, cycle is 28 days. Not on OCP or other medication for this. Never been sexually active		
	BMI 28, HR 70, BP 130/70. HS normal, chest clear, abdomen soft, non-tender, no masses		
	Needs blood test – to book in with phlebotomy, then GP appointment		
Investigations	None		
Household	None		

Ruth, Janine's carer, has requested a telephone appointment today.

Example Consultation **Mental Health and Learning Disability**

Open ☐ Hello, Ruth, I'm Dr Blount. It is a pleasure to meet you. You wanted to talk about Janine? Oh dear, I'm sorry to hear that. Can you take me back to the beginning and tell me what you have noticed about Janine? Anything else that has changed? Or changes in behaviour? Or communication? I'm wondering what Janine is like when she is feeling herself?

Curious ☐ Does Janine use any special ways of communicating? OK, so if she claps that means yes.

Experience ☐ Tell me what happened last time Janine needed a blood test. Oh dear, that sounds difficult.

History ☐ You asked what else might be causing her to look pale and be tired. How is Janine's appetite? Does she eat a good diet with protein and vegetables? How often is she opening her bowels? Any black sticky stools or bleeding from the back passage? Any blood in her wee? And please tell me about her periods. Any clots? How often are you needing to change her pads? Does she seem to be in pain? Is she sexually active?

Flags ☐ Has she lost any weight? Has her tummy been swollen? How is her sleep?

ICE1 ☐ Ruth – what are your thoughts about Janine's blood test?

ICE2 ☐ Is there anything else that you are worrying might be wrong?

Sense ☐ Ruth – you clearly care about Janine, she is fortunate to have you looking after her.

ICE3 ☐ Tell me what you thought I might say about how to enable her to have a blood test.

SummarICE ☐ To summarise – Janine looks pale and seems tired. Her diet is less good than usual, but no weight loss. Periods are very heavy with clots, which is unusual. You need to change her pads frequently. You know she needs a blood test for anaemia but worry about how this can get done. Janine hates needles and was distressed yesterday and you worry about her returning to the surgery. She has a good relationship with her ID nurse who visits at the care home.

Impression ☐ I am not entirely sure what is going on and that's why we need a blood test. From what you have said, the likeliest cause would be heavy periods, perhaps not helped by a slightly poorer diet. You asked about her tablets – carbamazepine and valproate. Whilst both of these can cause anaemia, it is not common at all, but we do need to check this out on the blood test.

InCludE ☐ You wondered about sedation – I'm not sure about that but I do wonder if we could make use of Janine's good relationship with her ID nurse and ask the nurse to come to the home to do the blood test? Also, I could prescribe some special numbing cream called EMLA which the nurse could rub into Janine's arm about 20 minutes before the blood test. Then she won't feel the needle going in. Would you be able to distract her?

Empathy ☐ I appreciate it is very difficult caring for Janine and being concerned about her, knowing that she needs a blood test and worried about how to go about this.

Options ☐ I can speak to the ID nurse and ask if she will do the blood test. Once we have this back, perhaps we could arrange to talk again? If, as I suspect, she is anaemic due to heavy periods, we could prescribe some tablets to take during her period to make the bleeding lighter, or start the OCP. We can also prescribe a course of iron tablets to treat the anaemia.

Empower ☐ Ruth – it would help if you encourage Janine to eat a diet rich in iron and green leafy vegetables. It's great that you can understand her needs through her clapping to indicate 'yes'. Could you point to parts of her body and ask her to clap if that part doesn't feel okay?

Future ☐ So, we will arrange for the ID nurse to take some blood tests to look at her blood count and vitamin levels as well as liver, kidney and thyroid function. I will send through a prescription for the EMLA cream to numb her arm.

Specifics ☐ Let's book a video call with Janine next week to review the blood tests and catch up.

Safety net ☐ If any new symptoms develop or Janine seems worse, please let me know.

Doctor's notes Janine Paton, 33 years. PMH: cerebral palsy, severe LD, constipation, UTIs and epilepsy – no seizure for 2 years. Medications: Laxido sachets 1 daily, sodium valproate 1 g daily, carbamazepine 400 mg BD.

Nurse appointment 2 days ago – seems tired and staff have noticed she looks pale. Eats reasonably well, bowels regular, no black stools. No symptoms of infection. No weight loss. Has heavy periods with clots – last 7 days, cycle is 28 days. Not on OCP or other medication for this. Never been sexually active.

Examination: BMI 28, HR 70, BP 130/70. HS normal, chest clear, abdomen soft, non-tender, no masses.

Needs blood test – to book in with phlebotomy, then GP appointment.

How to act You are the carer, Ruth. You are concerned about Janine and try to communicate this to the doctor.

PC *'I brought Janine to see the nurse yesterday. She needs a blood test, but I don't know how we are going to manage this – she is terrified of needles.'*

History Janine has been really tired recently and looks pale so you brought her to the nurse. The nurse asked lots of questions and found out that Janine has heavy periods and her diet has been a bit less good lately. Janine is non-verbal but can clap when she means 'yes'. Janine usually enjoys sitting in the lounge and watching television shows. She also likes it when music is on. However, over the past 2 months, she has not looked interested and stays in her room more. She seems 'weaker' because she has not got the same energy. She does not cry but sometimes makes a wailing sound.

Her urine does not smell abnormal. She is not vomiting. She has required more encouragement to eat her food and she often leaves a lot of it. She has not lost weight. Janine is opening her bowels once daily with Laxido. No rectal bleeding.

Janine has regular periods, the last one being 2 weeks ago. They are heavy with clots, lasting 1 week, and you need to change her pad at least 6 × per day.

Janine does not walk and transfers with the help of two carers between the bed and wheelchair. The carers have no information on Janine's family.

Social Janine lives in a home with several other residents cared for by the staff. Her learning disability nurse visits regularly and they seem to have a good relationship.

ICE You were worried something might be seriously wrong and hope the nurse is right that it is heavy periods. *'Could anything else be causing this?'*

But you are now concerned about how you can get Janine to have a blood test.

You also want to know why she might be anaemic. *'Could it be the medication for her epilepsy that is causing this?' 'Is it her diet?'*

You expect the doctor will tell you more about why she might be anaemic but have no idea what might be suggested to get Janine to have a blood test – though perhaps she could be sedated? *'Could she have sedation for the blood test?'*

In *Valuing People* (2001) 'learning disability (LD)' is defined as a 'significantly reduced ability to understand new or complex information, to learn new skills, reduced ability to cope independently, which starts before adulthood with lasting effects on development.'[1]

In the UK, the terms 'learning disability' (LD) and 'intellectual disability' (ID) are generally used interchangeably. The RCGP 2025 curriculum uses the term 'learning disability'.

As a GP, your role is to 'diagnose, investigate and manage people with learning disabilities, using history, examination, monitoring and referral where appropriate. Consider how differences can vary over time as well as between individuals.'[2]

The patient may struggle to express or verbalise their emotions. Helpful questions to consider include:

- Has there been a change in behaviour?
- Do they feel angry?
- Are there any changes to their routine – sleep or eating?
- Is there concern among family members?
- Can a collateral history be obtained?

'GPs should be able to recognise the following: atypical presentation of psychiatric or physical illness because of sensory, communication and cognitive difficulties.'[2]

Use language without jargon, seek a collateral history; however, also screen for risk of neglect and this includes seeing the patient alone.

Use open screening questions for physical and mental health problems and social challenges. Have vigilance and a high level of suspicion for atypical presentations of conditions.

Have a low threshold for suspicion of mental health problems and be proactive in enquiring about subtle changes and atypical presentations.

Other suggestions/tips to demonstrate the RCGP curriculum …

'coordinate care with carers and other organisations and professionals (including other health, education and social care services) and consider when and how best to share information'[2]

- Demonstrate your awareness of this by guiding where the patient can go to seek more information.

'Offer regular advice and support to patients, relatives and carers regarding prevention, prescribing, monitoring and self-management to address poorer health outcomes, reduced life expectancy and overall health inequalities.'[2]

- Tailor the examination to the condition and life stage. A complete assessment should also be performed in the annual health check.

- Signpost that, following your initial thorough examination and the investigation results, you may consider the help of the learning disability team.

'The care of people with learning disabilities is a multi-agency activity that involves the patient, their carers and professionals from health and social care. Your learning with other professionals is, therefore, very important to gain a better understanding of their roles and how best care may be delivered.'[2]

- Always ask about those who support or care for the patient. How are the relationships? Ask about the carer's health and concerns.

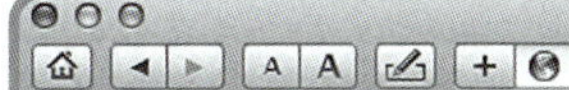

Doctor's Notes

Patient Raymond Styles 86 years M

PMH Ankle fracture placed in cast 3 weeks ago

Prostate cancer

Medications None

Allergies None

Consultations This morning, the carer called and the paramedic made a home visit. Notes:

'R leg pain and swelling. Suspected DVT. Refusing transfer to hospital. Examination findings: Sats 95%. RR 18. HR 108 bpm. Chest exam normal. Apyrexial. Left leg in cast. Right leg red and swollen, with tenderness in the calf and pitting oedema to knee. Calf circumference cannot be compared because left leg is in a cast.

GP to phone please'

Investigations 1 month ago – FBC, U&E and LFT normal

Household No household members registered

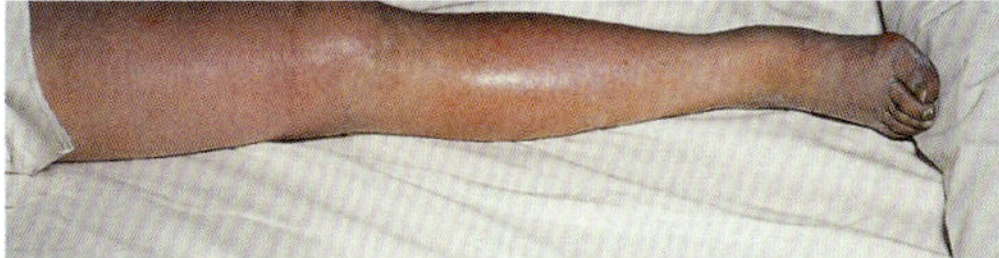

From: *Browse's Introduction to the Symptoms and Signs of Surgical Disease* (2021), CRC Press. With thanks to Kevin Burnand, Bijan Modarai and Ashish Patel.

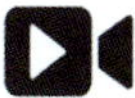

Example Consultation

Suspected DVT

Open ☐ I'm pleased your carer called. Tell me more about this pain and swelling. Is there anything else you have noticed?

ICE1 ☐ What do you think has caused the pain and swelling in your leg?

Flags ☐ Do you feel breathless? Are you coughing up anything? Any blood? Do you have any pain in your chest? Have you had a temperature?

ICE2 ☐ Is there anything you are worried it may be?

ICE3 ☐ Have you had any thoughts about what we might do today?

Sense ☐ You don't seem too concerned by this?

History ☐ How are you in general – your health? Are you otherwise well? Do you have family?

Curious ☐ Tell me more about your experience of hospital.

Impact ☐ Things must have been hard since you lost Maggie. How do you spend your days?

Empathy ☐ I hear that you do not want to have the same experience as your wife and will not go to hospital.

Empower ☐ No one will force you. I must explain to you what I think so you can make an informed decision, but you are in charge.

SummarICE ☐ Although you suspect the pain and swelling may be serious, you are clear that you don't want to go into hospital but might be willing to have treatment at home, so long as it is straightforward and doesn't need blood tests.

Impression ☐ I believe you almost certainly have a blood clot in your leg called a deep vein thrombosis, a DVT. There is a real risk that this could travel to your lungs and make you very ill – you could even die from this. Your broken leg has made you less mobile and having prostate cancer puts you at increased risk; therefore, I think this is most likely.

Recommend ☐ Usually in this situation, I would arrange for you to go to the hospital for a scan of your veins. At the hospital I would expect them to do a scan and a blood test so they could find out exactly what is wrong. I understand you're not keen on this; if I were to explain to the medical staff your previous experience and tell them you would want to come home as soon as possible, would this change your mind?

InCludE ☐ I respect any decision you make. Can I check that we have understood each other correctly? You are aware that I believe you should go to hospital for tests, and not going to hospital may mean ongoing pain in your leg or serious breathing problems and you could die from this. Can you repeat to me what we have just talked about so I can check you understand? Thank you.

Options ☐ If you won't go to hospital, would you take some tablets at home that would thin your blood? They make it less likely that any blood clot goes to your lungs. The downside of this tablet is it can make you more likely to bleed and, rarely, they can cause serious bleeding.

Explanation ☐ The tablet is called apixaban. You should take it twice a day and it's important to keep taking it and not stop it – otherwise your blood would soon start to clot again and this could cause serious problems. I can see you had a recent blood test that shows your liver and kidneys are working well so we can avoid doing another blood test today as you wish. Do you have any questions?

Future ☐ I suggest taking paracetamol, two tablets regularly, for pain relief. Don't take ibuprofen as this interferes with apixaban. I will e-consult with the doctors at the DVT clinic to explain about your situation and get advice about how long you should take the apixaban, but it is likely to be 3 months.

Safety net ☐ If you get short of breath, chest pain, cough up blood or your leg swelling or pain gets worse, please call the surgery, 111 if the surgery is closed or 999 if you have changed your mind about hospital. After starting the apixaban, if you notice any bleeding, please ring for advice straight away.

Patient's Story

Suspected DVT

Doctor's notes Raymond Styles, 86 years.

PMH: left ankle fracture placed in cast 3 weeks ago. Prostate cancer. Medications: none.

This morning, the carer called and the paramedic made a home visit: 'R leg pain and swelling. Suspected DVT. Refusing transfer to hospital. Examination findings: Sats 95%. RR 18. HR 108 bpm. Chest exam normal. Apyrexial. Left leg in cast. Right leg red and swollen, with tenderness in the calf and pitting oedema to knee. Calf circumference cannot be compared because left leg is in a cast. GP to phone please.'

Investigations: 1 month ago – FBC, U&E and LFT normal.

How to act Respectful and apologetic. Dismissive of your symptoms. Under no circumstances are you going to hospital for any tests. You will accept tablets to thin your blood but want as little fuss as possible.

PC *'Doctor, I'm sorry they called you. I'm fine now.'*

History You have prostate cancer. You were offered but declined hormone treatment for this but are currently not troubled by it.

Your carer called the doctor because she noticed that your right leg was swollen. You feel a little cross about this as you don't like to waste the doctor's time.

You first noticed your leg swelling and pain yesterday and have no chest pain or breathlessness. No fever. No confusion.

You have never felt this pain before. *'I must have pulled a muscle.'*

Social You live alone with carers attending four times daily at present, whilst your leg is in cast. You have no family.

ICE You do not know what has caused the pain and swelling. You suspect it may be serious.

If asked about any negative experiences: your wife, Maggie, died in the hospital and you do not want to have the same happen to you. Refuse to go to hospital whatever the doctor says. You will reluctantly accept tablets if the doctor persuades you but do not want injections or anything that needs frequent blood tests for monitoring, such as warfarin.

Learning Points

This case tests your ability to assess a patient with suspected DVT, and assess capacity.

Two-level DVT Wells score[3]

If you suspect DVT in a woman who is pregnant or has given birth in the last 6 weeks refer for same-day assessment and management. Otherwise use the two-level DVT Wells score: score 1 point for:

- Active cancer (treatment ongoing, within the last 6 months or palliative).
- Paralysis, paresis or recent plaster immobilisation of the legs.
- Recently bedbound for 3 days or more, or major surgery within the last 12 weeks requiring general or regional anaesthesia.
- Localised tenderness along the distribution of the deep venous system (such as the back of the calf).
- Entire leg is swollen.
- Calf swelling ≥3 cm compared with the asymptomatic leg.
- Pitting oedema present in symptomatic leg only.
- Collateral superficial veins (non-varicose).
- Previously documented DVT.

Subtract 2 points if an alternative cause is considered at least as likely as DVT.

Score ≥2 means DVT is *likely*, <2 means DVT is *unlikely*.

DVT pathway

For people who are *likely* to have DVT as assessed above:

- Follow local pathways to arrange an urgent USS of the leg – ideally within 4 hours.
- If this is not possible, arrange D-dimer and start anticoagulation and arrange proximal leg vein USS with results available in 24 hours.

For people who are *unlikely* to have DVT as assessed above:

- Offer D-dimer test first. If results within 4 hours are not possible then offer interim anticoagulation until result is available. This is likely to involve referral to haematology through your local VTE pathway.
- If D-dimer test is positive, arrange USS of leg.
- If D-dimer test is negative, stop treatment and consider alternative diagnosis.

If interim therapeutic anticoagulation is required:

- First line: apixaban or rivaroxaban (follow local formulary).
- Second line: LMWH for 5 days followed by dabigatran, edoxaban or LMWH + warfarin.
- Consider co-morbidities, contraindications and patient choice when selecting the anticoagulant.
- Check FBC, U&E, LFT, PT and APTT. Treat whilst awaiting results + review these promptly.

Assessing capacity

To do this you need to ensure that the patient understands the information, is able to remember this long enough to make a decision, can weigh up the risks and repeat these to the doctor, and can communicate their decision.

If a patient has capacity, is aware of the risk to life and all the risks of not following advice, and you cannot persuade them, you must respect the patient's autonomy. You should ask about involving family members and consider how else you can help the patient, including end-of-life and DNACPR discussions. However, you should not simply wash your hands of the patient because they have ignored your advice. Think about ways you can still help the patient, keep them safe and allow them the opportunity to change their mind.

Explore in detail WHY the patient refuses hospital. Explain what you expect would happen there. Learn about your local emergency care team (for patient who cares for others) and help for pets, e.g. Dogs Trust.

Doctor's Notes

Patient	Kirsty West	38 years	F
PMH	None		
Medications	None		
Allergies	None		
Consultations	None		
Investigations	None		
Household	Simeon West	42 years	M
	Rose West	11 years	F
	Toby West	6 years	M

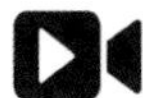

Example Consultation

Alcohol and Safeguarding

Open ☐ Please tell me the story from when this began.

History ☐ How is your husband's health? How is his mood? And how about you? Do you work? Do you have any close family or friends? Are they aware? Do you drink any alcohol? What has made you contact me today – has something happened?

Flags ☐ Does he suffer with low mood or anxiety? Is there any violence in the home? How have the children reacted? Does your husband drive? Does your husband take care of the children alone? Does he ever take drugs?

ICE1 ☐ What has been going through your mind?

Impact ☐ What impact has his drinking had on you? Your relationship? The children? How are you coping financially?

ICE2 ☐ What makes you feel most upset?

Sense ☐ I can hear how exhausting this is for you.

ICE3 ☐ Did you have anything in your mind that you thought we may decide today?

Curious ☐ You haven't asked your family for help – I'm wondering why that is. (Pause) Are you close to them? How may they react? Do you feel there is risk of violence if your husband knew you were speaking to me? What was his experience of the navy?

SummarICE ☐ To summarise, you are very concerned about the amount your husband is drinking and the impact this is having on your family. You are worried he won't find work and that home life will continue to be stressful. You are aware the children are having to make their own meals at times, and you have felt too embarrassed to inform your parents.

InCludE ☐ You were hoping I could speak to your husband. You don't know what else to do.

Empathy ☐ Kirsty, I can hear this is a really difficult situation. Running the home falls on you and you recognise your husband may be depressed and want to seek help for your family.

Impression ☐ It sounds as if your husband is drinking a harmful amount; he may be depressed too.

Options ☐ There is much we can do to help Simeon: support, medication, counselling and advice – I can call him to discuss. You may also wish to go to relationship counselling together, or you yourself could access counselling, perhaps also seeing me to discuss your health and wellbeing. Many others can also help, e.g. dedicated services for veterans. I wonder if your children need someone to talk to? I am concerned that they are having to make their own meals. When any children are involved, I have a duty to inform the safeguarding team, social services. I can hear you are upset; what is going through your mind?

Experience ☐ What do you know about social services?

Explanation ☐ This is not what you expected, but I believe it would be a positive step. This team will be able to provide you with support during this time of crisis. Social services aim to help families through difficult times and not take children from their parents. Your husband sounds unwell and it seems you would welcome additional help. Do I have your support to inform this team so they can contact you to make their assessment and offer help?

Empower ☐ Could you discuss our conversation with your husband? What do you think he'll say? If he will not talk to me on the phone, I could visit. I wonder if you need a work note so you can either leave work early or have time off work if you feel you need to relieve this pressure. We have identified many options today. Out of these options can you summarise how you would like to proceed? How do you feel about talking to your parents too, for their support?

Specifics ☐ We should talk again, ideally with your husband present, within the week. Which day would suit you? Let's book the appointment for a further video call now.

Safety net ☐ If ever you feel there is a risk to anyone, including your husband, contact the police, the surgery or 111.

Patient's Story

Doctor's notes Kirsty West, 38 years. PMH: none. Medications: none.

How to act Concerned. Articulate. You are mentally and physically well.

PC *'Doctor, I want to talk about my husband's drinking.'*

History He is in good health but has started drinking half a bottle of whisky every night.

He is a veteran and has struggled to find work since leaving the Royal Navy where he was a technician, was made redundant from his new job as a security guard last year and now can't find a job. You are worried and angry.

You were used to being on your own when he was at sea, and managed the home and children well, but now life has changed as he is back but has stopped interacting with the children and you feel the pressure. Your relationship is strained as you are often angry with him.

There is no violence in the home. You think he is depressed. His experience of the navy did not leave him with PTSD but he has been 'down' since he left the services.

You are looking after the children, running the home as well as bringing in the income. You are not depressed, *'just fed up with it.'*

Last night he fell over. He was not injured but the children started to cry.

Social You work full time in a pharmacy as an assistant and return home at 7 p.m. You drink no alcohol. Your children are 6 and 11 years old. You have no time for hobbies. Your family are close by. You've felt too embarrassed to tell your parents about the problem.

ICE *'I don't know what to do.'*

You are worried he will never get a job now and you can't see life getting better.

'Will you come to the house to see him? He may listen to you.'

If the doctor asks to arrange a phone call with your husband, you think this may be helpful.

If asked, you feel the children are starting to become withdrawn and spending more time in their rooms. He is not violent. He is home alone with the children after school and on Saturdays. He does not drive. The children return home on the school bus. He sometimes makes their tea but often the older child is making them beans on toast.

If the doctor mentions contacting social services, start to cry. Tell the doctor the children are safe. Then suggest you will inform your parents, who can look after the children. Plead with the doctor not to inform social services and be angry – you have asked for help!

If the doctor suggests a work note for altered hours for you whilst your husband seeks help, or they explain why social services need to be informed, agree you need help. You accept any suggestions offered. You believe your husband will accept help when he is aware of how serious this is.

Learning Points

Harmful drinking 'A pattern of alcohol consumption that is causing mental or physical damage.'[1]

Hazardous drinking 'A pattern of alcohol consumption that increases someone's risk of harm. Some would limit this definition to the physical or mental health consequences (as in harmful use). Others would include the social consequences. The term is currently used by WHO to describe this pattern of alcohol consumption. It is not a diagnostic term.'[1]

Alcohol dependence 'A cluster of behavioural, cognitive and physiological factors that typically include a strong desire to drink alcohol and difficulties in controlling its use. Someone who is alcohol dependent may persist in drinking, despite harmful consequences. They will also give alcohol a higher priority than other activities and obligations.'[1] For further information, please refer to *Diagnostic and Statistical Manual of Mental Disorders*, 5th edition (DSM-5-TR) (American Psychiatric Association, 2023)[2] and *International Classification of Diseases,* 11th Revision (ICD-11) (World Health Organization, 2022).[3]

Safeguarding

This case requires the doctor to negotiate speaking to the husband and the safeguarding referral. It can be difficult to decide when social services should be involved. If you are considering it, it is likely that a referral is required and, if safe to do so, make your thoughts known to the patient. You may signpost that you will seek advice from your safeguarding lead and be in touch with the patient/relative again.

Safeguarding teams ask that you gain consent from the parent before making the referral. You can also proceed without consent if this is not forthcoming.

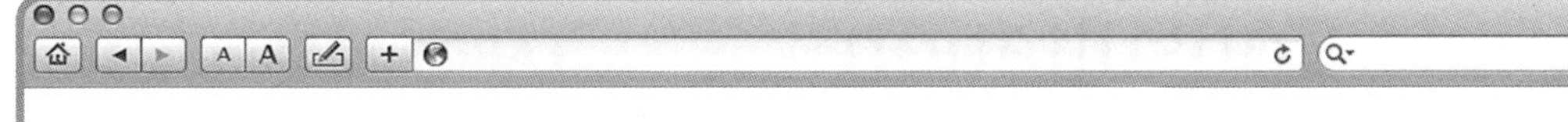

Doctor's Notes

Patient	Fedora Baros	38 years	F
PMH	None		
Medications	Ovranette		
Allergies	None		
Consultations	No recent consultations but has army medical records		
Investigations	None		
Household	None		

Example Consultation

LARC and Sterilisation

Open ☐ Please tell me about what has led to this decision.

History ☐ I'm interested to know more about you Fedora. Do you have any medical history? I see you were recently in the army. Please tell me about your service history.

Sense ☐ I'm sorry to hear about Afghanistan – that must have been very upsetting.

Flags ☐ How is your mood now? Any nightmares, flashbacks or anxiety? Please tell me what you experience. Are you getting any help for this, from the army or psychological services?

Risk ☐ Before thinking about sterilisation or other choices, I need to ask some personal questions: please tell me about your periods. Any abnormal bleeding between periods, after sex, or heavier bleeding or discharge? Any pain on intercourse or infections in the past 3 months? Are your periods manageable or painful? Do you have a partner? Any chance you might be pregnant?

ICE1 ☐ What thoughts have you had about contraception? What is right for you?

ICE2 ☐ Did you have any concerns about either procedure? How would you feel if you did fall pregnant? It sounds as if this would be stressful for you.

Impact ☐ Sterilisation is permanent. You should be at peace with it being irreversible.

Sense ☐ You were not expecting me to say that? Does this change things?

ICE3 ☐ What are your thoughts now about what we should decide today?

SummarICE ☐ To summarise, you once thought you would have children, but being in the army and witnessing traumatic events has cast doubt. Part of you is unsure. You've enjoyed your baby nephew. Also, you have flashbacks and nightmares, but have not had help. You're looking for work, money is tight and you are fed up with the pill. So, you requested sterilisation with the view to reversal in the future, but you didn't know it is permanent. We discussed regret; e.g. if you found work, life improved and you wanted children. Another option is the coil, but you don't want erratic bleeding and like regular periods.

Impression ☐ You would like reliable, hormone-free reversible contraception which you can forget about – perhaps the copper coil. You also want to be rid of the nightmares and flashbacks. Let's think about contraception first.

Options ☐ Condoms, a diaphragm or a copper coil avoid hormones. Or, you could continue with the pill or contraceptive injection or skin implant.

Experience ☐ What do you understand about how the coil, or IUD, works? And the risks?

Explanation ☐ The copper coil, with no hormones, usually gives regular periods, but perhaps heavier and longer. The hormone coil gives regular lighter bleeding, erratic bleeding or no bleeding at all. As your periods are manageable, you may be okay with a copper coil. No contraception is 100% but the coil is very reliable. But, if you fell pregnant, there is an increased risk of ectopic pregnancy, outside the womb, which is dangerous. There is a risk of infection when we fit the coil, so we take swabs first and use sterile equipment. When we fit it, it may briefly hurt, like a period cramp, or your BP may drop. There is a 1–2/1000 chance of the coil going through the womb and a 1 in 20 chance the coil may fall out, especially in the first few months.

For your nightmares and flashbacks – which are very common amongst veterans – help is available either through the NHS psychological services or dedicated veterans' support. I can give you contact details for both of these.

Empower ☐ Have you decided or would you like further information? Would you like to see our social prescriber to help you return to work, and tell you about support for veterans?

Empathy ☐ It is a lot of information and a big decision.

Specifics ☐ Please call me when you have decided about contraception or if you have further questions.

Patient's Story

Doctor's notes Fedora Baros, 38 years. PMH: none. Medications: Ovranette. Single.

How to act Very pleasant.

PC *'I would like to be sterilised please.'*

History You are an army veteran and have decided that the world is not a fit place for children.

You have a current partner but you are sure you don't want children and he does not mind if you do or don't. Some years ago, you thought that you would have a big family, but serving in the army has changed your views. *'The world doesn't need more children.'*

You are very well and have no medical history. You take no medicines apart from Ovranette.

Social You are currently unemployed. Being in the army was great and you served abroad including active service in Afghanistan. But this was also traumatic and you saw many hungry children and some who had lost limbs. You were also close to explosions and have recurrent nightmares. *'Those explosions – I keep hearing them, they wake me up.'* There are enough children in the world without you having more. But you are not sure and are wavering … your sister recently had a baby and you do enjoy being with her baby son. Money is currently tight and you are on benefits and looking for work. You spend your days cooking and looking after your home.

You are in a stable relationship with a male partner, Steve. He is a joiner.

You don't smoke or drink alcohol.

ICE You are fed up with taking the OCP. You don't want any hormones in your body. You have concerns about the coil as you have heard that it is painful, so you think you will be sterilised for now and then have it reversed if you change your mind.

In your mind, sterilisation can be reversed by putting the tubes back together. If asked about your risk of regret, you become unsure.

If the coil is suggested, your main concern is erratic bleeding. You like predictable monthly periods.

If the doctor explains how the coil is inserted and discusses the risks, you decide you feel comfortable about having this procedure.

You had not thought of getting help for your nightmares and flashbacks but are very interested if this is suggested.

Learning Points

Contraceptive implant[1]

Implant indication LARC or dysmenorrhoea.

How to take Insert in days 1–5 of cycle. Repeat within 3 years.

Side effects Acne, bleeding changes, mood or libido changes and headaches reported although 'no evidence of a causal association'.[1] No osteoporosis risk.

Bleeding risk Approximately 25% of people have regular periods, 33% infrequent bleeding, 20% no bleeding and 25% frequent/prolonged bleeding.[1]

Lost implant If impalpable implant, use additional contraception and arrange an USS.

Problematic bleeding Exclude pregnancy, chlamydia and malignancy (view cervix).

Consider an additional hormone off-licence (COCP or POP) for 3 months or a 5-day course of mefenamic acid.[1]

Use judgement: risks are unknown with longer use; see guidance.

Injection[2]

Side effects The same as other progesterone contraceptives and 'associated with weight gain'.[2]

Fertility Can be delayed for up to 1 year after discontinuation.[2]

BMD Small loss of BMD usually recovers after discontinuation. Review 2-yearly.[2]

Caution/CI Maximum recommended age of 50 years. Caution in CVD.[2]

IUS (Mirena)/IUD (copper coil)[3]

Indication IUS = LARC, progesterone cover for HRT and menorrhagia.

IUD = LARC and emergency contraception.

Mode of action IUS prevents implantation. IUD prevents fertilisation and implantation.

Risks Infection, perforation, failure rate, ectopic, expulsion and cervical shock.

Contraindications Must be 'reasonably certain'[2] she is not pregnant.

See also UKMEC guidance.[3]

Side effects IUS: erratic bleeding. Small risk of systemic progesterone side effects.

IUD may give longer/heavier periods. Tampons can be used.

Licensing of duration Mirena – now licensed for 8 years for contraception, but 5 years only for HRT.

Jaydess – licensed for 3 years for contraception only, not HRT.

Copper – depends on the device; it can be 5 or 10 years, so check the device.

Resources for veterans

Veterans Gateway provides information and support for veterans 24/7 including help with housing, finances and mental wellbeing (telephone 0808 802 1212).

Ministry of Defence Veterans UK provides support and compensation if appropriate (telephone 0808 191 4218).

Combat Stress provides clinical treatment and support for veterans with a focus on those with complex mental health issues (free helpline 24/7 – 0800 138 1619).

CHAPTER 9

ETHNICITY, CULTURE, DIVERSITY AND INCLUSIVITY

	Cases in this chapter	RCGP 2025 curriculum	Learning points
9.1	Squint	**Eyes and vision** 'Squint – childhood and acquired due to nerve palsy, amblyopia, blepharospasm'	Causes and management of squint Link to video of ophthalmologist describing squint and its treatment for patients/carers
9.2	Melasma	**Dermatology** 'Hyperpigmentation'	When to refer Treatment Melasma area and severity index
9.3	Education about Services	**Neurodevelopment conditions and neurodiversity** 'Difficulties with communication, social relationships or managing daily affairs'	Educating families with regard to how to use local services
9.4	Occupational Allergy	**Allergy and immunology** **Dermatology** 'Eczema – contact allergic, irritant (including occupational)'	Management of allergic contact dermatitis Taking an allergy-focused history Management of common allergic conditions Common and important allergic conditions
9.5	Sinusitis	**ENT, speech and hearing** 'Sinus problems including acute and chronic infection'	Management of sinusitis

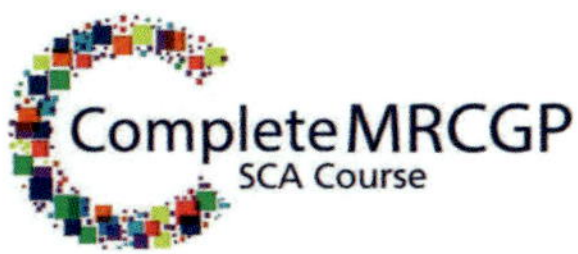

Links to the RCGP Curriculum

This broad blueprint group may feature clinical topics from throughout the curriculum and all life stages. In this chapter, the cases are drawn from the following clinical topic guides:

- Eyes and vision
- Dermatology
- Neurodevelopmental conditions and neurodiversity
- Allergy and immunology
- ENT, speech and hearing

And the following life stages topic guide:

- Children and young people

Scope of Conditions

Diversity involves recognising, respecting and valuing individuals' differences. Here are some examples of cases – this is not a complete list of all possibilities.

Examples from the RCGP website, curriculum area 'Equality, diversity and inclusion' include:

- Age, disability, gender reassignment, marital or civil partnership status, pregnancy and maternity, race, religion or belief, sex (noting that some people may not identify with either gender group, referred to as non-binary gender or non-gender) or sexual orientation
- Socioeconomic reasons (for example being homeless)
- Being a carer or being dependent
- Having a diagnosis with a potentially stigmatising condition (for example mental health or lifestyle-related conditions such as obesity or those caused by smoking, alcohol or drug use)
- Those with a criminal history, sex workers or those with different political views

Also for this blueprint group:

- Those with different healthcare expectations
- Ethnicity
- Culture

Skills and Pitfalls

In addition to the information in Chapter 1 'How to Demonstrate Skills: The Marking Scheme Made Easy' consider the following challenges for this blueprint group:

- Recognise that because, as doctors, we have authority and influence over colleagues and patients, it is particularly important not to discriminate against people.
- Recognise, respect and value differences.
- Empathise with individual situations and circumstances.
- Consider the person's challenge in the context of their life.
- Address the impact of the individual's challenges.
- Demonstrate your commitment to considering all the ways you can care for the person.
- Avoid making any assumptions. Avoid judgement.
- Respect and serve people with equal regard.
- Encourage diversity and equality.

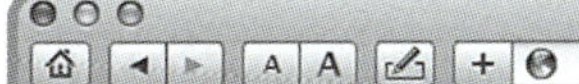

Doctor's Notes

Patient	Daniela Adamovich	4 years	F
PMH	None		
Medications	None		
Allergies	None		
Consultations	None		
Investigations	None		
Household	Ionna Adamovich	29 years	F

Photograph sent by parent yesterday requesting consultation.

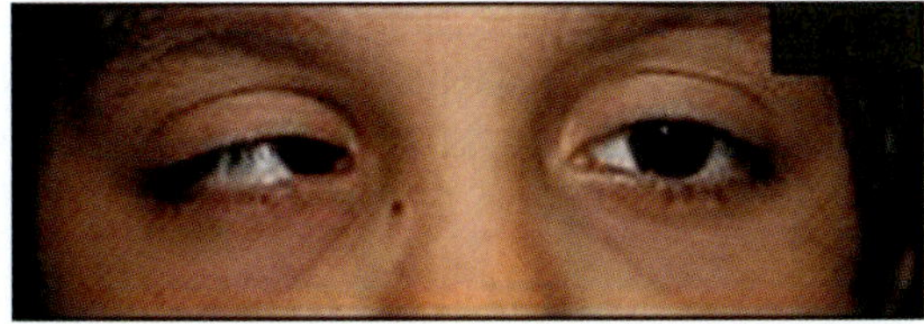

Reproduced from *Pediatric Clinical Ophthalmology* (2012), CRC Press. With thanks to Scott E. Olitsky and Leonard B. Nelson.

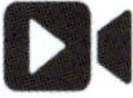

Example Consultation

Squint

Open ☐ How can I help?

History ☐ Oh I see. I'm very sorry to hear that. Please tell me more about her eyes. For example, how did you first notice this? How does her vision seem to you? And how is Daniela's health? Any previous illnesses? Does she take any medicines? What immunisations has she had? How has her development been with using her body and hands? How about her speech? And interacting with others? How is that?

Flags ☐ Has this stayed much the same or has it got worse? Does she seem to see okay? Can she run around without tripping and falling? Can she look at toys with you?

ICE1 ☐ Do you know anything about eye problems like this? Specifically, what has gone through your mind about Daniela's eye problems?

ICE2 ☐ Is there anything you've been particularly worried might be wrong? Are there any other health worries you have had?

Risk ☐ Has anyone in the family had eye problems? Did Daniela injure her eye as a baby?

Sense ☐ I sense you are worried about how she looks, about her eyesight and about whether not being able to get her to a doctor has made things worse.

Impact ☐ Tell me what's been happening in your life recently.

Curious ☐ I see you've only recently registered with us. How are you getting on in the UK?

ICE3 ☐ Is there anything specific that you hoped we might be able to do today to help?

SummarICE ☐ So, to recap, Daniela was fine at birth but, quite soon after she had an illness with a temperature, you noticed that her eyes were not straight and this has continued, not getting any better. You are worried about her vision and whether this can be corrected.

Empathy ☐ You must have been through such a lot in the last few months; I can't imagine how difficult it must have been for you. Especially on your own without your husband or family.

O/E ☐ Thank you for sending the photo. I can see what you mean as Daniela's right eye is turned in.

Impression ☐ Looking at the photo I suspect Daniela has a convergent squint.

Experience ☐ Can I check that you understand this word 'squint'? Have you heard about this before? Squints are very common; about 1 in 20 children have a squint and the good news is that we should be able to help. Convergent means pointing inwards.

Options ☐ I think we should get her eyes tested by the hospital eye specialists. They may suggest she needs to wear glasses or a patch on one eye to make the weak one stronger. This may be all she needs but she might need a small operation in the future to straighten the eyes. How do you feel about me making that referral for her?

InCLudE ☐ This is not your fault. There's nothing you've done wrong or neglected to do, it's just bad luck. You haven't left it too late for us to help Daniela.

Empower ☐ We can sort this out for you and there will be nothing to pay; NHS treatment is free. You can best help Daniela by taking her to appointments and following the treatment plan, e.g. ensuring she wears her glasses and uses an eye patch if that's what is recommended.

Future ☐ Julie, our health visitor, to get in touch? Is there anything else you need? You may be interested in a local organisation called Asylum Welcome. Also, you can meet other mums with small children at children's centres. I'll text you with the details. If ever you are unwell, we are here to help you. If we are closed, you can call 111.

Safety net ☐ If for any reason you are unable to get to her hospital appointment, please let us know. If her eyes change, or her sight seems to get worse, please contact a doctor or an optician. Opticians are available locally, usually at the shopping centres, and are also free for children – there is nothing to pay to have your child seen and tested.

Patient's Story

Squint

Doctor's notes Daniela Adamovich, 4 years. New patient. PMH: none. Medications: none. Photo sent to doctor of eyes.

How to act Worried, ground down, sad.

PC *'Her eyes are crossed, Doctor; she cannot look straight. Can anything be done?'*

History Daniela is your first child. She had lots of viral infections as a child. She has not had immunisations for a long time. There were no birth complications. No family history. You give Daniela no medication.

Social You were one of the first families to come to the UK from Ukraine when the war began. Your husband remained in Ukraine. You miss your husband, parents, brothers, sisters, nephews and nieces. You have a university degree and speak good English. You have recently moved out from the family you first stayed with and are now in temporary housing. A helper there suggested booking a GP appointment. You do not have a car so transport to the surgery is difficult this week. You therefore sent the photo.

ICE Daniela appeared normal at birth but developed 'crossed eyes' a few months after birth, after a febrile illness. You knew there was a problem but there were so many other priorities at the time. You fear that all the chaos of the war may have made it worse, especially a lack of vitamins because Daniela is such a picky eater and you did not give her vitamin drops. You are worried you have left it too late – that she will look like this forever and may not see straight. A friend said that, at 4, Daniela may be too old to have surgery and may not be able to see properly. You have little money and are unsure whether you will have to pay.

Ask the doctor *'Can anything be done?'*

'Is it my fault?'

'Can she see out of that eye?'

'Will an operation put things right?'

'Will I need to pay?'

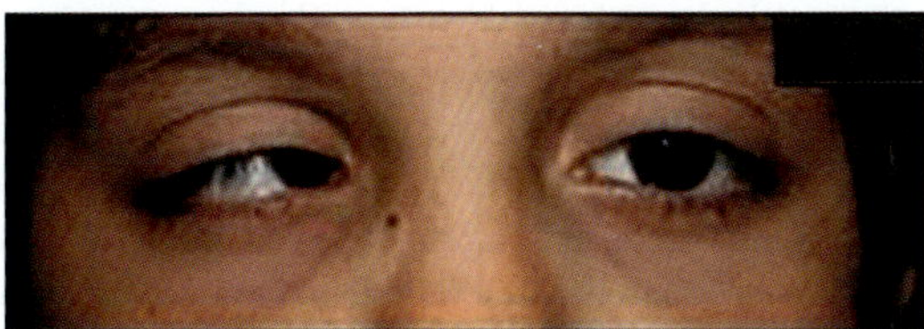

Reproduced from *Pediatric Clinical Ophthalmology* (2012), CRC Press. With thanks to Scott E. Olitsky and Leonard B. Nelson.

Learning Points

Terminology	Strabismus – any misalignment of the eyes. AKA 'squint'.[1]
	Amblyopia – decrease in vision caused by an abnormality of vision during eye development (i.e. first 2–3 years of life). Common causes are strabismus, congenital cataract and refractive error. AKA 'lazy eye'.[2]
Incidence	Squint (strabismus) is common – incidence about 1:20.[1]
Who to refer	It is 'normal' for eyes not to move together for a few weeks after birth but, if persisting longer than the age of 3 months, this needs a referral to a paediatric orthoptist.[1]
Cause[1]	Squint can appear from birth or may be acquired later.
	There can be a genetic link.
	Sometimes appears after febrile illness; however, would have happened anyway.
Complications[1]	Often associated with refraction problems such as long or short sight. Convergent squint is linked with long sight.

Treatment objectives[3]

1. Good sight in both eyes.
2. Both eyes working together (3D, stereoscopic vision).
3. Both eyes appear 'straight'.

Children often need glasses, then 'patching' of the good eye to make the weaker one stronger. If non-compliant, can use atropine drops to blur vision in the 'good' eye.[4]

Surgery is often needed to straighten the eyes. One or more muscles are tightened or detached/reattached. This is generally very successful day-case surgery and recovery is quick. The eye can feel itchy or sore for a few days afterwards. Treatment is best started as early as possible and, beyond age 6–7 years, it is difficult to achieve optimal results. 3D vision is essential for some occupations such as a fire fighter or airline pilot.

Social prescribing

Social prescribing recognises the positive impact that voluntary services can have on a patient or their family.

For example, a patient suffering with depression who is under housing, financial and emotional stress may benefit more from community advice and support than a doctor's pill. Social prescribing is a service becoming increasingly available in GP practices and the GP often refers to a social prescribing coordinator employed by the practice and commissioned by the PCN. The idea behind this is to recognise the social and psychological needs of the patient and direct patients to available community services with the aim of increasing quality of life. Local services may include: Citizen's Advice, Age UK, MIND, Asylum Services, Children's Centres, Women's Centres and hundreds/thousands more. A GP should be aware of the services available locally (community orientation).

The patient in this case is a Ukrainian who is not well versed in the structure and processes of the NHS. It is worth spelling out what may appear obvious to you but not to the patient – for example that NHS treatment is free. If the patient is worrying about cost, this may inhibit them from attending the specialist appointment.

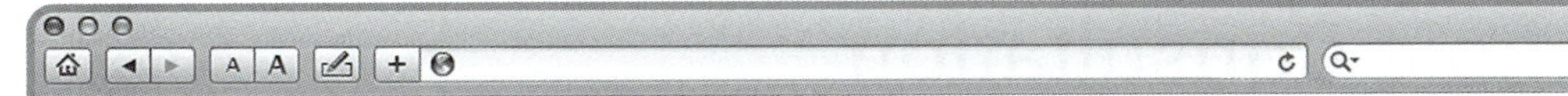

Doctor's Notes

Patient	Francesca Reece	32 years	F
PMH	None		
Medications	None		
Allergies	None		
Consultations	None		
Investigations	None		
Household	None		

Photograph sent into surgery from patient yesterday. Request for video call.

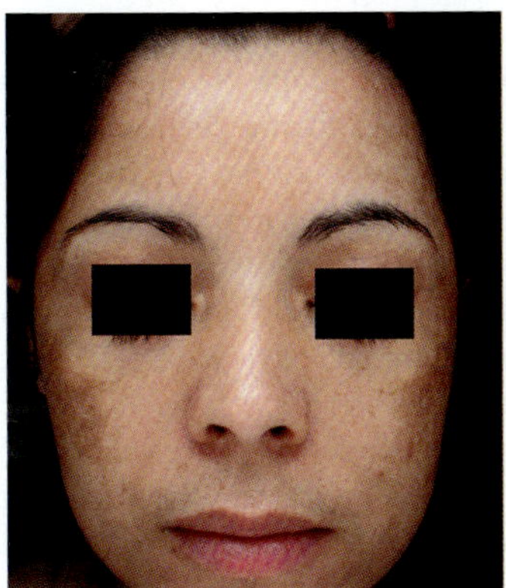

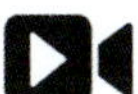

Example Consultation

Melasma

Open ☐ Tell me about this problem from the beginning. How would you describe the skin changes?

ICE1 ☐ What thoughts have you had about it?

Impact ☐ How has this affected you?

ICE2 ☐ And any particular worries that you have about your facial skin?

History ☐ Before a year ago, any problems with your skin at all? Have you any other symptoms or changes in your body elsewhere? Are you otherwise well? Any other medical conditions? Any family history of medical problems you are aware of? Do you take any medicines? Who is in your life? Do you live with anyone? So, this has been a big adjustment in your life. How are you generally? How is your relationship with your mum? How is your mood? Do you receive any support from a professional? I'll have a think about how I as your GP can help you with all the challenges you're having. How do you spend your days? What changes would you like to make for your future?

Empathy ☐ It sounds like you have had a difficult time; I'm sorry to hear that.

Risk ☐ How is your general health as a whole, as I'd like to help you in as many ways as possible? Do you drink much alcohol? Smoke? Or take drugs?

Sense ☐ It sounds like you are trying to think of positive changes you can make. That can take courage so I'm glad you came to see me today.

O/E ☐ Thank you for sending a photograph of your face. Looking at the photo, I can see some pale brown patches on your forehead and cheeks.

ICE3 ☐ I'll be sharing my recommendations; I'm wondering if there was anything specific you thought would be most helpful from me today?

Impression ☐ The skin changes on your face are called melasma.

Experience ☐ May I explain about melasma or do you already know about it?

Explanation ☐ Melasma is increased pigment in the skin. The exact cause is unknown but contributing factors are thought to be hormones, stress and sun exposure. There may be a family history.

InCludE ☐ It sounds like your hopes to make positive changes to your life, specifically rebuilding your relationship with your mum and finding work as a gardener, are important to you.

Options ☐ The sun can make melasma worse but, on balance, time outdoors sounds very therapeutic for you, so wear a hat that covers your face from the sun and apply factor 50 sun cream 2-hourly, throughout the year. By considering other things that can make melasma worse, you know what to avoid. If you use anything on your skin, make sure it is unperfumed. If, in the future, you require ibuprofen or hormone treatment, this may make melasma worse.

Recommend ☐ There are lots of creams for melasma. To start with, we could try azelaic acid 15% in the morning and adapalene at night. All creams can cause irritation, so give the skin a break for 1–2 days if this occurs. Perhaps start by using them on alternate days for a week. The risks of creams are that irritation can cause inflammation and make the pigmentation worse. What are your thoughts about this? If this doesn't help, we could try a different combination of creams. These suggestions may start to make a gradual improvement. How do you feel about the suggestions?

Empower ☐ I wonder if you would like to see my colleague who is called a social prescriber. They have wonderful knowledge of local resources, such as groups to help and support those returning to work. How would you feel about speaking to them?

Specifics ☐ Can you please make an appointment with me in 3 months so we can review your skin and how you are doing with your plans. If you are feeling frustrated, see me sooner.

Safety net ☐ If you ever notice any new skin lesions, see a GP straight away.

Patient's Story

Melasma

Doctor's notes Francesca Reece, 32 years. PMH: no information. Medications: none.

How to act Quiet, but make it clear that you would be grateful for the doctor's help.

PC *'My skin around my face looks brown.'*

History For the past year you have had discoloration around your face on the forehead and cheeks. You have not had skin changes before. You have had many chest infections or throat infections in the past but have no medical history.

Social If the doctor explores your background with specific or sensitive questions, explain that you were in prison for a year until 3 months ago. You do not wish to share the details of this if asked.

Your mental health is improving. You feel you were probably depressed before going to prison; however, this has changed now. You no longer feel low now the weather has improved and you are spending more time outdoors. You have moved back home with your mum whereas previously you lived with your partner, a relationship which has ended. Apart from a couple of friends you don't have anyone else in your life of significance. You are hoping to rebuild the relationship with your mum.

You have not worked for several years. You feel strong physically and enjoy the outdoors. You would like to become a gardener. You do not smoke or drink alcohol and have never taken drugs. You have not received any professional help.

ICE You are worried this will never go away. You do not want any medicine but would consider a cream.

Learning Points

Melasma

Ask	Family history (60% report a family history[1]).
	Sun exposure.
	Contraception.
	Impact on life and self-esteem.
	Medications can trigger a hyperpigmentation reaction, e.g. NSAID or minocycline.[1]
Blood tests	Thyroid levels if symptomatic.
	U&E if suspect Addison's disease.
Advice	Sun protection – hat and factor 50 sun cream, applied 2-hourly throughout the year.[1]
	Avoid perfumed cosmetics, deodorants or soaps.[1]
	All hormonal contraceptives can contribute, so discuss the risk/benefit of trying non-hormonal methods.
	Response to the advice and treatments can be slow.[1]
	Use make-up to disguise and camouflage the pigment.
Pregnancy	Usually melasma will start to fade a few months after pregnancy.[2]
Differential diagnosis	Post-inflammatory pigmentation.[1]
	Solar lentigines/lentigo.[1]
	Drug-induced pigmentation.[1]
	Naevus of Ota and naevus of Hori.[1]
	Addison's disease.
Severity	Melasma Area and Severity Index (MASI).[3]
Refer	For biopsy to confirm the diagnosis if uncertain.
	Consider dermatology email advice.
Treatment	'The most successful formulation has been a combination of hydroquinone, tretinoin and moderate potency topical steroid.'[1] This is available in combination as a private prescription called Pigmanorm.
	See DermNet NZ for the full list of treatments.[1]
Risks of treatment	Irritation – see BNF for individual treatment.
	Contact dermatitis and further post-inflammatory hyperpigmentation.[1]

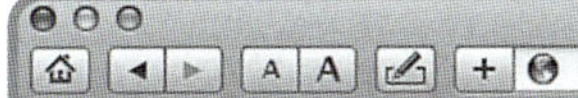

Doctor's Notes

Patient	Sara Azmeh	28 years	F
PMH	None		
Medications	None		
Allergies	None		
Consultations	None		
Investigations	None		
Household	Yusuf Azmeh	29 years	M
	Lilah Azmeh	7 years	F
	Najm Azmeh	5 years	M
	Akram Azmeh	4 years	M
	Rasha Azmeh	6 months	F

During a recent 'unplanned admission review' your practice has noted that this family have attended A&E and the out-of-hours services regularly. A letter has been sent inviting the parents to discuss the health of the family.

7 A&E attendances in 2 months with viral URTI symptoms between four children

1 A&E attendance with eczema (Akram)

1 A&E attendance with vomiting (Rasha)

1 out-of-hours attendance due to running out of salbutamol inhaler (Lilah)

1 out-of-hours attendance due to hay fever symptoms (Yusuf)

No admissions required, discharged back to GP care after each attendance

Example Consultation

Education about Services

Open ☐ Thank you for talking on the phone. As you have recently joined our practice, I wanted to discuss your family's health and offer help and support.

ICE3 ☐ Was there anything you were hoping for from our discussion today?

Open ☐ Could you tell me more about your family? Welcome to York. How are you settling in? What did you experience in Afghanistan? I'm sorry to hear what you've been through.

Impact ☐ How have you coped with the stress of the move? We are here to help your family.

History ☐ Are you well? How are you doing emotionally and mentally? And your husband? Have you made friends? Did you work in Afghanistan? Time to settle in is important, but do you have plans? Good luck with your studies! Are your children in school? Tell me about each family member: how they are coping and their health.

Sense ☐ I sense you are particularly worried about breathing problems in the children.

Curious ☐ Have you had any bad experiences with asthma or chest infections?

ICE1 ☐ How do you feel the children are at present?

ICE2 ☐ Do you have any particular worries about yourself, your husband or your children?

Experience ☐ Do you know where you can get help from if someone in the family is poorly?

SummarICE ☐ To summarise, your family have moved away from where you felt in great danger and it has been hard for you all. You feel exhausted and miss your loved ones; your husband has the stress of trying to find work and your children have been quiet. You feel this is from the shock of what they have experienced. You worry about Lilah's asthma, Akram's eczema and don't know where to get Rasha weighed. You would like some information about healthcare in England. Let's make a plan together.

Empathy ☐ I cannot imagine what you have been through, but I am glad you now feel safe.

Explanation ☐ In the UK, there are many different ways to seek help. For problems like hay fever or colds, you can go to a pharmacy to buy medications. Your local pharmacy is Brown's on the high street. Experienced pharmacists can give advice for these problems and are often a good first point of call. You may be able to sign up to 'Pharmacy First' to get free prescriptions for medicines like paracetamol for the children. Here, at the practice, we can offer emergency appointments if your family are unwell; please phone reception or book online. We also have doctors and nurses who manage long-term conditions like asthma or eczema. If the practice is closed and your problem cannot wait, you can phone 111, evenings, night-time and weekends. They can advise or arrange a GP appointment. If someone is very poorly or has a bad accident, you should go to A&E or call 999. This is a lot to take in. Any questions so far? It must be difficult when things are so different in a new country.

Recommend ☐ I recommend we book Akram in to assess his eczema and also see Lilah for her asthma. How do you feel about seeing us regularly so we can assess your family's health?

Specifics ☐ I'd also like to refer you to our health visitor service. Health visitors look after families with children under 5 years old and can advise you on minor problems and do health checks like weighing children. Would you be interested in seeing them? You can just turn up with Rasha to the health visitor's clinic once a week to get Rasha weighed. The health visitor can also put you in touch with other services like Sure Start which supports mums and runs mum and baby groups. We could arrange counselling for your children, what are your thoughts?

Empower ☐ Would you like me to email you an information sheet with the practice information? Helpful website addresses include NHS choices and patient.info.

Future ☐ Shall I book those appointments for you? I look forward to meeting your family.

Safety net ☐ If you are ever worried about a health problem, don't hesitate to give us a call.

Patient's Story

Education about Services

Doctor's notes Sara Azmeh, 28 years. PMH: no information. During a recent 'unplanned admissions review' your practice has noted that this family have been attending A&E and out-of-hours services regularly. You have sent a letter to the parents to ask them to book a telephone consultation to discuss the health of the family and the services available.

How to act Confused.

PC *'Hello, Doctor, you have asked me phone to discuss this letter I have received.'*

History You, your husband and four children moved to the UK 4 months ago. Your husband helped the UK armed forces in Afghanistan and you were granted asylum in the UK. You are unsure how the healthcare system works in the UK. You love your children dearly and get frightened when they are unwell. You and your husband are both well. Over recent years you have had very little access to healthcare in Afghanistan and worry about Lilah's asthma which isn't well controlled. You have had an inhaler from the practice which helps but she keeps running out. You also have trouble managing Akram's eczema; although you know it isn't life threatening, it often becomes sore and stops him sleeping. You are aware that you have been to A&E quite a lot but are unsure what else you should do when the practice is closed or if you can't get through on the phone. After you had been to hospital a couple of times, they told you to ring 111 next time, so you did when you required the extra inhaler for Lilah and they helped your husband when he had problems with his nose.

Social Your asylum request is being processed at present but you are very hopeful that it will be granted. Your husband used to work in local government in Afghanistan. Since having children, you have been a full-time mum but do hope to train as a nurse in the future. You have met a nice elderly woman who is your neighbour and has been helping to look after the children if you need to run errands. You hope your children can start school soon and your husband will find work.

In Afghanistan you were very frightened and your family walked for days to safety. You feel exhausted but you are thankful that you are safe. You cry when you think of home. You left your elderly relatives who were not able to travel. You lost contact with your parents but believe they are safe as they were with you until you crossed the border. The children have become very quiet since you left. You imagine they are shocked but you give them lots of love and tell them they will be okay now.

ICE You feel that if the children are poorly, you should take them to A&E where they can see a doctor and will be safe. You are concerned about Lilah's asthma and Akram's eczema. You also wonder where you should get Rasha weighed. You expect the doctor to tell you off for going to A&E too much but you worry about your children and didn't know what else to do. You hope that the doctor may help your children's chronic problems but you do not feel you should tell the doctor what to do. You knew a few babies in Afghanistan who died of chest infections as they didn't get seen by a doctor quickly enough, so you worry if any of the children start coughing.

Education about Services

Avoiding unplanned admissions and directing appropriate use of services can be quite difficult. It is important that patients are given as much information as possible to allow them to make the right decisions regarding their health.

Make sure you are aware of what is available in your area

- How do you access your health visitor/midwife/community nurses/community mental health services? How can patients access these in an emergency or out-of-hours?
- Does your practice offer extended opening hours or is there an NHS walk-in centre nearby?
- Do your patients know about the 111 helpline?
- Is 'Pharmacy First' available in your area? (Scheme running in certain areas to allow patients to receive prescription medicines for some conditions without the patient seeing a GP.)
- Do you have a social prescribing specialist or do you know the local services in your area?

Chronic conditions

In patients with chronic health problems such as asthma, COPD and heart failure, it is good practice to develop a care plan or action plan with the patient. For example, an asthma action plan would be based on symptoms and peak expiratory flow rate and include when the patient should go to see a GP or phone an ambulance. Likewise, does the COPD sufferer have clear instructions about when to start antibiotics or steroids? These care plans can be effective in reducing hospital attendances by empowering the patients to manage their condition themselves and giving them good advice about which signs and symptoms need routine, urgent or emergency attention. One of the most effective strategies for reducing admissions is continuity of care in primary care, so try to proactively providc this where possible.

Doctor's Notes

Patient	Lacey Archer	21 years	F
PMH	None		
Medications	None		
Allergies	None		
Consultations	None		
Investigations	None		
Household	None		

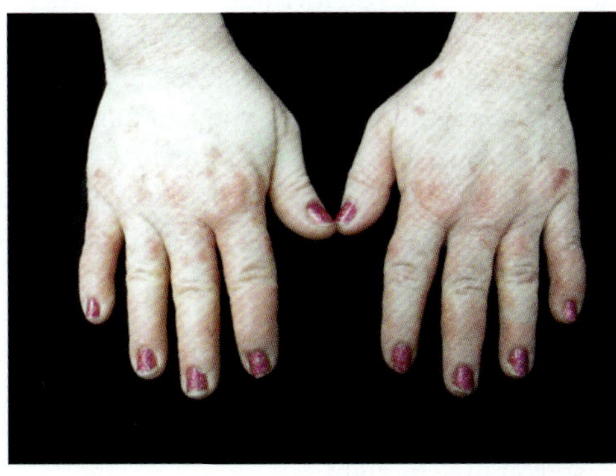

Reproduced from *Clinical Handbook of Contact Dermatitis* (2015), CRC Press. With thanks to Michael P. Sheehan, Monica Huynh, Michael Chung, Matthew Zirwas and Steven R. Feldman.

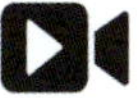

Example Consultation

Occupational Allergy

Open ☐ How can I help? I'm sorry you are having problems. What difficulties are you having with your hands? You mentioned a placement – where is this?

Sense ☐ I sense you seem worried about the rash; how has it been affecting you?

ICE1 ☐ Have you had any thoughts about the cause of the rash?

ICE2 ☐ What has worried you about it?

History ☐ When did you first notice the rash? What exactly do you do at the salon? How quickly does the rash come on? Does it itch? Is it sore? Any rash elsewhere? Any blisters? Has the skin been oozing? And your general health? Any medical history? Any medicines? Any family history of allergy, like asthma, eczema or hay fever?

Please tell me more about you. Do you live with anyone? I'm sorry to hear that – it must be really hard. Where do you sleep? Does anyone support you?

Risk ☐ Do you ever feel unsafe? How is your mood and mental health doing? Do you drink alcohol? Smoke? Or take drugs?

Summary ☐ Let me summarise. You've just started a hairdressing placement which you are enjoying, but have noticed that your hands become itchy and sore the next day. You wonder if it's from washing the hair dye pots, which is a worry because you love hairdressing – it's giving you motivation and keeping your mood stable at this difficult time. Since your family relationships broke down, you have stayed with friends but other times sleep outside.

ICE3 ☐ I'll be making some suggestions, but is there anything specific you had in mind?

Empathy ☐ It's really hard to go to work when you don't have a home at the moment.

Impression ☐ Let's talk first about your skin, as I see how important it is to you, then we can explore ways to help with the challenges since leaving home. Looking at the picture I can see areas of dryness and redness; I think this is contact dermatitis.

Experience ☐ Have you come across this term?

Explanation ☐ It means sore skin due to touching a chemical. Sometimes the chemical is an irritant, but sometimes the body is allergic to the chemical. Because your rash comes on after 1–2 days and is very itchy, I think it may be allergic and this fits with your personal and family history. Allergy to hair dye is quite common, so you may be right.

Options ☐ It is treatable, but avoiding the chemical is really important.

Empower ☐ How could you avoid touching the dye? Gloves? Perhaps speak to your tutor or mentor. Hair dye allergy is common so I suspect they will have come across it before.

Recommend ☐ Moisturising creams called emollients may help – apply them frequently to prevent the skin drying out. You can also use them instead of soap because soap is very drying. Because the rash is quite angry, I would also suggest a steroid cream, called Eumovate, nightly for a week. Use this sparingly, as it can cause skin thinning and be absorbed into the body. What are your thoughts? Did your sister use emollients and steroids for her eczema? You need to put two fingertips worth of steroid on each hand at night. Let it soak in, then apply the emollient 'Doublebase' on top – It will get better in time, but this may take weeks.

Future ☐ Could you speak with your tutor to explain about your allergy? Also, our social prescriber could help you with the challenges you've experienced since leaving home, e.g. local support groups. Would you like to see them? Great – I'll ask them to contact you. For the upset you've had with your parents, you could consider counselling, for you or together with a parent. What do you think?

Specifics ☐ I'll prescribe moisturiser and steroid cream to collect from the pharmacy. Please book to see me in 3–4 weeks. I'd like to keep in touch and see how you are. Any thoughts or questions?

Safety net ☐ If the rash doesn't improve after a week of steroids, or it becomes more painful, red or weepy, or if it spreads, please come and see us. If your mental health changes or life becomes harder, please book to see me or another GP.

Patient's Story

Occupational Allergy

Doctor's notes Lacey Archer, 21 years. No other information.

How to act Concerned.

PC *'It's my hands – I'm really struggling with this rash since I started my placement.'*

History You are a 21-year-old hairdressing student who has just started her first placement in a salon. To help out, you have been washing out hair dye bowls for the qualified hairdressers but have noticed irritation to your hands. At first you thought it was due to washing your hands so often, and perhaps because of the cold weather, but now you aren't so sure.

The rash tends to appear a day or two after you have been touching hair dye so you didn't make the link straight away. Usually, the following day you notice a strong itch, then the skin becomes red and can crack. This can happen at weekends and on college days when you aren't in the salon. You have tried E45, which soothes the skin a little, but it's getting worse. You haven't tried wearing gloves at work because no one else does and you were embarrassed to ask. You have started wearing gloves when you go out, more to hide your hands because the skin is no longer recovering before you go back to the salon.

Your mum has asthma and your sister had terrible eczema as a child, but this has improved since she has grown up. You do get bad hay fever in summer but manage this with over-the-counter medication. You haven't suffered with your skin before.

Social If the doctor explores your social history carefully, reveal you are using friends' sofas at the moment. Sometimes you have slept rough around the back of your friend's shop where you feel safe. You don't want to keep asking friends if you can sofa surf. The relationship with your parents broke down and now the job is all you have. Your mood is low but you don't feel depressed. The job motivates you to get up. There is a shower at work so you pretend you have been on a run and arrive early. You don't smoke, drink alcohol or take drugs. You are managing for food because of your wages and food banks. You hope to find a flat to rent but this is expensive. You have a couple of friends you can trust.

ICE You are starting to wonder if the chemicals you touch at work are causing the symptoms because, when the salon was closed for refurbishment for 2 weeks, your hands seemed better. But because the symptoms tend to appear a day or two later you weren't sure if this could be related. You are worried that if you can't do what other hairdressers do you will have to quit your course. This makes you upset because you love what you do. You hope the doctor can give you a cream which will help.

Examination findings See photograph.

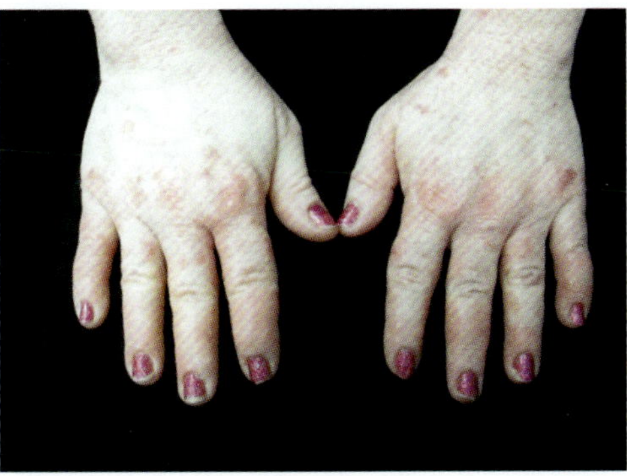

Reproduced from *Clinical Handbook of Contact Dermatitis* (2015), CRC Press. With thanks to Michael P. Sheehan, Monica Huynh, Michael Chung, Matthew Zirwas and Steven R. Feldman.

Allergic contact dermatitis[1]

Allergic contact dermatitis[1] is a type IV (delayed) hypersensitivity reaction due to repeated allergen exposure, commonly hair dye, cosmetics, nail varnish, nickel and cobalt (often found in jewellery), rubber, cement and plants. Therefore, high incidence in floristry, hairdressing, catering and metal handlers. Often delay of >24 hours before symptoms.

Acute irritant contact dermatitis typically occurs after a single overwhelming exposure or a few brief exposures to strong irritants. Itching prominent + symptoms in parts of body with no direct exposure.

Cumulative or chronic irritant contact dermatitis follows repeated exposure to weaker irritants, e.g. detergents, soaps, dust or low humidity air. Can be difficult to distinguish between allergic and irritant – may coexist.

Management[1]

Remove allergen. May take 8–12 weeks of avoidance before dermatitis settles. Apply emollients often and liberally +/– topical steroid; strength required dependent on rash severity. May need antibiotics if super-added infection. When allergen removal impossible, advise gloves, but remove frequently to prevent sweating. Wash hands with soap substitute, as water +/– soap can exacerbate.

Allergy – general points

Allergic conditions are becoming more common so may present in many consultations. Anaphylaxis is life threatening. Learn how to manage it in primary care. Also consider the following.

Taking an allergy-focused history

- When and how did symptoms start?
- Symptoms – oral, e.g. tongue swelling/tingling lips?
- Triggers?
- Getting worse on each exposure?
- Family history of allergy/atopy.
- Patient health belief.

Management of allergy immune conditions

- Investigation, e.g. patch test, skin prick, blood tests, challenge testing.
- Acute management – doses of adrenaline for different ages.
- Ongoing management – adrenaline devices, shared management plans (e.g. with school).
- Alert bracelets.
- Appropriate documentation of allergies in GP notes.

Common and important conditions

- Anaphylaxis including doses of adrenaline.
- Autoimmune conditions in primary care.
- Drug allergies and their mechanisms.
- Food allergies including milk allergy.
- Occupational allergies (latex, hair dye, metals, plants).
- Pollen food syndrome.
- Types of allergic reaction – immediate, delayed, possible mechanisms.
- Venom allergy.

Ethnicity, Culture, Diversity and Inclusivity – 9.4

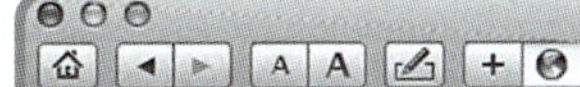

Doctor's Notes

Patient	Doran O'Brian	39 years	M
PMH	Upper respiratory tract infection		
	Hazardous alcohol use (recorded 6 years ago)		
	Smoker		
Medications	None		
Allergies	None		
Consultations	6 years ago – attended after episode of haematemesis following binge drinking at the weekend. Presented 4 days later. Given PPI and referred for urgent endoscopy. DNA the endoscopy appointment 10 days later		
	Cough 3 months ago, chest clear, amoxicillin prescribed		
	Sinusitis 2 months ago, doxycycline prescribed		
	Sore throat 1 month ago, viral infection diagnosed		
Investigations	BP 2 months ago: 102/60		
Household	Rosemary O'Brian	30 years	F
	Cian O'Brian	10 years	M
	Aoife O'Brian	8 years	F
	Caelan O'Brian	5 years	M

Example Consultation

Sinusitis

Open ☐ Hello, Mr O'Brian. Oh, I am sorry to hear that. Please tell me more about how your infection started this time and what symptoms you are getting.

History ☐ Tell me about the nasal discharge. Clear? Green? Any headaches – whereabouts? Has this happened before? Does your face feel sore to touch? Is the pain worse if you bend forward? Have you tried any medication for this? Please tell me about any medical problems in the past. I note you had trouble with your stomach after drinking quite a lot. Do you still drink alcohol? How much do you tend to drink? What about smoking?

ICE1 ☐ What conversations with doctors have you had about these infections? And what do you think?

Flags ☐ Does the light bother you? On a scale of 1–10, how bad are the headaches? Do you feel ill? Any double vision? Have you had a fever?

Sense ☐ You sound quite frustrated.

Impact ☐ How is the infection affecting you? How about at work?

Curious ☐ Tell me about your life. How do you spend your time?

ICE2 ☐ What worries you about the infection?

ICE3 ☐ As well as antibiotics, was there anything else you were hoping I could do to help?

SummarICE ☐ To summarise so far, you had a cold for about a week and now facial pain and discharge for 3 days which is not getting better with paracetamol. There's pressure in your face and this is affecting your ability to move bricks around on site.

Empathy ☐ Feeling lousy with facial pain and headaches must be pretty miserable, especially when you're trying to work.

Impression ☐ From what you've told me, I think you have sinusitis.

Explanation ☐ To be honest, it's far more likely to be viral than bacterial. The colour of the discharge and absence of fever is reassuring. There is no evidence that antibiotics make any difference for people who are normally fit and well. I appreciate you've been given antibiotics for this in the past; however, it may have been time that resolved your symptoms. Using antibiotics increases the chance of building up resistance. We want them to work for you when you really need them in the future. What are your thoughts?

InCludE ☐ I suspect that last time you got better despite the antibiotics rather than because of them. But there are some things which can help.

Options ☐ Shall I talk you through some self-help measures which should reduce the symptoms?

Recommend ☐ I recommend regular fluids and irrigating your nose with salt solution. Unfortunately, breathing in steam, warm facial compresses and decongestent sprays probably have no effect. So, you could try nasal douching or irrigation. People either love it because it flushes out the sinus passages or hate it because squirting salty water into your nose isn't pleasant. Ibuprofen may reduce inflammation and pressure, helping you through the next few days. Take it with food as it can irritate the stomach. It may be worth persisting with the paracetamol as well as ibuprofen.

Empower ☐ I'll text you a link to a PIL describing what you can do to help. Shall we talk about other ways you could become healthier, like reducing alcohol or stopping smoking? Is this something you've considered? Switching to vaping would be helpful in the long term, so that is certainly a positive step.

Future ☐ You should start to feel better soon and fully recover within 2–3 weeks. If not, please see me and at I would probably suggest a steroid nasal spray. If you change your mind about reducing alcohol or stopping smoking, please let me know.

Safety net ☐ If at any time you have bad headaches, blurred vision, a temperature or feel really ill, book to see me straight away. Out of hours, phone 111.

Patient's Story

Sinusitis

Doctor's notes Doran O'Brian, 39 years. PMH: URTI, hazardous alcohol use (recorded 6 years ago), smoker. 3 months ago: cough – amoxicillin given. 2 months ago: sinusitis – doxycycline given. 1 month ago: viral sore throat.

How to act Demanding. Get frustrated if you feel the GP is dragging the consultation out and not just giving you the antibiotics.

PC *'I won't keep you long, Doctor. I have an infection again – I just need antibiotics.'*

History Sore throat and runny nose for a week, self-medicated with paracetamol which has been 'useless' and you have not tried other treatment.

Last 3 days, increasing nasal discharge (clear, sometimes yellow) and facial pain especially if you press over your forehead and cheeks. Some headaches: frontal, worse when you bend your head forwards. You've had headaches for a few weeks anyway and think it is due to not getting much sleep.

You have a history of sinusitis; last time you were given antibiotics so you want these again.

Social Married with three children. You are part of the Irish travelling community. You split your time between Ireland and the UK. You have currently been back in the area around 3 months. You were previously registered at the practice 6 years ago when you attended with an episode of haematemesis following a weekend of binge drinking. The doctor gave you some pills and referred you to the hospital for tests but you had been moving around so never received the appointment letter. The symptoms settled so you didn't bother coming back. You do sporadic labouring work; you have a contact who is a builder and he sends work your way when you're around. You're currently supposed to be working on a building site but your symptoms are getting worse when bending to pick up and move bricks. You enjoy drinking with your extended family and friends in the evening (5–6 pints of lager most evenings). You smoke (15–20 a day).

ICE You believe infections require treatment with antibiotics, hence your request. You don't feel you drink too much; all your friends drink in this way. You do not wish to cut down and you do not want support or tests. You are aware smoking is bad for you; you would consider vaping but again do not want any referral or treatment to stop.

Ask the doctor Push the doctor for antibiotics – they worked last time. If refused antibiotics: *'What can you give me? My face hurts.'*

Acute sinusitis[1]

Diagnose if sinonasal inflammation lasts <12 weeks + sudden onset of ≥2 diagnostic symptoms:

- Nasal blockage/obstruction/congestion *or* nasal discharge (anterior/posterior nasal drip).
- Facial pain/pressure (or headache).
- Reduction (or loss) of the sense of smell.[1]

Usual management

If symptoms last <10 days and immediate referral is not indicated[1] explain that acute sinusitis is usually caused by a virus, resolves within 12 weeks and most people get better without antibiotics. Bacterial sinusitis is usually self-limiting and does not routinely need antibiotics.[1] Self-help includes:

- Paracetamol and/or ibuprofen (relieve symptoms by reducing pain and temperature).
- Consider irrigating nose with saline solution.
- NO evidence for intranasal or oral decongestants, though patients may wish to try (OTC)
- Note steam inhalations, antihistamines, mucolytics and warm face packs have no proven benefit.[1]

Antibiotics (refer to BNF and local guidelines)

Not needed if symptoms <10 days unless very unwell, has symptoms and signs of more serious illness, or is at high risk of complications.

Consider if symptoms >10 days – but remember adverse effects of antibiotics + make little difference to duration.

Adults: phenoxymethylpenicillin 500 mg QDS for 5 days or co-amoxiclav 500/125 TDS for 5 days, if systemically very unwell. Penicillin allergy? – Doxycycline or clarithromycin. Pregnant? – Erythromycin.

Children and young people <18 – as above, age-appropriate dose. No doxycyclineif <12 years.

Nasal corticosteroids (see NICE guidance for further details)

After 10 days of symptoms, consider prescribing high-dose nasal corticosteroid for 14 days, e.g. mometasone 20 mg BD (off-label use) in adults and children >12 years.

Rare but important complications needing admission[1]

- Severe systemic infection or signs of sepsis or reduced consciousness.
- Orbital involvement (double vision, oculomotor nerve paralysis, eyeball displaced, new ↓VA).
- Intracranial involvement with symptoms/signs of meningitis, severe headache or focal neuro signs.

Chronic sinusitis[1] – Associated with atopy, asthma, immunosuppression

Consider if nasal blockage/discharge with facial pain/headache and/or loss of smell for >12 weeks.

Manage with above measures but also consider 3 months of intranasal corticosteroids.

Consider referral to ENT if:

- No improvement in 6–12 weeks and/or doubt about diagnosis.
- The person is immunocompromised.
- Symptoms significantly affect quality of life.
- There is a suspected allergic or immunological cause.
- There is a co-morbidity complicating management, such as nasal polyps or asthma.
- Sinusitis is associated with an unusual or resistant bacteria.
- There are recurrent episodes of OM, or pneumonia, or suspicion of adenoid hypertrophy.

Ethnicity, Culture, Diversity and Inclusivity – 9.5

CHAPTER 10

NEW PRESENTATION OF UNDIFFERENTIATED DISEASE

	Cases in this chapter	RCGP 2025 curriculum	Learning points
10.1	Foot Pain – Plantar Fasciitis	**Musculoskeletal health** 'Soft tissue disorders such as bursitis, epicondylitis, Achilles tendon problems'	Differential diagnosis of foot pain Gout: • Causes • Management, including acute treatment and urate lowering therapy (ULT)
10.2	Neurological Symptoms – Multiple Sclerosis	**Neurology** 'Sensory and motor symptoms: weakness (for example foot drop), spasticity, paraesthesia' 'Multiple sclerosis and other demyelinating disorders such as transverse myelitis'	Multiple sclerosis: • Risk factors • Diagnosis and management
10.3	Rash – Lyme Disease	**Dermatology** 'Infections – spirochaetal, for example Lyme disease' **Infectious diseases and travel health** 'Tick borne diseases including Lyme disease'	Lyme disease: • Diagnosis and differentials • Management
10.4	Tired All the Time	**Metabolic problems and endocrinology** 'Tiredness and lethargy'	Tiredness: • Possible causes • Differentials
10.5	Bowel Symptoms – IBS	**Gastroenterology** 'Abdominal pain including the differential diagnoses from non-gastrointestinal causes (for example gynaecological or urological) … Bloating … Bowel issues including constipation, diarrhoea, changes in habit, tenesmus and faecal incontinence'	Irritable bowel syndrome: recognition and management

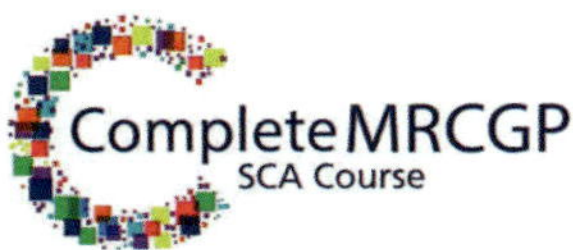

Links to the RCGP Curriculum

This broad blueprint group may feature clinical topics from throughout the curriculum and all life stages.

In this chapter, the cases are drawn from the following clinical topic guides:

- Musculoskeletal health
- Neurology
- Dermatology
- Infectious diseases and travel health
- Metabolic problems and endocrinology
- Gastroenterology

Scope of Conditions

Here are some examples of cases – this is not a complete list of all possibilities.

Virtually any condition can initially present as an undifferentiated disease. However, there are some common symptoms where it can be notoriously difficult to make a definitive diagnosis based on pattern recognition alone. Examples include:

- Tiredness
- Abdominal pain
- Pelvic pain
- Breathlessness
- Nausea
- Dizziness
- Tingling/numbness
- Blurred vision
- Persistent cough
- Chest pain
- Muscular aches and pains
- Weight loss

Consider how you would approach the above symptoms in your exam. If you're unsure of the scope of differentials attached to these symptoms, consider reading a 'Symptom Sorter' book.

Skills and Pitfalls

In addition to the information in Chapter 1 'How to Demonstrate Skills: The Marking Scheme Made Easy' consider the following challenges for this blueprint group.

To be able to arrive at the correct diagnosis when faced with an undifferentiated disease/symptom, excellent data-gathering and problem-solving skills are required. Pitfalls can include an unstructured or scattergun history and missed or unclear impression resulting in a vague or illogical plan. However, there are transferable skills that can be applied to each case which are likely to help you.

- Use plenty of open questions – listening to the answers carefully will allow you to look for familiar patterns and allow your brain time to process the information rather than constantly thinking of the next question.
- Ask about impact early – this can provide diagnostic information as often each differential will link to a different level of debility.
- Use the information provided – what does this information (e.g. age, sex, pre-existing conditions or drugs) tell you about the probability of each of your differentials?
- Ask your risk factor and red flag questions in groups relating to each differential to help you organise your evidence.
- If you're really stuck, consider a systems review to identity any further symptoms/clues.
- Don't forget ICE; although the patient may not be right, their ideas can often point you in the right direction or at least highlight a condition to rule out.
- It's okay for your impression to be a differential, but make sure you state which you think is most likely and base your plan around this.

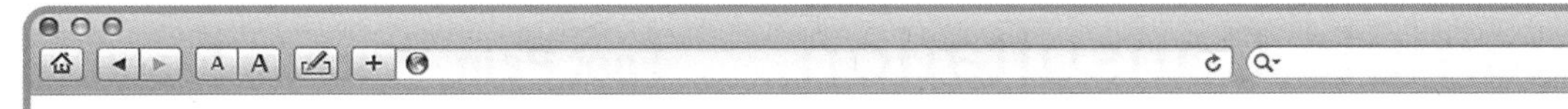

Doctor's Notes

Patient	Selina Richards	31 years	F
PMH	None		
Medications	None		
Allergies	None		
Consultations	None		
Investigations	None		
Household	Craig Richards	38 years	M
	Alexander Richards	8 years	M
	Maria Richards	6 years	F
	Amelia Richards	5 years	F

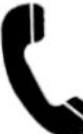

Example Consultation **Foot Pain – Plantar Fasciitis**

Open ☐ Please tell me how the pain first began. Anything else you have noticed?
Impact ☐ And since this problem started, what has the pain stopped you from doing?
History ☐ When does the pain come and go? Can you pinpoint where it hurts? Any medical problems? Have you tried any pain relief yet? Did it help?
Risk ☐ Have you ever had any injury in the past?
Flags ☐ Have you noticed any swelling? Can you move the ankle and foot normally? Any joints painful elsewhere in your body?
O/E ☐ Is there anything at all to see? Any redness or skin changes? Any differences to the other side?
ICE1 ☐ Have you had any thoughts as to what may be causing it?
ICE2 ☐ What worries you most about this pain?
Sense ☐ So this has come at a very difficult time for you?
Curious ☐ What did your friend suggest?
ICE3 ☐ Is there anything else you hoped we would arrange today?
SummarICE ☐ To summarise, you have told me that the pain in the right foot has been building over a month but especially in this past week. It has stopped you from walking the dog, something that you enjoy, but have had to do more since you separated from your husband. You wondered if it was gout.
Impression ☐ I think what is causing your pain is a plantar fasciitis. Have you come across this before?
Explanation ☐ The plantar fascia is a sheet of tissue that supports the bones of your foot. Sometimes it can become painful and inflamed. It may be triggered by an increase in physical activity.
InCludE ☐ I don't think you have gout as your foot is not red, hot or swollen and the site which hurts is typical of plantar fasciitis. X rays do not show this inflammation so are unlikely to be helpful.
Empathy ☐ This is an additional stress, especially as the dog is whining and you have three children to care for. I also hear that you are very fond of the dog. I appreciate why you feel you need to fix this problem straight away. The problem can unfortunately take many months to settle completely. However, for this common condition I have some suggestions.
Empower ☐ The ibuprofen could be changed for a tablet which is slightly stronger and lasts 12 hours, called naproxen. You take one tablet twice a day but, like ibuprofen, it can irritate your stomach lining so stop it if this becomes a problem. We don't tend to use colchicine for this problem. Exercises are useful. The exercises aim to stretch the tissue to help the repairing process. You can use a frozen 1 L drinks bottle to massage the plantar fascia by rolling your foot over it. The movement helps stretch the tissue and the ice helps reduce pain and swelling. The more you do, the sooner it will improve but, like any exercise, time is needed. Padded insoles can also help. Regarding the stress relief, could you do some non-weight-bearing exercise until your foot is better, e.g. swimming?
Options ☐ I could give you a PIL about PF? It also mentions steroid injections into the feet, which is an option but some do not find it effective and there are risks to injecting in the foot, such as infection or injury to the tendons there. We therefore don't recommend the injections as first line. What are your thoughts about what I have said?
Future ☐ How do you feel about trying this option for the next 6 weeks?
Specifics ☐ If you have seen no improvement after a month, please arrange an appointment to come back and we can think about either referring for formal physiotherapy or considering the injections.
Safety net ☐ Its unlikely but if you do notice any swelling or heat in the foot, please see the GP earlier.

Patient's Story

Foot Pain – Plantar Fasciitis

Doctor's notes Selina Richards, 31 years. PMH: none. Medications: none.

How to act Slightly pushy for the doctor to fix this problem.

PC *'It's a pain in my foot – it's a nightmare.'*

History You walk your dog every morning and have recently experienced pain in the right foot whilst walking. You have had no injury or swelling. There is nothing to see at all. The pain is particularly severe when you first get out of bed in the morning or if you have been resting. The pain improves initially with walking but then builds after a few minutes.

You started to notice this a month ago and over the past week you have had enough of this discomfort. You have always been well. Ibuprofen only helps slightly. You drink minimal alcohol and don't smoke.

Social You do not work. You have three children and a dog. Your children are all in primary school. Your husband has just left the marriage and he used to walk the dog in the morning.

You spend your days meeting your friends, doing housework, dog-sitting and food shopping for your mother. Financially you have always been very lucky and have never worked since you were married. You would like to have a job but don't know how or where to look. You are going to volunteer at the school with cooking classes.

ICE Your friend told you that the problem may be gout as she had the same thing and you have not had an injury. Therefore, you expect the doctor will give you colchicine, the tablet your friend was given. You would also like a blood test and an X-ray. You plan to pay for a dog walker, but will miss the time out of the house with the dog; this has helped with your stress whilst going through the divorce.

Impact The dog has been whining as you couldn't walk him and you need to get this sorted straight away. Apart from walking the dog, the pain has not stopped you from doing anything else.

You are coping well without your husband; he was always away on business anyway. The divorce proceedings, however, are stressful. You also want to keep the dog and fear your husband will want him if he is not being walked. You have never come across plantar fasciitis.

Examination You don't wish to attend the surgery for an examination, after all there is nothing to see and you can move your foot in all directions, none of this hurts. The pain is under your heel, sometimes spreading under the arch of your foot.

Differential Diagnosis – Foot Pain

Soft tissue	Chronic heel pad inflammation	'Warm dull throbbing pain over weight-bearing area of the heel … worse when first getting up.'[1]
	Acute synovitis	Throbbing pain made worse by movement.[1] Rule out systemic causes.
	Acute inflammation of anterior metatarsal heads	Common in women wearing slip-on/heeled shoes. Burning and throbbing on walking.[1]
	Plantar metatarsal bursitis	'Throbbing pain under the metatarsal head … persists at rest and exacerbated when the area is first loaded.'[1]
Bone	Fracture	Has there been impact? Use the Ottawa rules.[2]
	Stress fracture (march fracture)	Palpable tender lump.
	Osteoarthritis	Common at first MTP joint, tarsus joints and midfoot.[1]
	Rheumatoid arthritis	Swelling and deformity, may describe as walking on pebbles, due to swelling/subluxation.[1]
	Sever's disease	E.g. boys 8–13 years and exacerbated by jumping.[1]
	Hallux valgus	Great toe moves towards/overlies the second toe.[1]
	Bunion	Inflamed and painful metatarsal head.[1]
Red hot	Gout	Sudden, severe pain, often big toe. Joint is swollen and red with ↓movement
	Septic arthritis	Requires urgent aspiration/culture/Rx.
Nerve	Morton's neuroma	Burning and numbness … often the third/fourth toe.[1]
	Peripheral neuropathy	E.g. tarsal tunnel or 2° to ↓B12, alcohol or DM.
Arterial	Ischaemia	Absent pulses, signs of PVD and check ABPI.

Gout

Risk factors	Thiazides, ACE1, alcohol, obesity.
	Do not start allopurinol during an acute attack. But, if already taking allopurinol or febuxostat, do not stop this during an acute attack.[3]
Acute medication[3]	First line: NSAID at maximum dose, e.g. naproxen. Consider gastric protection.
	Second line: colchicine.
	Third line if NSAIDs contraindicated: consider short course of systemic corticosteroids, e.g. prednisolone 30–35 mg once daily for 3–5 days.
	When initiating allopurinol, offer colchicine to prevent flares, or NSAID or corticosteroid (both off-label use). Start with low dose 100 mg or less, adjust dose in 100 mg increments every 4 weeks according to urate level. Reduced dose in elderly or hepatic impairment.
Uric acid levels	Measure 4–6 weeks after an acute attack. Aim for normal levels of uric acid if the decision has been made to start allopurinol.
Self-management[3]	Rest, avoid trauma, keep the joint cool. Lifestyle: reduce alcohol, weight loss and dietary changes and avoid dehydration.

Doctor's Notes

Patient	Lydia Cooper	25 years	F
PMH	Tonsillitis – 3 years ago		
Medications	None		
Allergies	None		
Consultations	None		
Investigations	None		
Household	No household members registered		

A&E letter yesterday:

'Told to attend by optician. Has blurred vision and numbness/weakness of left leg of recent onset.

O/E – observations normal, urine dip normal. Loss sensation left lower leg, power 3/5, brisk reflexes.

Bloods (FBC, U&E, LFT, CRP) normal. Sent for CT head – no tumour, bleed or ischaemic stroke.

Impression – ?Atypical migraine ?Sciatica – for GP review'

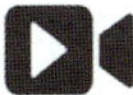

Example Consultation

Neurological Symptoms – Multiple Sclerosis

Open ☐ Tell me what led you to go to A&E. Can you take me back to when you first noticed a problem and talk me through the symptoms step by step? What happened at the hospital?

Sense ☐ I can see you are upset and very worried.

ICE1 ☐ Have you had any thoughts about what may be going on? What is going through your mind?

Flags ☐ Are you well usually? Has your speech changed? Does your leg still feel weak or floppy? Any worsening of symptoms since yesterday? Have you noticed a change in your coordination or balance? Have you noticed any difference in your control when going to the toilet? Have you lost weight? Any headaches or vomiting? Is your back painful? Have you had an injury? Have you had any recent illnesses or viral symptoms?

History ☐ Tell me more about you? Who are you close to? Do you work? Do you have hobbies?

Risk ☐ Has anyone in your family had similar symptoms in the past? Have you been abroad or noticed any insect bites? Have you ever had an infection through sex?

ICE3 ☐ Did you have any ideas about what I may say or suggest today?

Curious ☐ Tell me about your grandpa's experience.

Impact ☐ Have your symptoms stopped you from doing anything?

SummarICE ☐ To summarise, you have noticed unusual sensations now in both legs and your vision has been troubling you. You became very concerned when you realised you were wobbly on your feet. You fear it may be a similar problem to your grandpa's, but you are puzzled and worried by your symptoms as the A&E doctor wasn't sure what was happening. Is that correct?

Empathy ☐ I appreciate it's frightening when you have symptoms which you cannot explain, especially when they come together and it has made you wonder if this is similar to your grandpa's condition.

InCludE ☐ I don't believe it is the same as what happened to your grandpa as strokes are more common in elderly people and although CT scans aren't perfect, they do usually pick up significant strokes. I agree an MRI scan may be needed to get more information about what is going on.

Impression ☐ I think we need to ask a nerve doctor, a neurologist, to see you. I am questioning whether your nerves have become a little swollen, but the exact cause for why this has happened is not yet clear. This may be what the optician has seen.

Explanation ☐ Nerve swelling can occur for several reasons: following an infection, low vitamin B or where the nerve supply is irritated by something pushing against it. The body can also attack itself by mistake and affect the nerves so they become weak and lose their protective layer. Instead of this protective layer, scar tissue forms and it blocks the normal signals from the nerves, which can lead to strange sensations. This can be a condition called multiple sclerosis (MS). Unfortunately, I think this may be what's happening to you, but we need to do more tests to be sure. Have you heard of MS? Do you have any questions? You may find your symptoms go away and then come back again. Before we can give you the exact answer, we need to know what we are dealing with.

Specifics ☐ Would you be happy to have some extra blood tests to check your vitamin levels which were not done by A&E? I'll ask the nurse to do these now; meanwhile I'm going to give the nerve doctors at the hospital a call to ask if they want to see you today or in their rapid-access clinic.

Future ☐ At the hospital I expect they will examine you and they may arrange an MRI scan. There may still be further tests you need before we have the answer but if it does turn out to be MS, and there's still a chance it will not, there are effective treatments which I'm sure the team will discuss with you.

Patient's Story

Neurological Symptoms – Multiple Sclerosis

Doctor's notes Lydia Cooper, 25 years. PMH: tonsillitis – 3 years ago. Medications: none.

A&E letter yesterday:

'Told to attend by optician. Has blurred vision and numbness/weakness of left leg of recent onset. O/E – observations normal, urine dip normal. Loss sensation left lower leg, power 3/5, brisk reflexes. Bloods (FBC, U&E, LFT, CRP) normal. Sent for CT head – no tumour, bleed or ischaemic stroke. Impression – ?Atypical migraine ?Sciatica – for GP review.'

How to act Nervous and anxious.

Start to cry when you explain your symptoms.

PC *'I've got this strange feeling in my leg – it's the second time I've had it. The A&E doctor told me to see you.'*

History Six weeks ago you noticed your right foot was tingling within your shoe. You thought it must have been your tight trainers but you noticed it again in bed last week but this time on the left foot and lower leg and today it has gone above your knee. You feel wobbly when you walk today. You feel like you are going to fall over. Your coordination generally feels a bit off. A couple of months ago you realised that you needed glasses. Your right eye has been more blurry this week. You went to an optician yesterday who said the nerve at the back of your eye looked inflamed and you needed to see a doctor. You went straight to A&E. The doctor there examined you and said there was some slight weakness in your left leg and reduced sensation. Your observations were normal and your urine was clear. You had a CT scan of your head; there was no tumour or sign of stroke so you were discharged and told to see your GP for follow-up.

No headache or weight loss.

No urinary symptoms. Your bowels are normal. No other symptoms on systemic enquiry.

Social You live with your boyfriend of 1 year. You are looking for work. You left college aged 16 years. Since then you've found temporary work in offices.

You smoked in your teens. You do not drink alcohol.

ICE You don't know what may be causing it. The doctor in A&E mentioned the leg symptoms could be coming from your back or unusual type of migraine but did not seem sure. This has left you worried. Could they have missed a stroke? You read online that not all strokes are picked up on CT and you may need an MRI. The doctor didn't explain the blurred vision.

Your grandpa had a stroke 2 years ago; he lost all movement on the right side and his speech was different and he lost part of his vision.

You don't know what the doctor will say today. You hope they may refer you for an MRI.

Ask the doctor *'Will it get better?'*

Learning Points

Neurological Symptoms – Multiple Sclerosis

MS may take the course of relapsing-remitting, primary or secondary progressive.[1] It is usually a progressive disease. Relapses may be triggered by infections, stress and post-partum.[1,2]

Epidemiology	Incidence F>M; common in young adults.
Risk factors[2]	Genetic.
	EBV infection.
	Smoking.
	Obesity in adolescence.
	Low levels of vitamin D.
Symptoms[1]	Visual changes, e.g. acuity, colour vision, visual fields (optic neuritis).
	Reduced vision, loss of vision or double vision.
	Hearing loss.
	Facial weakness.
	Altered sensations.
	Limb weakness, gait problems.
	Bladder and bowel control may be affected.
	Altered temperature regulation, e.g. sweating.
	Altered sexual function/impotence.
	Lhermitte's phenomenon: the feeling of electricity down the spine on neck flexion.
	Cerebellar symptoms: ataxia, nystagmus, dysarthria, vertigo.
	Cognitive dysfunction (late symptoms).
Diagnosis	Relapsing, remitting: ≥2 demyelinating lesions in the brain/spinal cord occurring in different places at different times.[2]
	Primary progressive: progressive deterioration over 12 months.[2]
Investigations	These may include MRI, lumbar puncture and visual evoked potentials.
Differential diagnosis[1]	Sarcoidosis.
	Spinal cord compression.
	Vitamin B12 deficiency.
	Neurosyphilis.
	SLE.
	Cerebrovascular disease.
	SOL/tumours.
	Lyme disease.
Blood tests	FBC, U&E, LFT, calcium, glucose, TFTs, ESR, CRP, vitamin B12, ANA, HIV ± syphilis.

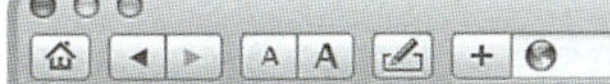

Doctor's Notes

Patient	Paul Haydock	21 years	M
PMH	None		
Medications	None		
Allergies	None		
Consultations	None		
Investigations	None		
Household	Nicola Jones	21 years	F
	Tomash Komosa	24 years	M
	Gavin Thompson	22 years	M
	Tareeq Khan	23 years	M

Photo supplied by patient:

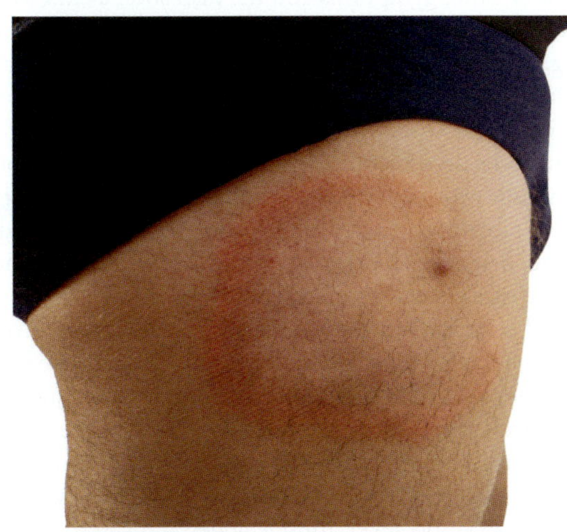

Credit: Shutterstock.

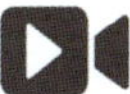

Example Consultation

Rash – Lyme Disease

Open ☐ Yes, of course. I'm sure we will be able to treat this. How did you first notice it?

History ☐ How has the rash changed since you first noticed it? Has it been itchy, sore or even painful?

ICE1 ☐ What's gone through your mind about the rash? What made your girlfriend think of ringworm? Did you have any other thoughts?

Curious ☐ Tell me about yourself – what are you doing in your life? And who do you live with?

Risk ☐ Have you been away from home in the last 3–6 weeks? Tell me about your trip to Scotland – in particular about any activities outdoors such as camping or hiking.

Flags ☐ How have you felt in yourself? Any aches and pains or fatigue? Shortness of breath? Eye soreness or blurred vision? Have you checked your temperature?

ICE2 ☐ Has anything particularly worried you about this rash?

Sense ☐ I sense you haven't been too worried yourself about this, but your girlfriend is concerned she might catch it from you.

ICE3 ☐ After discussions with Nicola was there anything specific you were hoping for?

Examination ☐ I've had a look at the photo you sent, thank you.

Impression ☐ I don't think this is ringworm, although the rash is similar. I think it may be Lyme disease which is an infection that may be caused by tick bites.

Experience ☐ Have you heard of Lyme disease or known anyone who has had this? I'm sorry to hear about your friend's experience, but that isn't common. Most people get a rash like yours, rather than tiredness or other symptoms and the rash soon clears with antibiotics.

Explanation ☐ Lyme disease is caused when you are bitten by a tick that has already been infected with a bacterial bug. The bug is passed on in the tick saliva and infects the skin giving this rash, which is called erythema migrans. Erythema means 'red' and migrans means 'spreading', so the name describes what the rash does if untreated.

Recommend ☐ There is no need to do a blood test because the appearance of the rash is so typical. Are there any antibiotics you can't take or are allergic to? Good, I suggest one called doxycycline. Please take one tablet twice a day for 3 weeks. You may get mild tummy symptoms such as loss of appetite, nausea or diarrhoea – these are common, ignore them if you can. If you have any severe side effects, let me know.

InCLudE ☐ You mentioned a cream, but that won't work for this rash – you need to have a course of antibiotics. I appreciate you were not expecting this. (Pause for response.)

Empathy ☐ I agree that 3 weeks is a long time and I completely understand your hesitation about antibiotics but it's important that we completely get rid of the bug that's causing the rash, and this can take time. May I prescribe the antibiotics for you? Any other thoughts?

Empower ☐ If there were 100 people like you starting antibiotics for Lyme disease, about 16 would feel worse at first, for example fever, muscle aches and sweating. This shows that the immune system and the antibiotic are working. If this happens, carry on with the treatment. Thankfully, you can't infect anyone else, so no-one can get the rash from you. Avoiding tick bites is the best way to prevent recurrence. Despite having the infection, you won't be immune and can catch it again if bitten. I recommend long trousers when you are walking or working in places where there may be deer, and always check your skin for ticks at the end of the day. Tuck your socks into your trousers so the ticks can't get in. You can safely remove ticks using fine-pointed tweezers and a steady pull. The UK-based Lyme Disease Action website has a video about how to do this.

Future ☐ Symptoms can persist following treatment. If you feel well after completing the antibiotics, there's no need to see me again, but if you have concerns, let me know.

Safety net ☐ If you start to feel very unwell soon, get a rash like nettle rash, or notice eye, breathing or nerve problems such as tingling or weakness, please contact a doctor. Also see a doctor if you start to feel tired, weak or unwell in the next few weeks.

Patient's Story

Rash – Lyme Disease

Doctor's notes Paul Haydock, male, 21 years. No PMH, drugs or allergies. No recent consultations.

How to act Initially you are unconcerned. You become anxious if Lyme disease or 3 weeks of antibiotics are mentioned.

PC ***'Can I have some cream for a rash on my leg? I sent you a photo.'***

History Two weeks ago you noticed a red mark on your right leg. Since then, it has grown and seems to be spreading. The middle part has improved but it's growing in a ring. You do not feel unwell and the rash is not itchy or sore. Three weeks ago, you went on a field trip to Scotland when you were camping in an informal campsite. If asked, you did not notice a tick bite or remove a tick from your skin. You were wearing long trousers when outside but did not tuck them into your socks.

Social You are a geography student at Leeds University in your final year. You live with four other students in a shared house, including your girlfriend, Nicola, who is a medical student. ***'Nicola thinks it's ringworm.'***

ICE Nicola has told you that she thinks this is ringworm and that you should get some cream to treat it. She is concerned she might catch a fungal infection from you. If the doctor suspects Lyme disease, you become alarmed. A fellow student got this and had to leave the course because they became so ill with fatigue. You ask for investigations and become concerned if the doctor prescribes antibiotics without doing tests. ***'Can I have a blood test or something to be sure that's what it is?'*** You are shocked at the length of antibiotic course: ***'3 weeks! That seems a long time. I thought antibiotics were bad for you.'***

O/E Checked own temperature – 37.0°C. Girlfriend checked HR 68 bpm regular. No other skin rashes.

Learning Points

Rash – Lyme Disease

Cause Body's response to infection with spirochaete *Borrelia burgdorferi*, transmitted from deer ticks.[1]

Pathophysiology Once bitten by an infected tick, there are several possible responses:

- Infection cleared by host defences (no symptoms but seropositive).
- Direct invasion of the skin causing typical rash, erythema migrans.
- Immune response with clinical symptoms, but no rash, e.g. neurological, MSK, etc.[1]

Epidemiology More common in many areas of southern England, Thetford Forest, Lake District, North Yorkshire moors and Scottish Highlands.[1] Grassy and wooded areas including gardens and parks.[2] Most tick bites do not transmit Lyme disease – prompt removal of tick reduces risk.[2]

Incidence Estimated 3000 cases per year in the UK. All ages and genders. 15% acquired abroad.[1]

Presentation *Erythema migrans*: red rash that increases in size, not itchy, hot or painful. Usually appears 1–4 weeks (range 3 days to 3 months) after bite. May also get local reaction – usually develops and recedes within 48 hours of bite, more likely to be hot, itchy and/or painful. This is inflammation/infection with common skin pathogen, not *Borrelia*.[2]

Consider Lyme disease as possible cause of fever and sweats, swollen glands, malaise, fatigue, neck pain or stiffness, migratory joint or muscle aches and pain, cognitive impairment, such as memory problems and difficulty concentrating ('brain fog'), headache and paraesthesia.[2]

Lyme disease is an uncommon cause of: neuro symptoms, e.g. facial palsy or unexplained cranial nerve palsy, mononeuritis multiplex, rarely encephalitis; inflammatory arthritis affecting one or more joints; cardiac problems, e.g. heart block, pericarditis; uveitis or keratitis; or skin rashes such as acrodermatitis chronica atrophicans or lymphocytoma.[2]

History Ask about activities that might have exposed patient to ticks and travel to areas of high prevalence.[2]

Consider possibility even with no clear history of tick exposure.

Investigations Diagnose and treat erythema migrans without investigating further:

- If suspicious but no rash, offer ELISA test and treat with antibiotics until results.[2]
- If ELISA positive or equivocal, request immunoblot test and consider antibiotics. Further details can be found in the NICE guidance *Lyme disease*.[3]

Information for patients Lab tests have limitations with false positives and false negatives. If symptoms persist and tests are negative, other diagnoses will be considered. Symptoms such as tiredness, headaches and muscle pain are common and a medical cause may not be found.[2]

Treatment

1. Emergency referral if CNS infection, uveitis, cardiac complications.
2. Specialist advice if:
    - <18, unless single erythema migrans lesion only and no other symptoms.
    - Adult with focal symptoms (e.g. to infectious diseases, rheumatology, neurology).
3. Lyme disease without focal symptoms (i.e. typical rash only) – no investigations needed. Treat with antibiotics promptly:
    - First choice: oral doxycycline 100 mg BD or 200 mg OD for 21 days.
    - Alternative: oral amoxicillin 1 g TDS for 21 days.
    - Second alternative: oral azithromycin 500 mg daily for 17 days.

See NICE CKS *Lyme disease*[2] for doses for children.

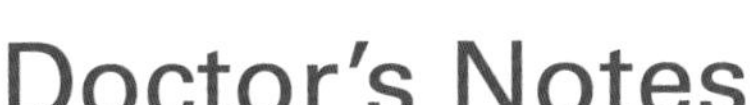

Doctor's Notes

Patient	Jayne Fitzpatrick	56 years	F
PMH	None		
Medications	None		
Allergies	None		
Consultations	None		
Investigations	None		
Household	Michael Fitzpatrick	59 years	M

Example Consultation

Tired All the Time

Open ☐	Please take me back to when you first began feeling tired? Can you pinpoint any trigger?
Impact ☐	How does the tiredness affect you day to day? Does it prevent you from doing anything?
ICE1 ☐	Have you had any thoughts as to what may be causing you to feel tired?
ICE2 ☐	This has been going on a while; have any worries crossed your mind about what it could be?
History ☐	Do you feel you have a healthy lifestyle? Do you manage to do any exercise? Do you drink much caffeine? Do you feel you're getting enough sleep? Can you talk me through your bedtime routine? Do you snore? Or wake in the night?
Flags ☐	Have you noticed any other symptoms? A change in your bowels or bladder? Any weight changes? Any breathlessness? Any flutterings of your heart or dizziness? Any fevers or sweats? Do you feel you look more pale than normal? How is your mood? Any memory problems?
Risk ☐	It looks from your records like you're normally fit and well, is that correct? Any family history of anything in particular? What stresses are you under at present?
Sense ☐	It sounds like you've had a lot on your plate recently.
ICE3 ☐	When you've been thinking about this tiredness and today's appointment, was there anything in particular you were hoping I'd suggest?
SummarICE ☐	So you've been feeling tired for around 6 months, though you can't really pinpoint when it started. You've always been an active person so not having the energy for your usual activities is a concern for you. At the back of your mind you're worried it could be something serious, but also feel it could just be your age/menopause. You wondered if some blood tests would be helpful.
Explanation ☐	Tiredness is a very common problem, but unfortunately we don't always find a specific, treatable cause. It can often be a consequence of our busy and stressful lives. However, there are some conditions which we can usually rule out which can present as tiredness, such as anaemia, thyroid problems, diabetes, vitamin deficiencies or chronic inflammation, which can have many causes.
Impression ☐	At the moment, it's not clear what is causing your tiredness symptom as there are no other symptoms to guide us. I wonder if it could be a combination of the various stresses you have been under, a reduction in physical activity which can perpetuate feelings of tiredness and menopause, as you suspected.
InCludE ☐	Thankfully, there are no symptoms that point to a worrying underlying cause but I agree some blood tests are likely to be helpful.
Options ☐	How would you feel about having some blood tests initially to look for the problems I mentioned, then we could arrange a follow-up appointment to talk through the results?
Empower ☐	In the meantime, you may find building up your activity levels again helpful, often the less we do, the less we feel like doing. Do you think you could start swimming again? Or perhaps go for a walk to destress after work? You could drag your husband along to help with his blood pressure. I'd also recommend cutting out caffeine as this can cause tiredness and poor sleep. It may be worth making some slight changes to your bedtime routine, e.g. reading downstairs rather than in bed to help you fall asleep faster. I can send you a leaflet which includes more tips about quality sleep.
Future ☐	How do you feel about trying these things and us having a catch up in around 4 weeks? If you're no better and your bloods are normal, perhaps we can think more about the role of menopause?
Safety net ☐	If we pick up anything unexpected on your blood tests we will let you know straight away. Could you let us know if you notice any new symptoms?

Patient's Story

Tired All the Time

Doctor's notes Jayne Fitzpatrick, 56 years. PMH: none. Medications: none.

How to act Fed up.

PC *'Doctor, I'm just so exhausted all the time, I don't know what's wrong with me.'*

History Over the last 6 months or so you have been feeling tired all the time. Subtle onset, no specific trigger. You have no specific symptoms, no weight loss, you've gained a few pounds, no change in bowel habit or urination, no excess thirst, no SOB or palpitations. No tremor or hair/nail changes. You sleep reasonably well, though not as well as you did pre-menopause. You usually go to bed at 10 p.m. and read for 30–60 minutes before falling asleep. It does often take you a little while to drop off. You get up once in the night to pee then usually wake around 6 a.m. Your LMP was 5 years ago. You're no longer particularly troubled by vasomotor symptoms though get them occasionally. You did get some generalised aches and pains. Your mood is fine. You drink alcohol occasionally. You have never smoked. You do enjoy a nice cup of tea (caffeinated). You used to go swimming but got out of the habit due to being busy at work and now feel like you don't have the energy. You also used to walk the dog regularly but sadly he had to be put down last year. You always used to be so active and on the go; it's not like you to want to sit around in the evenings and weekends.

Social You work in accounts in a busy manufacturing firm. The job can be stressful, particularly at month end when you have to ensure everyone's pay is correct. This can lead to long hours. You feel your brain isn't as quick as it used to be so stay late to double check your work at times. You wonder if this is another consequence of the menopause. You live with your husband; he is pretty well though does have high BP which you feel cannot be helped by his stressful job and inactivity. You do worry about him. You have two grown-up daughters; your youngest is having relationship problems which is also a worry for you. She has just asked her partner to move out as she discovered he was having an affair. She has a 2-year-old so you suspect you'll be called upon for more child care support too.

ICE You worry there is something wrong, an underlying condition making you feel like this though you're not sure what. You also wonder if it's to do with the menopause. You have no specific expectations other than *'perhaps some blood tests?'*

Impact The tiredness is stopping you exercising and you feel it is impacting your concentration at work which means you're staying late to double check your figures; this isn't helping your overall satisfaction with life at present.

Learning Points

Tiredness is a common symptom, but unfortunately often no underlying cause is found. Detailed history taking can point to either a lifestyle cause or an underlying disease process. When faced with a case of feeling tired all the time, remember our motto 'Common things are common, but what mustn't I miss?' Use your list of differentials to frame your questions; a systems review may be helpful too.

The list of conditions that can cause tiredness is endless but below are some to consider:

- Anaemia of any cause – ?pallor, risk factor for bleeding/active bleeding, cancer red flag?
- Chronic diseases, e.g. COPD, heart failure, renal disease, liver disease.
- Any chronic inflammatory condition including diabetes.
- Vitamin deficiency, e.g. vitamin D, B12, folic acid, iron – ?dietary, malabsorption or loss.
- Obstructive sleep apnoea – nocturnal waking, snoring, gasping (described by partner).
- Thyroid abnormalities – weight, skin, hair, nail changes, palpitations, oedema.
- Cushing's disease – weight gain, high BP, striae, central adiposity.
- Addison's disease – low BP, dizziness, electrolyte disturbance.
- Mental health problems.
- Menopause/perimenopause.
- Medication, e.g. beta-blockers, opiates, benzodiazepines, mirtazapine, amitriptyline . . .

The above can be whittled down through consideration of the clinical notes provided (?pre-existing conditions or medications), associated symptoms, risk factors and red flag questions. If none seem likely, focus on life events, stress, lifestyle and sleep habits to see if there are any clues there to the cause of tiredness.

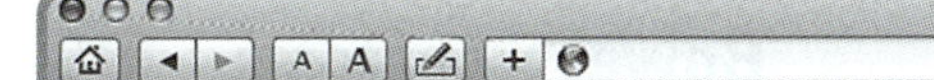

Doctor's Notes

Patient	Hamza Khan	19 years	M
PMH	None		
Medications	None		
Allergies	None		
Consultations	None		
Investigations	None		
Household	None		

Out-of-hours note: seen by ANP 3 days ago

'Diarrhoea over the weekend, some cramps. No vomiting. No travel. Student. Examination normal including PR. Obs stable. Probably viral, advised fluids, paracetamol and see GP if not settling'

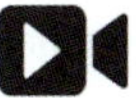

Open ☐ Sorry to hear that, what problems have you been having?

History ☐ Tell me how the problem first started? Any changes in your life around then? Any other symptoms you have noticed? Pain for example? Any times when it's difficult to open your bowels? Any mucus? Is there any pattern to when the symptoms are worse? Have you seen anyone about this before? What did she say? Tell me about yourself – what are you doing in life at the moment? How is the course? What do you do to relax?

Impact ☐ How do these symptoms affect you day to day? Have they stopped you from playing cricket or attending lectures?

ICE1 ☐ What do you think is the most likely cause?

Sense ☐ I sense the unpredictable nature of the symptoms has been causing you a lot of worry.

ICE2 ☐ Have you also been worried about what could be causing it? What else has worried you about the symptoms?

Risk ☐ Have you noticed any link to food? Is there any FH of food allergy or bowel problems? Do you drink alcohol? Or smoke?

Flags ☐ Have you ever noticed any blood when you've been for a poo? Any weight loss? Any nausea or vomiting? Any fevers?

ICE3 ☐ After hearing about the student who passed away, were you hoping for any particular tests today? Anything else you were hoping for?

SummarICE ☐ So you've been struggling with diarrhoea, bloating and pain for about a year; you thought it was probably a food allergy but because of what's happened at university recently you're worried it could be bowel cancer so you hoped I could tell you what's wrong. You'd like to get it sorted so you can worry less about playing sport and completing your studies.

Impression ☐ Lots of things can cause diarrhoea and tummy pains. You're right – these include food allergies or intolerances, bowel inflammation and, yes, bowel cancer too. Thankfully, you've had none of the other symptoms that would make me worry about bowel cancer or inflammation, such as passing blood or weight loss. I think it's more likely you have a condition called irritable bowel syndrome, IBS.

Experience ☐ Have you heard of irritable bowel syndrome?

Explanation ☐ IBS is a common condition which causes a mixture of diarrhoea, constipation, bloating and tummy cramps. The exact cause is unknown, but it relates to the interaction between the gut and the brain. This is why it can be made worse by stress as well as certain types of food. This link to foods is not the same as a true allergy though.

Recommend ☐ There is no specific test for IBS, but it's helpful to do tests to rule out other things, such as bowel inflammation or infection, specific allergies (e.g. to gluten) and bowel cancer. We can do this with a combination of blood tests and stool tests.

InCLudE ☐ You mentioned allergy and bowel cancer – would you be happy to have these tests?

Empower ☐ IBS is usually managed by dietary changes, e.g. adjusting fibre and reducing foods containing complex sugars. You've already thought about your diet; could you try this? I can send you a PIL from the Association of UK Dietitians with examples of foods that are good for IBS and ones to avoid. Medication, e.g. Buscopan or peppermint oil which are available from the chemist, may help with cramping pain. You could also use occasional loperamide to stop diarrhoea. Perhaps consider this on days when you're playing cricket or have an exam? But watch out for constipation.

Future ☐ Please book in with reception for your blood test, and collect 2× stool pots (1 for infection, 1 for inflammation) as well as a FIT kit – this is the test which helps rule out bowel cancer. Could we catch up again next month to go through your results and see how you've got on with the low FODMAP diet?

Safety net ☐ If you do notice any blood when opening your bowels or your symptoms worsen, particularly if you develop severe pain or fever, please contact us again straight away.

Patient's Story

Doctor's notes Hamza Khan, 19 years. M. No PMH, drugs or allergies.

Out-of-hours note: seen by ANP 3 days ago

'Diarrhoea over the weekend, some cramps. No vomiting. No travel. Student. Examination normal including PR. Obs stable. Probably viral, advised fluids, paracetamol and see GP if not settling'

How to act Anxious

PC *'Doctor, I'm troubled by my bowels.'*

History For the last year you have been experiencing intermittent diarrhoea and bloating. You can also become constipated at times. Some days you experience cramping pains, which can be quite severe, but do usually settle after opening your bowels. When you have diarrhoea, you often get urgency symptoms which worry you. You have never seen any blood, though sometimes notice mucus. The symptoms started just before you began university. No weight loss, no vomiting, occasional mild nausea. You have not noticed any particular foods that make the symptoms worse, though have made the food you cook less spicy. You get migraines now and then, usually when you're stressed. You had another bout of diarrhoea and cramps last weekend; you went to the out-of-hours service and saw a nurse practitioner. She examined you and said all was normal on examination, including PR. She thought you probably had a tummy bug.

Social You are a politics student in your first year at university. You live in halls of residence. You have friends and like to socialise but you do not drink alcohol so sometimes get frustrated with the noisy students who get drunk and keep you awake at night. You enjoy playing cricket but get anxious when playing as you can be out on the field for a long time and not able to get to the toilet easily. You've also had to rush out of lectures occasionally due to needing to go to the toilet. You're worried about your upcoming exams; one is 4 hours long and you're not sure how you'll manage if your symptoms flare up – they do seem to be worse around exams and stressful periods. You have a supportive family at home, no significant FH.

Impact The biggest impact is around worry about not getting to the toilet and this impacting on your enjoyment of cricket and your ability to concentrate in lectures.

ICE You recently heard about a university student who died of bowel cancer, as a group of fellow students have been fund raising in her name. You're worried it could be something serious like cancer and it's this that has prompted you to book an appointment after so long. Initially, you were embarrassed so didn't attend and put it down to some sort of food intolerance, though you're not sure what. You hope the doctor can tell you it's nothing to worry about; you wouldn't mind having some tests to be sure.

Bowel Symptoms – IBS[1]

IBS is a common, chronic, often debilitating condition of the gut–brain axis. It is unknown what exactly causes it.

Symptoms

Bloating, pain, diarrhoea/constipation or change in bowel habit (CIBH), pain worsened by eating or relieved by opening bowels, passage of mucus.

Symptoms should have been present for 6 months or more. IBS does not usually cause nocturnal symptoms.

Main differential diagnosis

IBD, coeliac disease, abdominal cancers (e.g. bowel or ovarian).

Secondary care diagnostic criteria

ROME IV criteria: recurrent abdominal pain, on average, at least 1 day per week in the last 3 months (with symptom onset at least 6 months prior to diagnosis) which is associated with two or more of the following:

- Related to defaecation.
- Change in frequency of stool.
- Change in stool form.

Patients are subgrouped according to predominant Bristol stool type:

- IBS with diarrhoea (IBS-D).
- IBS with constipation (IBS-C).
- IBS with mixed bowel habits (IBS-M).
- IBS unclassified (IBS-U).

Investigations

NICE recommends:

- Bloods – FBC, CRP + ESR, coeliac screen.
- Faecal calprotectin.

You may wish to consider other tests such as FIT, stool MC&S or bloods (U&E, LFT, TFT) to help rule out other causes.

Management

Dietary adjustments are usually required and can significantly reduce symptoms in some patients. Adjusting fibre and reducing certain foods/drinks (e.g. alcohol, caffeine, fizzy drinks, fatty/fried foods) and limiting fresh fruit to three portions a day can help.

NICE recommends that strict restrictions on diet (e.g. excluding FODMAPs) should be done under dietitian supervision as prolonged dietary restriction can result in inadequate nutrient intake and alteration of the gut microbiome.

Medications – depend on symptoms but could include laxatives (except lactulose), loperamide, antispasmodics such as mebeverine, alverine, peppermint oil, hyoscine butylbromide, amitriptyline, SSRIs.

CHAPTER 11

PRESCRIBING

	Cases in this chapter	RCGP 2025 curriculum	Learning points
11.1	Dyspepsia/ Reflux	**Gastroenterology** 'Dyspepsia, gastro-oesophageal reflux disease (GORD)'	Dyspepsia: assessment, diagnosis and management Upper GI malignancy: referral for suspected caner
11.2	Chronic pain	**Musculoskeletal health** 'Chronic pain (such as complex regional pain syndrome)'	Chronic pain: assessment and management
11.3	High Cholesterol	**Cardiovascular health** 'Principles of primary, secondary and tertiary prevention of disease'	NHS health check Assessing cardiovascular risk Lipid management
11.4	Hypertension	**Cardiovascular health** 'Hypertension: essential (and its classification into stages), secondary and malignant … Cardiovascular health screening'	Hypertension: definition, assessment and management
11.5	Migraine	**Neurology** 'Headaches including tension, migraine, cluster, raised intracranial pressure including idiopathic intracranial hypertension'	Migraine: • Assessment • Red flags • Differential diagnosis • Management

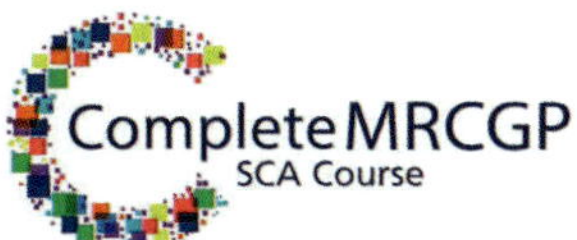

Links to the RCGP Clinical Curriculum

This broad blueprint group may feature clinical topics from throughout the curriculum and all life stages. In this chapter, the cases are drawn from the following clinical topic guides:

- Gastroenterology
- Musculoskeletal health
- Cardiovascular health
- Neurology

Prescribing in the SCA – Skills and Pitfalls

Prescribing is a core GP skill, and a good knowledge of medications and prescribing guidelines is essential. Within the SCA, you will probably need to prescribe medication in one or more cases, managing potential interactions with current medications, and recognise when to deprescribe.

The BNF is no longer allowed during the exam, so you must learn the names, doses, actions, side effects and normal regimes of common medications. You are not expected to know details of uncommon drugs but, for example, you should be able to explain to a patient how to take a weekly bisphosphonate tablet.

Check the case notes for any drug history and consider if this might affect the consultation or interact with something you might prescribe. You might notice that an older patient is prescribed an NSAID such as diclofenac on repeat with no clear reason and no gastric protection. Their PMH may include heart disease. You would be expected to recognise that this is potentially both unsafe and inappropriate and, whatever the presenting problem, flag it up in the consultation.

If, from the case notes, you can anticipate the need for medication, e.g. test results showing hypothyroidism or osteoporosis, use your 3-minute preparation time to think about what to prescribe. If you are unsure of the dose or frequency for a medication, say that you will confirm details after the consultation and will write these clearly on the prescription. Do give as much information as you can about the medication but don't bluff – if you don't know, be honest and say so.

If medication is required, remember to give the following details and check the patient is happy to proceed:

1. Name
2. Why you recommend this drug (benefits).
3. How to take it (route, number of times a day and for how long).
4. Potential side effects (risks).

Be alert for cases where your first-choice 'new' medication might interact with the patient's regular medication. You may also get a case where the patient is already taking two or more medications that could interact and which may need addressing.

There may be a consultation where the key is not to prescribe, e.g. pressure from patient to prescribe antibiotics, opiates or another controlled drug. Make sure you have a strategy to tackle this. Emphasising the potential risks/harms and exploring an alternative approach is a good place to start.

Prescribing and Medical Complexity

Prescribing is a common and important area where medical complexity may feature. Be vigilant, and ready to problem-solve, working with the patient. Uncovering information in DG will alert you to possible dilemmas that may otherwise, less helpfully, emerge in CM. Where might the complexity lie?

Medical notes

Everything in the patient's notes will be relevant to the imminent consultation, with no unnecessary or redundant information. Therefore, details in the notes may alert you to potential prescribing issues. Note these on your white board so you do not overlook them during DG, and are prompted to incorporate them in management.

- **PMH.** A previous DVT or migraine becomes highly relevant if a patient asks about starting the OCP, because these are contraindications to the combined OCP.
- **Current medication.** With a long list of tablets, consider polypharmacy and drug interactions, and any additional risks with any drug you consider prescribing.
- **Deprescribing.** Why is an older patient taking regular high dose co-codamol? Do they need this regularly or only intermittently? Is it appropriate? Are there side effects – drowsiness, confusion or constipation?
- **Common drug interactions.** Learn some common interactions, as these may explain why a drug that should be effective is either not working or is causing problems or side effects. Examples:
  - A young woman starts iron tablets for anaemia, and finds that doxycycline, prescribed for acne, is less effective. Explanation – oral iron reduces the absorption of tetracyclines by up to 90%.
  - A man taking simvastatin was prescribed clarithromycin for a chest infection last week and now has muscle aches. Explanation – clarithromycin increases blood levels of simvastatin and makes side effects more likely.
- **Potentially harmful drugs.** Some drugs, commonly prescribed in the past, are now known to cause harm. For example, look out for drugs that increase the cholinergic burden and may not be needed. Examples might include amitriptyline and oxybutynin. Other drugs are of limited clinical value, such as quinine sulfate for leg cramps – consider stopping these after discussion with the patient.
- **Known side effects of drugs** may present as symptoms. E.g. Ramipril (persistent cough) or amlodipine (swollen legs). Similarly, if a drug has been prescribed inappropriately, e.g. beta blocker in a patient with asthma, you are expected to identify and tackle this.
- **A patient's chronic illness** may limit what you might prescribe. A patient with significant asthma, on regular inhalers, describes acute situational anxiety, where you might otherwise consider beta blockers. Or a young woman with epilepsy treated with phenytoin asks about using Desogestrel for contraception – not a suitable choice because phenytoin will reduce contraceptive effectiveness.

  Explore these dilemmas during DG. For example, you could explore other strategies for anxiety management, asking, '*What have you tried already? What has helped?*' Or you might ask the young woman why she particularly requested the POP and what other contraception she has tried or thought about.
- **Drug allergy** – e.g. penicillin or aspirin. You are expected to incorporate this into your plan. '*Normally we would prescribe penicillin, but I can see you are allergic to this, so an alternative would be...*'

Data gathering and diagnosis

During DG, further issues may emerge. Listening carefully and checking expectations (ICE3) will yield helpful information ready for prescribing in CM. For example, you might hear:

- '*Someone at work also has [a similar condition] and s/he has been prescribed X.*' Explore this and check with the patient if this is an expectation – something they are also hoping you might prescribe.

Prescribing and Medical Complexity

- Asking expectations, you may well learn what medication or treatment the patient is hoping for. This might be appropriate, completely inappropriate or even dangerous. Being patient-centred does not, of course, mean acceding to this request, however unreasonable. Instead, acknowledge their thoughts and address these later in your CM. '*You hoped I might prescribe morphine, which is a very strong painkiller and has many side effects. As you have not yet tried anything else, I suggest we start with something I think will help but without all the risks and side effects.*'
- You may hear a strong 'always/never' statement such as, '*I never take antibiotics, they'll poison my gut microbiome*'. If the patient may need an antibiotic, you will need to explore their health beliefs. In CM, negotiate alternative strategies if appropriate.
- Remember to ask about OTC medications. With a new diagnosis of AKI, it is highly relevant that a patient takes regular OTC ibuprofen for headaches.
- Compliance. Never assume that the patient complies with medication! Ask, non-judgementally, about their experience of taking the tablets and whether they are taking them. Avoid leading questions '*You are taking the tablets, aren't you?*' and ones where it is difficult for the patient to answer 'no' such as '*Do you always remember to take the tablets?*' Instead, use an open question, '*How are you getting on with the medication?*'

Clinical management

If you have read and assimilated the notes, listened carefully during data gathering, explored and found out the patient's expectations, there should not be too many unanticipated challenges in clinical management. You can incorporate the possible dilemmas into your explanation. For example:

'*You wondered if the same medicine that your brother is taking would work for you too. Let me explain why I think a different approach might be better.*'

'*I appreciate you wanted antibiotics and that these have always worked before. May I explain to you why I don't think we should use them on this occasion?*'

'*Normally we would prescribe drug X but, on this occasion, I think we should use something different because…*'

However, you may find that challenges appear unexpectedly, and it is important to think how you will manage this emergent medical complexity.

If the patient disagrees with what you suggest – they refuse the medication, or strongly request something different, how you will approach this? If the patient 'closes the door' no amount of pushing is going to open it. Avoid insisting that you know best and that the patient should do as they are told. This will be ineffective and not gain marks. The examiners are looking for skilled negotiation, not confrontation. If you are challenged, take a step back and do not react with frustration. Instead, think what you may have missed. Ask, '*Tell me what makes you think that*' or '*That's interesting. What is your previous experience of [the drug]?*'

Be prepared to be creative and flexible. Emphasise any risks and harms that may be caused by the patient's preference and look for an alternative. This is a place to earn good marks in the domains of both CM&C and RTO.

Conclusion

This area has the potential for you to gain great marks or lose them! Read the notes carefully, explore ICE and previous experience of relevant medications in DG, and be ready to negotiate rather than argue.

Finally, take every opportunity to learn about common drugs, their side effects and interactions in your everyday consultations.

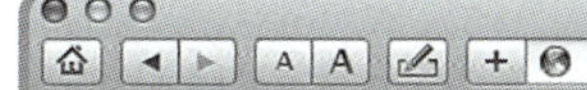

Doctor's Notes

Patient	Daniel Hernandez	38 years	M
PMH	None		
Medications	None		
Allergies	None		
Consultations	New patient check last week with HCA. Smoker 15/day, alcohol 25 units/week. BP 124/75, BMI 32. Mentioned tummy pain, abdomen checked by practice paramedic before leaving, soft non-tender, no masses. Advised to book with GP to discuss abdominal pain further		
Investigations	No recent investigations		
Household	No household members registered		

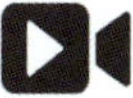

Example Consultation

Dyspepsia/Reflux

Open ☐ Can you tell me more about this pain? When did you first notice it? Is there a pattern?

History ☐ What brings it on? Does anything make it worse? Or better? Where do you feel the pain? Does it go anywhere else? How have your bowels and waterworks been?

Impact ☐ How has this pain affected you? Has it stopped you doing anything? Where do you work? A food magazine – do you eat a healthy diet, would you say? Have you noticed any particular meals which make the pain worse? Have you noticed a cough at night or first thing in the morning?

Risk ☐ Do you smoke? Drink any alcohol? Is there a family history of stomach problems? Have you been taking any painkillers, for example ibuprofen, for anything?

Flags ☐ Have you lost weight? Vomited blood? Passed black stools? Does it cause any other symptoms like nausea, sweating or breathlessness? Have you had any difficulty swallowing?

ICE1 ☐ You've had this pain a while now; what do you think it could be?

Curious ☐ Tell me about your mum's experience.

Sense ☐ I sense you are anxious about what happened to your mum.

ICE2 ☐ What worries have crossed your mind? Have you been worried about needing an operation?

ICE3 ☐ Given your mum's experience, was there anything you hoped I may suggest today?

SummarICE ☐ So, you have been getting pain in your upper tummy for 2 months; it is worse at night and after large meals or alcohol. You thought it could be due to gallstones as your mum had this problem. You are worried about needing an operation or blood tests as you really don't like needles.

Impression ☐ From listening to your symptoms it seems you have acid reflux rather than gallstones. Thankfully there are no worrying symptoms.

Experience ☐ Have you heard of reflux? Do you know anything about it?

Explanation ☐ Reflux is when stomach acid comes out of the stomach and into the food pipe. This causes pain as the acid irritates the food pipe. It can go all the way up to your throat and cause soreness there too.

Empathy ☐ Reflux is common but can be uncomfortable and I see it's affected your enjoyment of food.

Options ☐ Thankfully, reflux is treatable. How do you feel about trying a medication called omeprazole which reduces stomach acid and usually makes the symptoms better? You would take it each morning for a month then come back for a review. With short-term use there are usually few side effects though some people notice changes to their bowels such as constipation or diarrhoea.

Future ☐ In most cases the symptoms will settle but, if not, there are other investigations we can do. For example, some people have a bacterial bug in their stomach which can cause this. If your pain is still there after the treatment, I would suggest testing for this. Blood tests can sometimes be helpful, but as you've had no worrying symptoms, I think we can avoid these for the time being.

Empower ☐ There are some things that you can do to help too. Adjusting your eating habits to avoid large meals in the evening and reducing fatty, spicy and acidic foods, caffeine and alcohol also tends to help. Keeping to a healthy weight helps prevent reflux too. You mentioned that you smoke – is this something you have considered stopping? We have a stop smoking service; would you like the details?

Safety net ☐ I would like to see you in 4 weeks to see how you are but if you start vomiting, the pain worsens or you pass blood or black stools, please arrange to come to the surgery to see me straight away. If the pain has gone and all is well, you can cancel the appointment, but let me know if it flares up again.

Patient's Story

Dyspepsia/Reflux

Doctor's notes Daniel Hernandez, 38 years.

New patient HCA consultation last week. BP 124/75, smoker 15/day, alcohol 25 units/week. BMI 32. Mentioned tummy pains, checked by practice paramedic prior to leaving – abdo SNT, no masses, advised to see GP. No investigations. No household members registered.

How to act Relaxed but anxious if tests are mentioned.

PC *'Doctor, I have a pain in the stomach.'*

History For the last 2 months you have been getting stomach pains intermittently. The pain can be sharp or burning and is located in your upper abdomen/lower chest. The pain starts in the lower chest but radiates up, sometimes to your throat. You feel you have been belching more too. The pain is worse at night after a large meal. It tends to be worse at the weekends when you have been out with your friends.

You have not been sick, you have normal bowel motions and no black stools. You have not lost any weight, although you have been trying to.

You have tried Gaviscon which did help a bit. You have since been trying to avoid foods you would normally enjoy. You have taken no other medicines.

Social You came to the UK from Spain 20 years ago to study at university.

You got a good job as a graduate journalist so decided to stay and now write for a food magazine, enjoying going out for meals. You will often have a few glasses of wine with your meals. When you saw the nurse she told you that you were drinking too much, so you have tried to cut down. You do smoke but know you should stop! You're thinking about trying an e-cigarette.

You live alone but have some good friends and colleagues with whom you socialise.

ICE You are worried about gallstones. Your mother had an operation to remove her gallbladder and you remember her getting abdominal pains when eating. She still lives in Spain so you haven't had a chance to ask her more about her symptoms.

You have a needle phobia so worry you may need blood tests or surgery.

You expect the doctor will possibly want to order blood tests.

Learning Points

Dyspepsia/Reflux[1]

Assessment

Ask about:

- Frequency, pattern, duration and impact.
- Red flag symptoms – dysphagia, weight loss, vomiting/haematemesis, melaena.
- Risk factors – FH, obesity, alcohol, smoking, caffeine, spicy/acidic foods, anxiety, meds including OTC.

Examination:

- BMI.
- Signs of anaemia.
- Abdominal masses/tenderness.

Tests:

- FBC (anaemia + raised platelets → suspect malignancy).
- *Helicobacter pylori*.

Differential diagnosis

- Upper GI malignancy or ulcers.
- Hepatobiliary disease, e.g. gallstones, cholecystitis.
- Pancreatic disease, e.g. pancreatitis (acute or chronic).
- Intestinal – IBS, coeliac disease, lactose intolerance, small intestine bacterial overgrowth.
- Cardiac pain, AAA.

Management

- Advise about modifiable lifestyle factors – timing of meals (evening meal 3–4 hours prior to bed), size of meals, foods to avoid/reduce (e.g. fatty, spicy, acidic, caffeinated), reduction in alcohol, stopping smoking, weight loss where required, stress/anxiety reduction.
- Medication review – recommend OTC antacids. Advise stopping NSAIDs, may need to stop/alter other medications if likely to be exacerbating symptoms.
- Consider full-dose PPI for 1 month or testing for *H. pylori* (i.e. omeprazole 20–40 mg, lansoprazole 30 mg, esomeprazole 20 mg, pantoprazole 40 mg or rabeprazole 20 mg).
- *H. pylori* eradication examples (check local guidance), 7 days triple therapy:
  - Full-dose PPI **twice** daily + amoxicillin 1 g twice daily.
  - Either clarithromycin 500 mg twice daily or metronidazole 400 mg twice daily.

Suspected cancer referral oesophageal/stomach cancer[1–3]

Refer if either:

- Dysphagia, or:
- Age ≥55 years + weight loss and any of the following:
  - Upper abdo pain.
  - Reflux.
  - Dyspepsia.

Non-urgent direct-access endoscopy if haematemesis, or:

- Age ≥55 years with one of the following:
  - Treatment-resistant dyspepsia
  - Upper abdo pain + low haemoglobin.
  - Raised platelets + any of the following: nausea, vomiting, weight loss, reflux, dyspepsia, upper abdo pain.

Doctor's Notes

Patient Rachel West 43 years F

PMH Back pain, IBS

Medications Mebeverine 135 mg TDS

Tramadol 50–100 mg QDS as required. Last issued 14 days ago by practice (4 week supply)

Medicines management notes:

6 weeks ago – early issue due to holiday

10 weeks ago – extra script due to lost medications

Allergies None

Consultations 2 weeks ago saw GP in out of hours. 'Request for tramadol for back pain, states ran out and couldn't get hold of own GP due to phone lines engaged. Suffers with chronic back pain, no neurology, examination normal. 7 days tramadol given, advised to see own GP if needs more'

Investigations MRI lumbar spine 6 months ago – minor degenerative changes, nil else

Household No household members registered

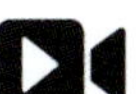

Example Consultation

Chronic Pain

Open ☐	Can you tell me more about what you use the tramadol for?
Impact ☐	Tell me which areas of your life are affected by the back pain. Has the pain stopped you doing anything? How do you manage the pain day to day? Are you working at present?
History ☐	You've been struggling with this pain for some time; what have you been told about it in the past? Have any other painkillers helped? Have you tried exercises or physiotherapy before?
ICE1 ☐	When you were told there was not much wrong with your back, what did you think?
Flags ☐	Have any of your symptoms changed? Anything new or unexpected? Before you haven't had any pain in your legs, weakness, numbness or difficulty going to the toilet; is that still the case?
Curious ☐	Thinking back to when the pain first started, what was happening in your life then?
ICE2 ☐	Is there anything that you are especially worried about? How do you feel about the future?
Sense ☐	Looking at your record, I'm picking up some suggestions that you may be struggling to manage the pain with the current treatment.
Risk ☐	Sometimes when pain is bad, patients feel the need to take extra doses of medication; this can leave them short each month and result in them asking for prescriptions early or getting more from other places like out of hours. Has that ever happened to you?
Empathy ☐	It must have been hard managing this pain for such a long time.
ICE3 ☐	You've mentioned needing the tramadol; is there anything else you feel will be helpful? Can you tell me how you're taking the tramadol at present?
SummarICE ☐	So overall, you accept that the doctors can't find a serious cause for the pain, but wonder why your back is so painful. You would like more tramadol tablets to reduce the pain.
Impression ☐	From what you have told me, I'm worried that your body has become addicted to the tramadol. This shows from your need to take more to get the same benefit and running out of tablets early. Do you agree this is a possibility? How does this make you feel?
InCludE ☐	You're right that it is odd that there is no significant problem with your back, but it still hurts a lot; however, there is an explanation for this experience.
Explanation ☐	After 3 months, your body has usually healed as much as it is going to so pain should subside. However, for some, the pain does not settle, as the nervous system has become oversensitive and overprotective. Our brain generates all pain sensations; this may be helpful to protect us, but sometimes it is not helpful and stops us getting on with our lives. We don't always know what causes chronic pain, but it can be linked to your emotional state at the time the pain started. You've mentioned a difficult time personally when the pain began. Chronic pain is complex, and painkillers don't always work well. Patients like you commonly have problems with medication, through no fault of their own. That's why we try to help people move away from painkillers, and all the side effects and problems they cause. How would you feel about trying to come off the tramadol?
Recommend ☐	I would recommend slowly weaning down off the tramadol, reducing by 1 tablet every 2–4 weeks. To help you, I will switch you to weekly scripts to reduce the temptation to take more. I would like to refer you to our health coach who can help you learn other ways to manage pain through gentle exercise and strategies. I have some useful resources on chronic pain, a video and website, which explain it well.
Future ☐	Often patients feel better off the tramadol, but if you did get more pain, we could consider using a non-addictive painkiller such as duloxetine or amitriptyline to see if that helps?
Empower ☐	Although recovering from chronic pain may be a long journey, it is certainly possible with the actions we've discussed already.
Specifics ☐	I'd like to see you again in 2–3 weeks; would that be okay? In that time, perhaps you could think about some goals you'd like to achieve, such as taking up a hobby or getting back into work, which we could discuss further next time?

Patient's Story

Chronic Pain

Doctor's notes Rachel West, 43 years. Back pain, IBS.

Medications: mebeverine 135 mg TDS, tramadol 50–100 mg QDS as required. Last issued 14 days ago by practice (4-week supply). Medicines management notes: 6 weeks ago – early issue due to holiday; 10 weeks ago – extra script due to lost medications. No allergies.

Consultations: 2 weeks ago saw GP in out of hours. 'Request for tramadol for back pain, states ran out and couldn't get hold of own GP due to phone lines engaged. Suffers with chronic back pain, no neurology, examination normal. 7 days tramadol given, advised to see own GP if needs more.'

Investigations: MRI lumbar spine 6 months ago – minor degenerative changes, nil else.

How to act Relaxed initially, but agitated if think won't get what you want. Can be talked round though and calmed if doctor uses appropriate interpersonal skills.

PC *'Hi, Doctor, quick one for you, I just need my tramadol tablets.'*

History You have suffered with back pain since your late teens; it is something you have just had to deal with over the years. You have been prescribed medication to help, initially ibuprofen, then co-codamol and now tramadol. Each painkiller has helped at first but over time becomes ineffective. You take 8–10 tramadol tablets per day, and are aware this is more than advised. You've had physio and tests before such as an MRI; no-one can explain why your back is so painful. The pain started during a difficult time in your life – your parents were going through a divorce and your grandmother, whom you were close to, had died. The pain is in the middle of your back at the bottom which can radiate into your buttocks. There are no neurological symptoms. Ibuprofen upsets your IBS. Co-codamol doesn't work. You would try a neuropathic agent if offered.

Social You're unemployed. You have tried a few jobs (e.g. bar work and being a carer) but you generally find the jobs make your back pain worse. You're claiming benefits at present due to your back pain. You live alone. You have some friends locally. No exercise. Limited alcohol. Non-smoker. You find the back pain limiting; you don't want to go out but sitting around at home doesn't help either. You feel you haven't achieved as much in your life as you could have done due to the pain.

ICE You expect the doctor to give you another prescription for tramadol. If they question your use of tramadol, initially try to explain away the extra prescriptions. Deep down you know you're addicted to the tramadol; you don't want to be. You believe the doctors when they say there is nothing significant wrong with your back, but you don't know why it should continue to hurt. If the doctor is non-judgemental and able to explain chronic pain to you, you would be willing to try to cut down on the tablets.

Learning Points

Chronic Pain[1]

Chronic primary pain Pain with no clear underlying cause or pain disproportionate to the pathology.
Chronic secondary pain Long-standing pain with underlying pathology.

Assessment

Once red flag symptoms have been ruled out, adopt a person-centred approach. Identifying the impact of the problem on the person's life, and how their life affects the problem is key to understanding the situation. There is often a significant emotional component to chronic pain, so identifying stress, anxiety, depression or history of traumatic events can shed light on the origin of pain or current deteriorations.

Follow a SOCRATES approach to obtain a description of the pain, the site and severity and any changes over time. This helps to identify the type of pain, e.g. neuropathic, nociceptive or mixed.

Using a biopsychosocial approach to history taking, pay particular attention to history of mental health problems, substance misuse, social isolation, traumatic events or stressful life events.

Exploring ICE is also extremely important – identifying the patient's thoughts about the cause of the pain, their expectations for the future and expectations of any possible treatments can be key, as there may well be unhelpful health beliefs, e.g. there must be something serious wrong or the purpose of pain relief is to remove all pain, which need to be tackled. Careful management of expectations and reframing of what successful treatment looks like may be necessary.

Management

A significant portion of management will revolve around information giving. Patients may not be aware of the difference between acute and chronic pain. There are some excellent videos explaining this such as 'Understanding pain in less than 5 minutes'[2] which are worth watching to help you find the language to describe chronic pain to patients. These videos can also be shared with patients as well.

Dos and don'ts for chronic primary pain

Do:

- Provide a holistic approach.
- Offer supervised group exercise.
- Offer CBT or acceptance and commitment therapy (ACT).
- Consider acupuncture.
- Consider antidepressant – duloxetine, amitriptyline or SSRI – taking into account risks and benefits (off-label use).
- Encourage deprescribing medications listed below if currently in use.

Don't offer:

- Biofeedback.
- Interferential therapy.
- TENS or ultrasound.
- Nabilone, dronabinol, THC, cannabidiol (CBD), except as part of a clinical trial.

Don't initiate:

- Gabapentoids, ketamine, antiepileptics.
- Corticosteroid trigger point injections.
- Local anaesthetics.
- NSAIDs, opioids, paracetamol.

Chronic secondary pain

Use clinical judgement and shared decision making about management options.

Prescribing – 11.2

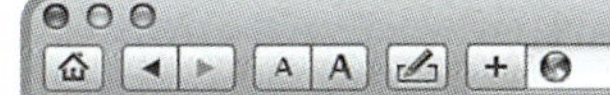

Doctor's Notes

Patient	Vincent Riley 60 years M
PMH	Hypertension. Ex-smoker
Medications	Amlodipine 10 mg daily
Allergies	None
Consultations	Nurse appointment for bloods and blood pressure
	Letter to patient: 'Dear Mr Riley. Thank you for having your blood tests for your medication review. I would be grateful if you could please make an appointment with the doctor to discuss your cholesterol'
Investigations	BP 139/80
	Height 185 cm
	Weight 70 kg
	BMI 20.4
	Cholesterol/HDL ratio 5.8
	QRISK 15%
Household	No household members registered

Example Consultation

High Cholesterol

Open ☐ Thank you for calling, it's good to have an opportunity to find out more about you and discuss your recent blood results.

ICE1 ☐ When you read the letter we sent, what went through your mind? As well as the results, is there anything else that you would like to talk about today?

History ☐ So – your cholesterol is a little high but what we do about this depends on your general health. How do you feel your health is? You have an active lifestyle. How often do you exercise? When did you stop smoking? How much alcohol do you drink? Who is in your life?

Flags ☐ A couple of specifics – do you ever become breathless or have any chest or leg pains?

ICE2 ☐ I sense you are not too worried but are you interested in discussing ways to prevent problems down the line?

Risk ☐ Do you have a FH of angina or heart disease in relatives when they were <60 years old?

Sense ☐ I sense you feel this is a waste of time but, if there is anything we can do to protect you from having angina, a heart attack or stroke, I want to offer help.

ICE3 ☐ Do you have ideas about what we might discuss today to help with this?

Curious ☐ Tell me more about how you have come across statins?

Impact ☐ It sounds as if you are healthy but is there anything more you can try, do you think, to improve your diet? Do you avoid saturated fats in your food?

SummarICE ☐ To summarise, you feel well and your blood pressure is well controlled. Your cholesterol is slightly high. Your friends have had bad experiences with statins.

Empower ☐ I want to ensure you have the information you need to make an informed decision.

Impression ☐ We can put this information into a calculator. It is not perfect but it is based on research, so we can share with you, if you wish, your predicted risk of having a heart attack or a stroke in the next 10 years. Are you interested to know? We take into account if your vessels may have been affected by cigarettes or require BP treatment. Your predicted risk is 15%. If there were 100 people like you, about 15 of them would have a heart attack or stroke in the next 10 years. This is not extremely high but we want to do everything we can to bring that down. Your cholesterol was 5.8; it could be better. If your risk is greater than 10%, you may benefit from a statin. What are your thoughts?

Empathy ☐ I appreciate I am being pessimistic when talking about events like heart attacks and strokes, which is not what you want to hear when you do all you can for your health. I understand this is a big decision as it involves taking a tablet every day.

Experience ☐ What do you know about statins? Do you know how they work?

Explanation ☐ Over time, our arteries can develop plaque that sticks to the vessel walls. This is more likely if you smoke, have high cholesterol or a FH. If part of the plaque breaks off, it can travel down the vessel and get stuck, causing a heart attack or stroke. Statins lower cholesterol, but have extra benefit above what we would expect from this, potentially stabilising or even reversing furring of the arteries. Because you already lead a healthy lifestyle and have stopped smoking, what we can do to reduce your risk is to lower your cholesterol. Guidance suggests we start atorvastatin 20 mg. Like all tablets there are potential side effects which can include feeling unwell with stomach and muscle aches and, rarely, muscle breakdown. Statins can also affect the liver; however, we monitor this and if this occurs we stop the statin. Many people feel well on statins and usually they do lower cholesterol. Whether you choose to take the statin or not will depend on your own perception of the risk versus the downsides of taking a daily tablet.

Options ☐ What do you think? You are always welcome to phone and discuss this again and we will continue to invite you for an annual health check. Are you interested in reading material to go through at home? Do you have any questions?

Future ☐ I respect your decision. Thank you for taking the time to listen to me today. If you ever want to talk again, please don't hesitate to make another appointment.

Patient's Story

High Cholesterol

Doctor's notes Vincent Riley, 60 years. PMH: hypertension and ex-smoker.

Medications: amlodipine 10 mg daily.

Consultations: nurse appointment for bloods and blood pressure. Letter to patient. 'Dear Mr Riley. Thank you for having your blood tests for your medication review. I would be grateful if you could please make an appointment with the doctor to discuss your cholesterol.'

Investigations: BP 139/80, height 185 cm, weight 70 kg, BMI 20.4, cholesterol/HDL ratio 5.8, QRISK 15%.

How to act Apprehensive about why the doctor has called you in today.

PC *'I had a letter asking me to contact you to talk about cholesterol treatment.'*

History You feel very well. Apart from well-controlled high blood pressure you have no other medical history.

Social You are a semi-professional golfer but are starting to spend more time helping around the clubhouse. You remain active, usually playing a few rounds a week and you also enjoy running and cycling. You eat a healthy diet. You are divorced and have a new female partner since last year. Things are going well and you are very happy. You used to smoke until the age of 48 years, on average 10 cigarettes a day. You drink 1–2 beers a couple of nights a week.

You have three children with your ex-wife and they live in different parts of the world.

ICE You are not concerned about your health. You feel very fit and active.

You ask the doctor: *'Is this a box-ticking exercise, Doc?'*

You have heard about statins. Several of your friends have tried them and felt awful on them.

You are interested to hear what the doctor has to say but you do not accept any cholesterol treatment.

NHS health check

All patients between 40 and 74 years of age who do not have pre-existing CVD should be invited for an NHS health check every 5 years. This should include BP check, BMI, lifestyle discussion and blood tests including lipids to allow a QRISK to be calculated.[1] Patients with calculated risks greater than 10% should be offered a statin medication – atorvastatin 20 mg once a day.

QRISK should not be used for patients with type 1 diabetes, CKD3/4/5 (eGFR <60 mL/min/1.73 m^2) or familial hyperlipidaemia as they are automatically considered high risk so statin therapy should have been offered.

Use clinical judgement for patients ≥85 years.

Lipid management

Prior to starting medication request baseline bloods: non-fasting lipids, LFTs, U&E, HbA1c, TFT, CK (if patient has generalised muscle pain).

Repeat LFTs and lipid 3 months after commencing treatment.

Primary prevention – aim for 40% decrease in non-HDL cholesterol. If target not reached, then consider increasing dose of statin.

Secondary prevention – first-line treatment atorvastatin 80 mg. Aim for cholesterol/non-HDL ratio of 2.6 or less.

If a patient declines a statin or is not reaching their lipid target on maximum tolerated therapy you can consider additional medication:

- Ezetimibe.
- Bempedoic acid in combination with ezetimibe if targets not reached or statin declined.

Don't miss the opportunity to discuss lifestyle factors!

Familial hypercholesterolaemia

Consider if total cholesterol >7.5 mmol/L + FH of early CVD.

Refer for assessment if:

- Total cholesterol >9.0 mmol/L or cholesterol/non-HDL ratio >7.5.
- Triglycerides >20 mmol/L (not due to alcohol or poorly controlled diabetes) – urgent referral.
- Triglycerides 10–20 mmol/L (after repeat fasting test 5–14 days after first test).

Be aware in those with triglycerides between 4.5 and 9.9 mmol/L that the CVD risk may be underestimated.

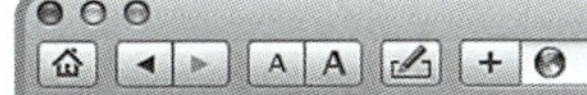

Doctor's Notes

Patient	Richard Turner	57 years	M
PMH	None		
Medications	None		
Allergies	None		
Consultations	Nurse appointment for blood pressure – BP 162/102 right arm, 160/102 left arm. Advised to complete ambulatory BP – average ABPM 151/96 Height 181 cm Weight 80 kg BMI 24.4		
Household	Gillian Turner	56 years	F

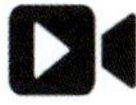

Example Consultation

Hypertension

Open ☐ What led you to have this tested? Do you know your readings?

ICE1 ☐ When you saw the 151/96 figure what went through your mind?

History ☐ How is your general health – do you have any medical conditions or take any medication, prescribed or OTC? Do you work? Please tell me about your job – that sounds very active. Is it stressful? And home – do you live alone or with anyone? How is your relationship? And your lifestyle? Do you take any additional exercise? Do you smoke or drink alcohol? Please tell me about your diet. What do you eat in a typical day? Do you cook from scratch or buy ready meals or takeaways? Do you add salt when cooking or at the table?

Risk ☐ Has a family member had a heart problem, high BP or a stroke? A very personal question if I may – there can be a link between erectile dysfunction and raised BP. Is that something you experience or not?

ICE2 ☐ Of course your father-in-law is not a direct relative but it must have been a shock when he had a stroke. Is that something you worry about happening to you?

Sense ☐ So this has come out of the blue? How do you feel about being told your BP is raised?

Flags ☐ When talking about BP, I usually check that people haven't suffered with any headaches? Or any chest or calf pains? Does your heart ever feel like it is beating too fast?

Curious ☐ You mentioned your wife was helping you test it and she wanted you to have a check; what does she think? Why do you think she is worried?

ICE3 ☐ What did you think I was going to say?

SummarICE ☐ So to summarise, you've been very well and therefore you were surprised when your BP was high. You were hoping that I'd say we'll keep an eye on it but your wife wants you to take tablets, especially with her father's experience. Is that right?

Empathy ☐ I can see you take this seriously and your wife is concerned as her father had high BP.

Impression ☐ Your diagnosis is stage 2 hypertension, which is the medical word for high BP. It is stage 2 because the top number is >150 and the bottom >95.

Experience ☐ What do you understand about why we treat high BP?

Explanation ☐ High BP can increase your risk of a stroke, angina or a heart attack, so it's important to control it. It can also harm your kidneys and eyes. Stage 2 hypertension is not dangerous, but it suggests that we should be treating the BP with tablets as well as lifestyle advice.

Recommend ☐ Whether to start treatment is your decision. There are several types of BP medication, but my recommendation would be to start a tablet called amlodipine 5 mg each morning. This is the favoured medication for someone your age. Amlodipine helps to relax the blood vessels to decrease the pressure. Like any tablet there may be side effects, such as the possibility of ankle swelling, tummy upset or headaches, in which case we could consider a different tablet. How do you feel about taking the tablet? I also suggest you see your optician and inform them that you are now receiving BP medication. Rarely, eyesight can be affected. However, if they see small changes from the effects of BP this is useful for us all to be aware of, so do let me know if this is the case, please.

Empower ☐ Although you already have a healthy lifestyle, if you can increase exercise, reduce alcohol and restrict salt in your diet, these are all likely to help. A 6 g reduction in salt each day reduces your BP number by 10. Do you feel these suggestions will be possible?

Future ☐ Thinking ahead, I would recommend doing routine tests with the nurse to check your general health including an ECG, which is a heart tracing, and blood tests including cholesterol, diabetes screen and kidney function. It's also helpful to send a urine sample to check your kidneys. How do you feel about that?

Specifics ☐ So to summarise, you will start a morning tablet, make an appointment with the nurse for a heart tracing, blood test and urine test, and see me in a month. Please also see an optician. If you're having problems with the tablet or any concerns, please let me know.

Patient's Story

Hypertension

Doctor's notes Richard Turner, 57 years. PMH: none. Medications: none.

Last consultation: BP 162/102 right arm, 160/102 left arm (practice nurse). Average ambulatory BP reading 151/96.

How to act Interested in your health.

PC *'I've called to find out what I need to do about my blood pressure.'*

History You feel well. No PMH or FH.

You were at a friend's house for dinner, and they had purchased a BP machine, so you checked yours.

'My wife wanted me to go to the nurse to check it again.'

The nurse found that your BP was raised and gave you a machine to check it at home. You discussed the average BP, 151/96, with the nurse and have been told to phone the doctor.

Social Very healthy. You enjoy squash and consider yourself to be a healthy eater.

You drink alcohol occasionally and have never smoked.

You work as a gardener so are active during the day. You enjoy your work, and do not find it stressful.

You have a good relationship with your wife. You do not have ED.

ICE You thought 151/96 was high but thought you'd be told to keep an eye on it. You are worried the doctor will want to start a tablet. You are not keen as this will make you feel old, but it won't otherwise impact on your life.

You thought you had no CV risk factors, so you were quite shocked to hear about your BP and the doctor's suggestions.

You understand that it was your father-in-law's BP that led to his stroke.

You are happy to take the tablet, once its importance has been explained. You are also interested in other ways to decrease your BP.

Do not tell the doctor your wife is worried unless the doctor asks. You have mentioned your wife twice already. It is your wife who is worried. Her father was always talking about his BP before his stroke. She would like you to take tablets.

Learning Points

Refer to full NICE Guideline NG136 *Hypertension in adults: diagnosis and management.*[1]

Investigations	Bloods: lipids (for QRISK) and HbA1c (co-morbidity), U&E, eGFR (baseline for Rx), FBC (anaemia) and TFT (cause). ECG (ventricular hypertrophy, arrhythmia), ACR (microalbuminuria/CKD) and fundi (retinopathy).
Diagnosis	Check BP in both arms; if difference >15 mmHg persists use the arm with higher readings. Ambulatory monitoring (best): two measurements/hour during waking hours. Home BP monitoring: twice/day (two readings 1 minute apart) for 4–7 days. Discard first day's reading and average remaining.
Stage 1 HTN	Clinic BP ≥140/90 and home BP ≥135/85. Treat if any of the below apply: Adult <80 years with persistent stage 1 hypertension **and** ≥1 of: • Target organ damage. • Established cardiovascular disease. • Renal disease • Estimated 10-year risk CVD ≥10%. Use clinical judgement if frailty or multi-morbidity.
Stage 2 HTN	Clinic BP ≥160/100 and home BP ≥150/95. Start treatment.
Stage 3/severe HTN	Clinic SBP ≥180 or DBP ≥110. Treat immediately.
Accelerated HTN	Papilloedema or retinal haemorrhage. Admission. Suspected phaeochromocytoma. Admission.
Aims of clinic	BP: <140/90 if <80 years or <150/90 if >80 years with treated HTN. <140/80 if type 2 DM or <135/85 if type 1 DM. <130/80 if DM and either CKD or retinopathy or cerebrovascular disease.
Treatment	Check you have stopped the OCP! A = ACE inhibitor, B = β-blocker, C = calcium-channel blocker, D = thiazide-like diuretic. If <55 years start with ACE1. If required, add C and D, i.e. A + C + D. If >55 years or people of Black ethnicity and of African/Caribbean descent start with C. If required, add A and then D, i.e. C +A + D. NB: Always check compliance before adding new drug.
Secondary causes of HTN	Primary hyperaldosteronism, phaeochromocytoma, CKD and sleep apnoea. Ask about UTIs as a child. Investigations: urinary normetadrenalines, USS kidneys + referral to exclude fibromuscular dysplasia of the renal artery.

Prescribing – 11.4

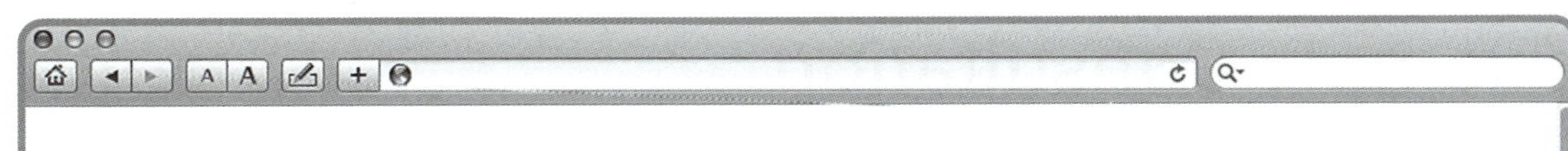

Doctor's Notes

Patient	Yasmin Small	23 years	F
PMH	Migraine		
Medications	Sumatriptan 50 mg PRN		
	Desogestrel 75 mcg OD		
Allergies	No known drug allergies		
Consultations	Pill review 3 months ago, no issues with pill. BP 110/75, HR 75, BMI 21. Migraines occurring 2–3 times per month but coping. Fundi normal. Normal neurology. Swap ibuprofen (no longer effective) for sumatriptan 50 mg PRN		
Household	No household members registered		

Example Consultation

Migraine

Open ☐ Tell me more about your headaches please. Can you talk me through a typical headache episode? Any other symptoms you've noticed? Thank you.

History ☐ Is there one type of headache? A pattern or relation to periods? How often are they occurring? What time of day do they start? Do they wake you? Where on the head? What does it feel like? Severity from 1 to 10? What makes it worse? Or better? Does lying down help? Any medical problems? Sinus trouble or increased headache leaning forward? What medicines are you taking at the moment? Do they help? Any changes in your life that may have triggered them? Are work and home okay? Any stress?

Impact ☐ How does it feel living with all these headaches? You mentioned anxiety?

Curious ☐ You've had these headaches a long time, what prompted you to arrange to discuss this today?

ICE2 ☐ Have you worried you could have a brain tumour?

Flags ☐ Any visual disturbance? Do the arms or legs feel different or weak? Any weight loss? Nausea? Vomiting? Are you ever confused or unusually sleepy? Has anyone said your behaviour has changed? Do you now struggle with anything you could easily do a few months ago? Any fevers? Does the light bother you? Any neck stiffness? Any head injury?

Risk ☐ Any FH? Do you have much alcohol, caffeine, cheese, chocolate or citrus fruits? How is your sleep? Do you have much screen time? Do you drink plenty of water?

ICE3 ☐ Have you read much about migraines or talked to anyone? What did your friend say? Were you hoping I may prescribe topiramate? Anything else you'd wondered about?

SummarICE ☐ Your headaches affect your life and this is frustrating. You have anxiety and worry about a serious cause like a brain tumour and would like specialist advice. Sumatriptan helps but you want to prevent their onset. Your friend suggested topiramate. Anything I've missed?

Empathy ☐ I appreciate why you want to check that this frequent headache is nothing serious.

Impression ☐ I agree with you and the previous GP that these headaches are migraines. I suspect the change in frequency may be to do with the change in management at work.

Experience ☐ What do you know about migraines? Do you know anything that can trigger them?

Explanation ☐ A one-sided headache which takes you to bed is typical of a migraine. The cause of the migraine is not completely known but theories include chemical and blood vessel changes.

InCludE ☐ You thought a specialist may help to find the cause and exclude a tumour. You have no symptoms of a brain tumour so it's unlikely further assessment will change anything. Your nerves were fine when my colleague examined you; this is all reassuring.

Recommend ☐ A few different medications may help prevent migraines. Topiramate is an option but we'd need to change your contraception as it can cause serious problems in pregnancy. We could try amitriptyline or propranolol as alternatives. You have to get up early in the morning; given amitriptyline can cause morning grogginess, propranolol may be the best option; it may help your anxiety too. Side effects can include tiredness, but most people feel fine. We can start at a low dose. Thoughts? May I check, have you ever had asthma or used inhalers? Let's start with 40 mg daily to make sure there are no side effects and after a week increase to 40 mg twice daily. Meanwhile, could you keep a headache diary? The features/timing and triggers for headaches would be very helpful.

Empower ☐ Please try to avoid caffeine, citrus, chocolate and alcohol. Be prepared for rebound headaches at first when stopping caffeine. Regular healthy meals, a good sleep pattern, and exercise and relaxation exercises may also help.

Future ☐ Next time we'll discuss other ways to help your anxiety if it doesn't improve with the propranolol, e.g. talking therapies. If we're not winning with the headaches, we could consider a head scan.

Specifics ☐ I'll send the prescription to your pharmacy; could you book a review in 4 weeks?

Safety net ☐ If at any time you start vomiting, feel unwell, have any new symptoms or the headaches wake you, see a GP as we would have to reassess your migraine diagnosis.

Prescribing – 11.5

Patient's Story

Migraine

Doctor's notes Yasmin Small, 23 years. PMH: migraine.

Medications: desogestrel 75 mcg daily, sumatriptan 50 mg PRN.

Last consultation: 3 months ago, pill check, all fine. BP 110/75, HR 75, BMI 21, migraines 2–3 per month, fundi normal, neurology normal, swap ibuprofen (no longer effective) for sumatriptan 50 mg PRN.

How to act Concerned.

PC *'I keep getting headaches.'*

History You have suffered with migraines for years, but they started becoming more frequent 3 months ago. Now they occur at least twice a week. It is always the same headache. Left side or frontal. Onset usually mid-afternoon. It develops over an hour and reaches 8/10 severity. Apart from occasional nausea, only during the headache, you have no associated symptoms. You can't think of any triggers. If asked about work, can mention on reflection change of management at work.

You are not consciously stressed or depressed.

The headaches are not related to your periods.

You have no medical history. Your mum had migraines.

You don't take any other pain relief, just the prescribed sumatriptan which has helped.

When the headache comes on you lie down in a dark room and sleep it off.

Social You work in a clothes shop which you enjoy, though you now have a new store manager who is stricter than the one before and you worry she doesn't like you as she's always getting at you and giving you the worst jobs. She started around 3 months ago.

You live with your boyfriend of 2 years. You drink a couple of glasses of wine weekly. You do not smoke. At work you take it in turns to buy each other a coffee and chocolate.

You have had to have time off work. Your health anxiety has also been running wild with the headaches happening so frequently. The anxiety stops you from focusing on tasks.

ICE *'Well, I suppose you always worry you may have a brain tumour, don't you?'*

You saw a programme 3 nights ago about a girl who had a brain tumour.

Your friend told you that you should be on topiramate; she takes this and finds it works.

You would like to see a specialist, your reason being that the headaches keep coming back and you want to know what is wrong.

You are open to discuss preventative medicines; you have to get up at 6 a.m. so you don't want anything which may make you tired in the morning.

You don't really know anything about migraines other than they are bad headaches.

Learning Points

Migraine[1]

Red flags

Neurological or raised intracranial pressure symptoms or seizures.

Changes in behaviour, memory or skills.

Unilateral deafness or pulse synchronous tinnitus.

Drowsiness or loss of consciousness.

Ataxia.

Sudden visual loss.

Migraine with aura using OCP.

Diagnosis

See NICE guidelines for full details.[1] Can diagnose migraine without aura if there are at least five attacks that fulfil criteria (duration, characteristics, associated symptoms, photophobia/phonophobia, no other explanation). Diagnose migraine with aura if there are at least two attacks that fulfil criteria (typical fully reversible symptoms, characteristic features of aura, no other explanation for headache).

Differential diagnosis

Tension headache.

Trigeminal autonomic cephalgias, e.g. cluster headache.

Primary cough headache and cold-stimulus ('ice-cream') headache.

Secondary headache, e.g. from trauma to head or neck.

Subarachnoid haemorrhage: 'thunder-clap' headache – severe, sudden onset.

Subdural haemorrhage: risk factors include alcohol, being elderly and falls.

Temporal arteritis: >50 years + pain on chewing or combing your hair? Temporal artery: 'absent pulse, beaded, tender or enlarged'.

Exposure to, or withdrawal from, substances: carbon monoxide, cocaine, alcohol. Also medication-overuse headache.

Infections, e.g. ear, sinuses, meningitis, encephalitis, cerebral abscess.

Hypoxia/hypertension – including pre-eclampsia and eclampsia.

Head/neck problems such as angle closure glaucoma or temporomandibular joint dysfunction.

There are many more – see guidance for the full list.[1]

Migraine management options to consider

Medication options

Ibuprofen.

Aspirin.

Metoclopramide or prochlorperazine. Migraines cause gastric stasis so patients are likely to benefit from prokinetic treatment (with acute therapy) to assist absorption and decrease nausea. There is a risk of extrapyramidal side effects.

Triptans; sumatriptan first line, try others if sumatriptan is ineffective. Avoid if uncontrolled HTN and vascular disease. Check licensing: >60 years and children.

Migraine prophylaxis

Propranolol, amitriptyline or topiramate. Remember highly effective contraception is required in women of child-bearing age if using topiramate (e.g. injectable contraception, implant, IUS, COCP + barrier). In this context, POP is not regarded as being highly effective.

CHAPTER 12

INVESTIGATION/RESULTS

	Cases in this chapter	RCGP 2025 curriculum	Learning points
12.1	Hypertrophic Cardiomyopathy	**Cardiovascular health** **Genomic medicine** 'Cardiomyopathies: primary and acquired, including dilated, hypertrophic obstructive' 'Autosomal dominant conditions'	HCM/HOCM Exercise in HCM/HOCM Other genetic conditions and how to explain them
12.2	Myeloma	**Haematology** 'Haematological malignancies such as acute and chronic leukaemias, lymphomas (including Hodgkin's and non-Hodgkin's lymphomas, gut and skin lymphomas), multiple myeloma'	When to suspect Investigations Management Secondary care treatment
12.3	Acute Kidney Injury	**Renal and urology** 'Acute kidney injury'	Acute kidney injury Sick day rules
12.4	PSA Test Result	**Renal and urology** 'Prostatic problems such as acute and chronic prostatitis, benign prostatic hyperplasia, prostatic carcinoma'	Prostate cancer: • PSA testing • PSA levels – by age
12.5	Atrial Fibrillation	**Cardiovascular health** **Urgent and unscheduled care** 'Arrhythmias including conduction defects such as atrial fibrillation and flutter, heart block, supraventricular tachycardia, ventricular rhythm abnormalities'	Atrial fibrillation: • When to suspect • Management • Rate control CHA_2DS_2VASc score

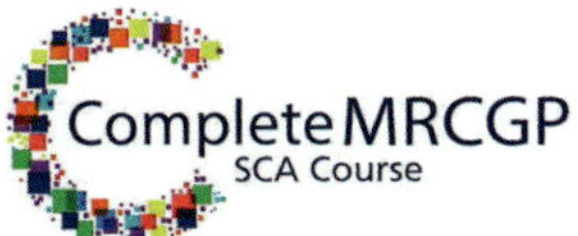

Links to the RCGP Curriculum

This broad blueprint group may feature clinical topics from throughout the curriculum and all life stages.

In this chapter, the cases are drawn from the following clinical topic guides:

- Cardiovascular health
- Genomic medicine
- Haematology
- Renal and urology
- Urgent and unscheduled care

Giving Results in the SCA – Skills and Pitfalls

In the exam you can expect at least one case where you need to interpret and communicate results to a patient. The results will be in the case notes. Take time to carefully read the results, checking for a final page of information; you may need to scroll down to see the full results. With this type of case, you will know what is coming. Once you have interpreted the results, and potentially found an abnormality, use your 3 minutes wisely to think how to manage the case.

Things to consider:

- Avoid the pitfall of jumping into giving the test result and missing data gathering.
- Is this likely to be received as bad news? If so, make sure you leave plenty of time for management.
- Can you rehearse your explanation? Practise out loud to ensure you are fluent.
- Will you need to prescribe? If so, do you know the dose and prescription information?
- Can you start to map a management plan? We can never predict the twists and turns of the case, or what the patient will want, but you could jot down pointers to help you structure your plan.

When to give results

The timing of when to give results can significantly affect your consultation. Done at the right moment, the rapport will flourish, and the consultation will flow. Done at the wrong time, the patient may become overanxious or restless, or potentially distracted by the result, preventing proper data gathering. Knowing when to give the result takes practice, but it is often helpful to initially give a short summary of the result, complete your data gathering, then go through the result in more detail.

For example:

> '*We've picked up a slight abnormality on your liver function test; this may be nothing to worry about but it would be helpful to know a little more about any symptoms you have been having to help me work out the likely cause* (take history of what has led up to the test, symptoms, risk factors and red flags). *Thank you, that's really helpful. Now we have a full picture, it seems likely that the abnormalities are caused by fat in your liver …*'

In some cases the patient will be relaxed, for example following a routine test where the patient was not expecting any abnormality to be identified. In these cases, it is likely to be easier to do your traditional data gathering first. If, however, the patient is concerned about the result, it is generally better to be upfront – either put their mind at ease if their fears have not been realised or break the bad news carefully. Do remember to go back and take some history. This may be around any changes in symptoms since their last visit (double check red flags), and thoughts, worries or expectations since their previous consultation and of course the impact the problem is having. Given the focus of these cases is generally on management, it is not necessary to spend too long in data gathering; have confidence to move on to the priority of the case. Don't forget though that you need to understand ICE and impact to create a shared management plan.

Doctor's Notes

Patient	Jason Wright	26 years	M
PMH	None		
Medications	None		
Allergies	No known drug allergies		
Consultations	Six weeks ago, presented with intermittent chest pain with shortness of breath, ECG did not show any ischaemic changes but large QRS complexes noted. Examination revealed soft systolic murmur. Patient referred to cardiology		
Investigations	ECG – sinus rhythm, large QRS complexes suggestive of left ventricular hypertrophy		
Household	None		

Letter from cardiology:

Dear GP,

Thank you for referring this 26-year-old gentleman, who had noted some chest pain during football, to our rapid access clinic. His ECG in primary care was suggestive of left ventricular hypertrophy and he was referred for further assessment. He underwent an ECHO in clinic which confirmed LV hypertrophy. The working diagnosis is one of hypertrophic cardiomyopathy. He has been referred for a cardiac MRI and genetic testing. We will contact you with the results in due course.

Regards,

Dr A. Cardiologist

Example Consultation **Hypertrophic Cardiomyopathy**

Open ☐ It sounds like you've been through a lot; can you tell me what has happened so far? How have you been feeling since you saw the cardiologist?

History ☐ What did the cardiologist say?

ICE1 ☐ What did you think when you were told the news?

Impact ☐ How has this news affected you? Have you stopped doing anything following the news?

Sense ☐ I sense you are worried about what will happen next.

ICE2 ☐ What worries have crossed your mind?

Risk ☐ Have you been advised to stop any activities? Are you aware of anyone in your family with the same condition, or anyone who died suddenly without explanation?

Flags ☐ Have you had any further chest pain since you started resting? Any fluttering in your chest or light-headed spells?

ICE3 ☐ Did you have any specific questions you hoped I would be able to answer today?

Summary ☐ You've been told you may well have HCM, which worries you as your life and career revolve around sport. You also worry about the implications if you wanted to have children in the future.

Empathy ☐ I can see how this must be a huge worry for you and your family.

Impression ☐ You'd like to know more about the condition and what may happen in the future.

Experience ☐ What have you found out about the condition so far?

Explanation ☐ HCM is a genetic condition that causes the heart muscle to become too thick. This affects how well the heart can squeeze and can also cause electrical faults with the heart. The condition usually passes from parent to child, with a 50% chance of it being passed down. Occasionally it happens due to a new mutation and no-one else in the family is affected.

Options ☐ Though it can be a dangerous condition, now we know about it, there are likely to be medicines you can take to help. Your specialist may also suggest that you have a defibrillator or pacemaker implanted into your chest to protect against dangerous heart rhythms.

Future ☐ It's likely that the genetic heart condition specialist will want to check your parents and sister for the condition. Given your Dad's brother died unexpectedly, it's possible this could have come from his side of the family. Once the genetics team has confirmed if this is a genetic condition, they can talk you through the risks going forward, though if it is the usual type there would be a 50% chance of you passing the condition to any children you had. Regarding sport, if you have been advised to take it easy for now, please do. However, with treatment you may be able to get back to some form of sport in the future, how intensive will depend on your results. Perhaps you could consider being involved in sport in some other ways too such as doing a coaching qualification?

Empower ☐ Are you able to speak to your club medical team to explain the situation? They may be able to liaise with your specialist about what is safe to do to maintain your fitness whilst you're awaiting more input from the hospital.

Safety net ☐ Hopefully, nothing will change between now and your specialist follow-up but if you do experience severe chest pain, sustained dizziness, breathlessness or fluttering in your chest, please ring 999.

Investigation/Results – 12.1

Patient's Story

Hypertrophic Cardiomyopathy

Patient's notes Jason Wright, 26 years old. PMH/DH/allergies: none.

Consultations: 6 weeks ago, presented with intermittent chest pain with shortness of breath, ECG did not show any ischaemic changes but large QRS complexes noted. Examination revealed soft systolic murmur. Patient referred to cardiology.

Investigations: ECG – sinus rhythm, large QRS complexes suggestive of left ventricular hypertrophy.

Letter from cardiology: 'Thank you for referring this 26-year-old gentleman, who had noted some chest pain during football, to our rapid access clinic. His ECG in primary care was suggestive of left ventricular hypertrophy and he was referred for further assessment. He underwent an ECHO in clinic which confirmed LV hypertrophy. The working diagnosis is one of hypertrophic cardiomyopathy. He has been referred for a cardiac MRI and genetic testing. We will contact you with the results in due course.'

How to act Anxious.

PC *'Doctor, I have been told I have HCM and I'm not sure what it all means.'*

History You have been experiencing occasional chest pain, mostly associated with intensive sport. You are a semi-professional footballer. You didn't tell your coach about it as you were worried about them dropping you from the team but you thought you better get it checked out. You saw your GP at home who examined you and did a heart tracing and then referred you to a specialist. You were pleased to be seen quickly. The consultant told you at the appointment that your heart scan was not normal and that you likely had a condition called hypertrophic cardiomyopathy (HCM). After being told there was something wrong with your heart, you found it difficult to take in what else was said. You remember something about genetics and avoiding sport.

Social You live with team mates from the same football club. You have only confided in your best friend that there is a problem though you have spoken to your parents. You are very health conscious given your dream to become a full-time professional footballer. You do not smoke or drink and have a healthy diet. When you are not playing football you work part-time in a leisure centre.

ICE You believe the diagnosis will be the end of your career and you will have to give up sport entirely. You worry about what this means for the future. You're also worried about the implications for your family and any children you may have in the future. You would like the doctor to answer your questions: *'What causes the condition?' 'What may happen to me in the future?' 'Will I be able to play sport again?' 'Will my children get it too?'*

Learning Points

Hypertrophic Cardiomyopathy

'If you have HCM, the muscular wall of your heart (the myocardium) becomes thickened which can make the heart muscle stiff. This can make it harder for your heart to pump blood out of your heart and around your body. How thick your heart muscle is and how much of your muscle is affected, is different for everyone. The left ventricle ... is almost always affected. The septum ... can also be affected.'[1]

Genetics Usually autosomal dominant.

Symptoms May be none at all until critical event, e.g. arrhythmia. Chest pain, dyspnoea, palpitations and dizziness may occur.

Complications Arrhythmias (e.g. AF, heart block, VT, VF) heart failure or endocarditis. Risk of sudden death from arrhythmia.

Investigations ECG, echocardiogram, exercise stress test, cardiac MRI. Genetic testing may be done.

Management Medication depending on whether heart failure, arrhythmia, etc., are present. Implantable defibrillator or pacemaker may be required.

Exercise with HCM/HCOM

Patients with HCM were formerly discouraged from taking part in exercise due to the perceived risk of sudden cardiac death so that only 45% of patients met minimal guidelines for exercise and many intentionally reduced exercise on diagnosis.[2] A less restrictive approach has been developed based upon risk stratification for individual patients. This is based around the LVOT gradient, BP and ECG response to exercise. The American Heart Association has developed an online calculator.[3]

Other genetic conditions

Autosomal dominant	Autosomal recessive	X-linked recessive	X-linked dominant	Chromosomal
• Familial adenomatous polyposis (FAP) • Polycystic kidney disease (PCKD) • Hereditary non-polyposis colorectal cancer (HNPCC) • Factor V Leyden thrombophilia • Ehlers–Danlos • Gilbert's syndrome • Hereditary haemorrhagic telangiectasia • Von Willebrand's syndrome • Prader–Willi syndrome	• Cystic fibrosis • Haemochromatosis • Wilson's disease • Sickle cell • Thalassaemia	• Haemophilia • Becker and Duchenne muscular dystrophy	• Fragile X	• Down syndrome (trisomy 21) • Edward's syndrome (trisomy 18) • Patau's syndrome (trisomy 13) • Turner's syndrome (XO) • Klinefelter's syndrome (XXY)

It is worth practising how to explain genetically inherited conditions as these are common cases. A useful analogy to explain genetics is that of an instruction manual: the words are genes; the chapters are the chromosomes. Put it all together and you have a plan to build a body and make it work.

Doctor's Notes

Patient	William Jefferies	65 years	M
PMH	None		
Medications	Paracetamol 1 g QDS		
	Naproxen 500 mg BD		
	Codeine 30 mg 1–2 tablets QDS		
Allergies	None		
Consultations	Several consultations for backache over the last 3 months. Prescribed paracetamol and naproxen. Had private physiotherapy		
	1 month ago – HbA1c and PSA normal		
	1 week ago 'Continues to c/o low back pain. No neurological symptoms or signs. Full examination of the back and neurology of legs normal. Blood tests arranged'		
Investigations	FBC:	Hb 110 g/L – normocytic, normochromic picture	
	ESR:	90	
	U&E:	Urea 11.3 mmol/L (2.5–7.8)	
		Creatinine 162 μmol/L (59–104)	
		Sodium and potassium normal	
		eGFR 54 mL/min/1.73 m^2 (CKD3)	
	Bone:	Calcium 2.8 mmol/L (2.1–2.6)	
		Other results normal	
	LFT:	Total protein 120 mg/dL (60–80). Comment – sample sent for electrophoresis, results to follow, please send urine for Bence Jones protein. Rest of LFTs normal	
Household	Mary Jefferies	65 years	F

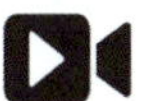

Example Consultation

Myeloma

Open ☐ Hello, Mr Jefferies. Yes, I do have your results. But, as we haven't spoken before, it would help me to find out more about you first. Please tell me what symptoms led to the tests?

History ☐ Tell me more about the backache, e.g. where is it and when do you notice it most? Any other symptoms such as tiredness or weight loss? Constipation? How is your mood?

Impact ☐ You said the backache interferes with gardening. Does it stop you doing anything else?

Curious ☐ What does Mary think? You mentioned you are retired. What was your work? How do you spend your days in retirement?

Flags ☐ Has anything changed since last week? Have you had weakness or numbness in your legs?

ICE1 ☐ What's gone through your mind?

Risk ☐ Has any relative had similar symptoms?

ICE2 ☐ You sound worried – what's your worst fear?

SummarICE ☐ So, for the last 6 months or so you have been having troublesome low back pain, not getting better with either physiotherapy or painkillers and interfering with your ability to look after your garden, play golf and drive to see your grandchildren. You are worried it might be prostate cancer. You had blood tests last week and are here for the results.

ICE3 ☐ As well as giving you the results, is there anything else you were hoping I might do today?

Empathy ☐ This has been a worrying time for you and you can't spend your retirement how you wish.

InCludE ☐ Thankfully, I don't think this is prostate cancer as you had a normal PSA test and the symptoms don't fit. Your blood test results appear to explain many of your symptoms so I'm hopeful you will be able to get back to gardening very soon.

Explanation ☐ You are slightly anaemic, which will tend to make you tired. Your kidneys are not working as well as usual. We have also found more protein in your bloodstream than is usual, your calcium is a little high and it is possible that you may have a condition called myeloma.

Experience ☐ Have you heard of myeloma or known anyone with this?

Explanation ☐ Myeloma is a condition where some of the cells in your bone marrow, called plasma cells, start to be more active than they should be and produce too much of a particular protein called immunoglobulin. The cells start to crowd out other cells in the bone marrow, so the body can't make its normal red and white cells, making you anaemic. These excess proteins can also block up small tubes in the kidneys so they can't work as well.

Options ☐ I would like to get an urgent urine test done to measure how much protein is passing through the kidneys. This and a further blood test may confirm the diagnosis. If so, I would then suggest you see a blood specialist called a haematologist who will be able to start treatment. We would arrange this within 2 weeks. Do you have any questions at this stage?

Explanation ☐ No, this isn't leukaemia, although it is a type of blood cancer. At the hospital I expect the doctors will examine you and take more blood tests. They may want to take a sample of your bone marrow, look at this under the microscope and do a scan to look at all your bones. This will guide treatment, which may be chemotherapy, steroids or other drugs to bring this under control.

Empower ☐ There are some things you can do. Please stop the naproxen as this may affect your kidneys. Paracetamol and codeine are safe. Drink plenty of fluids so you are well hydrated and to help your kidneys. Exercise will help – perhaps a daily walk; build up the distance slowly.

Future ☐ May I book you an appointment for next week so we can talk through the rest of your results, and I will answer any questions you have? We will also need to discuss immunising you against pneumonia and what to do if you get any infection.

Specifics ☐ If you begin to feel very thirsty, sick, tired or have increased aches and pains, your calcium levels may be too high. So please ring us, asking for the duty doctor, or 111 if we are closed.

Safety net ☐ If you get numbness around the back passage, lose that feeling of your bladder being full or get weakness of the legs, you must contact a doctor at once, even at night or the weekend.

Patient's Story

Myeloma

Doctor's notes William Jefferies, 65 years. PMH/allergies: none.

Medications: paracetamol 1 g QDS, naproxen 500 mg BD, codeine 30 mg 1–2 tablets QDS.

Consultations: several consultations for backache over the last 3 months. Prescribed paracetamol and naproxen. Had private physiotherapy. 1 month ago – HbA1c and PSA normal. 1 week ago: 'Continues to c/o low back pain. No neurological symptoms or signs. Full examination of the back and neurology of legs normal. Blood tests arranged.'

Investigations: FBC: Hb 110 g/L – normocytic, normochromic picture. ESR: 90. U&E: urea 11.3 mmol/L (2.5–7.8), creatinine 162 μmol/L (59–104), eGFR 54 mL/min/1.73 m^2 (CKD3). Bone: calcium 2.8 mmol/L (2.1–2.6). LFT: total protein 120 mg/dL (60–80). Comment – sample sent for electrophoresis, results to follow, please send urine for Bence Jones protein. Rest of LFTs normal.

How to act In discomfort with your back – it hurts when you walk and even sitting is uncomfortable. Worried.

PC *'I've phoned for my blood test results – does it explain why I've been getting back pain?'*

History For the last 3 months you have had troublesome back pain. Initially you thought you had done too much on the allotment. You took some paracetamol and ibuprofen, which did not help, and then went to a private physiotherapist. He gave you exercises and you have been following these but with no real improvement. The back pain is getting worse; you can no longer play golf. You are now in pain all the time and it's keeping you awake. You have lost a little weight without trying. You have been more tired than usual, and your muscles seem weak (e.g. when gardening). You have also been constipated and drinking more. The doctor thought you might have diabetes but a fasting blood sugar and HbA1c were completely normal. A week ago, you saw a different doctor who did a full examination of your back and legs (normal) and arranged some more blood tests. You are here for the results.

Social You are a retired businessman and enjoy gardening as a hobby. You have always been fit and well and played sport including golf. You live with your wife who is also retired and have two grown-up children who live about 100 miles away and four grandchildren. Driving to see the grandchildren is really uncomfortable so you are going less often and miss these visits.

ICE Your good friend had backache which turned out to be secondaries from prostate cancer. Your wife is worried about this too. The blood test may have shown something to explain the back pain.

'Could this be cancer? Is it going to get better? What can you do to help me get back to my gardening?'

You hope the doctor will have found out what is wrong and you hope it's nothing serious like cancer.

You have never heard of myeloma and will ask the doctor what it is if this is mentioned. If 'blood cancer' is mentioned, ask *'Is it leukaemia?'* A friend's son had this and died when he was 6.

Investigation/Results – 12.2

Myeloma[1,2]

What is it? A blood cancer arising from plasma cells. Represents 2% of all cancers. Patients mainly aged >65 years although can be much younger.

When to suspect Adults, especially if >60 years with:

- Unexplained back pain, especially thoracic or lower back.
- Fatigue (30%).
- Symptoms of hypercalcaemia (30%), e.g. pain (bone, abdominal), low mood, confusion, muscle weakness, constipation, thirst, polyuria.
- Weight loss (25%).
- Hyperviscosity symptoms, e.g. headache, cognitive impairment, visual disturbance, mucosal bleeding (7%).
- Cord compression symptoms.
- Fever (1%).
- Onset often gradual, may be picked up following pathological fracture or recurrent infection.

Examination Normal or hepatomegaly (4%), splenomegaly (1%), lymphadenopathy (1%).

Blood tests FBC – normochromic, normocytic anaemia.

U&E – renal impairment (50%).

Bone profile – hypercalcaemia (15%).

Raised ESR, serum protein or globulin.

Management Blood tests – FBC, serum calcium, ESR, U&E.

Consider X-rays of painful areas to rule out pathological fractures.

Arrange urgent plasma and urine protein electrophoresis (ideally within 48 hours) – be aware these are negative in 1–2% of people with myeloma.

Urgent admission if suspected cord compression, corrected calcium >2.9 or AKI.

Otherwise – haematology urgent suspected cancer referral.

Secondary care Bone marrow aspiration and trephine biopsy (monoclonal plasma cells).

MRI to detect extent of bone disease. Low-dose CT scan if MRI unsuitable or declined. Plain X-ray of spine, skull, chest, pelvis and upper limbs if MRI and CT unsuitable or declined.

Treatment Chemotherapy, steroids, anaemia treatments, bisphosphonates for pain, immunomodulatory therapy. Stem cell transplant.

Ongoing primary care

- Treat infections promptly.
- Manage pain, e.g. paracetamol ± codeine (avoid NSAIDs).
- Offer flu and pneumococcal vaccination.
- Monitor mental health and offer help where needed.
- Support and advise family and carers, e.g. advise exercise and adequate hydration.
- Discuss role of palliative care, when appropriate.
- Advise re DLA, PIP payments.

Doctor's Notes

Patient	Alexander Dickens 78 years M
PMH	Chronic kidney disease, osteoarthritis and heart failure
Medications	Furosemide 20 mg 2 tablets daily
	Spironolactone 50 mg daily
	Indapamide 2.5 mg daily
	Ramipril 5 mg daily
	Bisoprolol 5 mg daily
	Paracetamol 500 mg PRN
Allergies	No information
Consultations	Last week seen by GP. Pitting oedema to knees. Sats 95%
	Crepitations at lung bases. JVP 3 cm. Agreed to increase furosemide to 40 mg daily. BP 162/72. Ramipril increased from 2.5 to 5 mg
Investigations	Blood test 1 week ago: eGFR 51 mL/min/1.73 m^2, creatinine 92 µmol/L, potassium 4.8 mmol/L, sodium 143 mmol/L
Household	Dorothy Dickens 74 years F

Message from biochemistry:

'AKI stage 1 warning

eGFR 32 mL/min/1.73 m^2, creatinine 180 µmol/L, potassium 5.5 mmol/L, sodium 142 mmol/L'

Example Consultation

Open ☐ Mr Dickens, I'm calling about your blood tests which show that your kidneys are struggling more than usual. I'd like to talk to you about what may be causing this so we can put them right again.

History ☐ Tell me the story about what led the doctor to see you last week. What medication changes did you both make? How have you been since the doctor last saw you? Do you feel more tired at all? Are you passing urine normally? Who is at home with you? Is Mrs Dickens well? And to understand more about what's important to you, how do you spend your time?

Flags ☐ Any fevers, any pain passing urine or going more frequently? Any loose stools or vomiting recently? Do you have any problems with the flow of your urine or getting up at night?

Risk ☐ You started taking furosemide last week. What dose are you taking each day? And can I check which other medicines you take?

Curious ☐ You mentioned your knee plays up. Do you ever take anything for that?

ICE2 ☐ Is there anything that keeps worrying you?

ICE1 ☐ Anything else you have wondered?

Impact ☐ How active are you generally?

ICE3 ☐ Is there anything else that you would like or would find helpful?

SummarICE ☐ To summarise, you have been very worried that your breathing is getting worse, as it did 6 months ago, when you needed to go into hospital. You have been well on 80 mg furosemide previously. Your main concern now is balancing the kidneys with the breathing.

Impression ☐ When your kidney blood tests worsen suddenly, we call this acute kidney injury.

Experience ☐ Have you had problems with your kidney blood tests before?

Explanation ☐ I think what has caused it is a combination of factors that all impact on the kidney. The recent diarrhoea made you more dehydrated and increasing the ramipril and furosemide at the same time was just too much for the kidneys. The ibuprofen is also contributing to this, unfortunately.

Sense ☐ You sound very disappointed.

Empathy ☐ I appreciate it must be very disheartening going from one problem to another.

InCludE ☐ This is a common balancing act, but I am sure we can make tweaks to prevent you going back into hospital.

Options ☐ Have you taken your medicines this morning? I would suggest you hold off taking them for now. Initially, I would suggest repeating the test as it may have already begun to improve now the diarrhoea has settled. I will ask the team to squeeze you in tomorrow for the repeat blood test and ask them to check your blood pressure whilst you are here. Please stop the ibuprofen tablets; perhaps we could try a gel instead which won't affect your kidneys? Maybe we could also try physiotherapy for your knees; what do you think?

Future ☐ I wonder whether, to help monitor your breathing, we could involve the heart failure nurses?

Empower ☐ You mentioned your weight has changed. Monitoring your weight is helpful to detect warning signs and guide your medications. The heart failure nurses will explain about regularly weighing yourself to help guide your medicines. I also have some information to give you which includes a card telling you what you can do when you feel unwell; it's called a medicines sick day rule card. For example, if you're poorly with diarrhoea or vomiting, we would advise not taking your ramipril or water tablets until you're eating and drinking again normally.

Specifics ☐ Can you attend the blood test walk-in clinic tomorrow? Then I can give you a ring when we have the result back to let you know if you can restart your tablets.

Investigation/Results – 12.3

Patient's Story

Acute Kidney Injury

Doctor's notes Alexander Dickens, 78 years. PMH: chronic kidney disease, osteoarthritis and heart failure. Medications: furosemide 20 mg 2 tablets daily, spironolactone 50 mg daily, indapamide 2.5 mg daily, ramipril 5 mg daily, bisoprolol 5 mg daily, paracetamol 500 mg PRN.

Last week seen by GP. Pitting oedema to knees. Sats 95%. Crepitations at lung bases. JVP 3 cm. Agreed to increase furosemide to 40 mg daily. BP 162/72. Ramipril increased from 2.5 to 5 mg. Blood test 1 week ago: eGFR 51 mL/min/1.73 m^2, creatinine 92 µmol/L, potassium 4.8 mmol/L, sodium 143 mmol/L.

Message from biochemistry:

'AKI stage 1 warning.

eGFR 32 mL/min/1.73 m^2, creatinine 180 µmol/L, potassium 5.5 mmol/L, sodium 142 mmol/L.'

How to act You are surprised when the doctor calls.

PC *'Hello, Doctor, what can I do for you? … I'm very well thank you.'*

History The doctor saw you last week. You were last in hospital 6 months ago when the fluid was on your lungs. This was frightening. Since then, you have been *'not too bad'* but you started to feel the fluid coming back last week so called the doctor. You had noticed you were not moving around the house as easily with your breathing. When the doctor suggested taking 40 mg furosemide, initially it didn't seem to help so you increased it to 80 mg. They have given you 120 mg in hospital before, so you thought 80 mg would be fine. You can tell your fluid is going as your breathing is better and you have lost a little weight. You feel fine. Last week, however, your grandchild came around and you had a couple of days with diarrhoea. You feel fine now. You are passing urine normally. You have no symptoms of a UTI. You have no fever. Your knee arthritis does 'play up'. If asked, tell the doctor you buy ibuprofen OTC for this. Otherwise, you take only the prescribed medicines. You have not yet taken this morning's medication.

Social You live with your wife. Your son lives around the corner with your grandchildren. You have a good circle of friends and don't let your medical conditions get you down. You have noticed a general decline in your health over the last few years.

ICE You have never heard of the diagnosis 'acute kidney injury'.

You become very apologetic that you have changed the dose yourself without consulting the doctor and apologise to the doctor for causing an inconvenience to them.

'Oh dear, Doctor, I am worried about my breathing … now my kidneys. I just can't win.'

You are hoping the doctor will be able to advise about how best to manage the heart failure/breathing problems. You're happy with any options the doctor suggests.

Investigation/Results – 12.3

Warning system for AKI[1]

Labs now often automatically report AKI stage when results are sent so this does not necessarily need to be calculated by the GP.

Stage 1: Creatinine ≥1.5× baseline.

Stage 2: Creatinine ≥2× baseline.

Stage 3: Creatinine ≥3× baseline.

Baseline taken from lowest creatinine value within last 7 days or if not available, lowest or mean creatinine in last 12 months.

Management

Management depends on clinical circumstances and the suspected underlying cause. Determining probability of a genuine AKI can be assessed based on known circumstances, e.g. were the blood tests done during acute illness or after medication changes? Or was the test routine, e.g. QOF/health check?

	Acute management
Stage 1	Manage underlying cause. Offer advice about maintaining fluid balance. Review medications and temporarily stop/reduce dose of specific medications.[3] Regularly monitor creatinine clearance – even small increases in serum creatinine may be significant. Reconsider hospital admission.
Stage 2	Discuss with a general physician or nephrologist if there is uncertainty about management, e.g. moderate hyperkalaemia (K^+ of 6.0–6.4 mmol/L), depending on clinical judgement.
Stage 3	Urgent admission or same day referral if likely Stage 3 AKI, no identifiable cause, sepsis, risk of urinary tract obstruction. (See NICE guidelines[1] for full list.) Discuss with consultant nephrologist within 24 hours if likely Stage 4 or 5 CKD, specialist treatment needed, inadequate response in primary care, or past renal transplant.

Admission may be required for any stage if the suspected cause needs hospital treatment, e.g. suspected retention/urinary obstruction, pyelonephritis/UTI/sepsis, neutropenic sepsis, renal/ureteric calculus or if there is a complication such as hyperkalaemia or fluid overload.

Risk factors for development of AKI[1]

- Age over 65 years
- Specific meds in last week, e.g. NSAIDs, ACE inhibitors, ARBs
- Cancer
- Previous AKI
- Chronic kidney disease
- Reliance on carer
- Hypovolaemia
- Sepsis or infection (e.g. urine)
- Vomiting
- Urological obstruction
- Nephritis
- Heart failure
- Diabetes
- Liver disease
- Severe diarrhoea
- Oliguria (UO <0.5 mL/kg/h)
- Iodinated contrast used in past week
- Hypotension

Sick day rule card

The sick day rule card was originally developed by NHS Highland to advise patients which medicines to stop when they become unwell with either 'vomiting or diarrhoea (unless only minor), fever sweats or shaking unless only minor'.[2]

Medicines to stop include: ACEIs, ARBs, NSAIDs, diuretics and metformin.[2]

Investigation/Results – 12.3

Doctor's Notes

Patient	Remigio Sanchez	50 years	M
PMH	No medical history		
Medications	No medications		
Allergies	No information		
Consultations	3 weeks ago. Concerned about prostate cancer due to family history. No symptoms. Examination: prostate smooth, normal size. Abdomen soft, non-tender. PSA in 2 weeks then review		
Investigations	PSA 4.6 ng/mL		
Household	Perla Sanchez	48 years	F
	Sosimo Sanchez	16 years	M
	Manuela Sanchez	14 years	F
	Pilar Sanchez	10 years	M

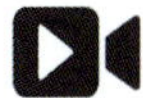

Example Consultation

Open ☐ What has led to this test being taken?

Experience ☐ Tell me more about your father's and brother's experiences. What is your understanding of the PSA test? Has a doctor explained?

Sense ☐ I can see you are keen to know the result.

ICE1 ☐ Is there anything specific which has been on your mind?

Impression ☐ The result is slightly raised. This doesn't necessarily mean you have prostate cancer; activities such as running, cycling, ejaculating or intercourse can all increase this result. In the week prior to the test, did you do any of these activities? That is helpful to know.

History ☐ Thinking about other possible causes for a raised PSA, are you well in yourself? Any medical problems? You told the last GP that you hadn't had any symptoms; may I just check, have you noticed any changes at all in the flow of your urine or how often you go, day or night? Any pain? Any fever? Do you have to wait because it dribbles at the end or feel your bladder isn't quite empty? Any problems with erections?

Flags ☐ Have you seen any blood in the urine? Have you noticed any new back pain? Have you lost weight? I'm pleased you have no symptoms.

Curious ☐ You mentioned ***'I haven't got time to be ill.'*** What's happening in your life at the moment? Is there anything else important to you?

ICE2 ☐ What worries you most? When you saw the doctor a couple of weeks ago, did you think prostate cancer was likely?

Impact ☐ Coming for a result can be worrying. How did you feel prior to coming today? Had you had thoughts about how it may affect you if the result was abnormal?

ICE3 ☐ What did you think I might suggest today?

Empathy ☐ I appreciate that, with your family history and fear of the impact a diagnosis may have on your life, this result is very important to you.

SummarICE ☐ So to summarise, your brother and father have prostate cancer and you have arranged this test in the hope that if there was a cancer you are catching it early. You fear how a diagnosis of prostate cancer would impact on your health and ability to provide for your family. This has been very stressful for you.

Impression ☐ As I mentioned earlier, the result was slightly raised, but this could be due to the exercise you did prior to the test. We generally don't rely on one result before making a decision if it's only a little raised.

InCludE ☐ However, I agree, given your family history and result we do need to be more suspicious.

Explanation ☐ The PSA level can be raised in prostate cancer. But it can also be raised in harmless growth of the prostate. PSA is an imperfect test as its common to have an abnormal result and not have cancer, but also it's possible to have a normal PSA and have cancer.

Options ☐ I feel the best next step is to repeat the test, but please avoid sex, ejaculation and exercise for 48 hours before the test. The repeat test should be done 2–4 weeks after the first. Given your family history and worries, shall we repeat it after 2 weeks rather than 4? If the result comes back raised again, I recommend referral to a specialist under the suspected cancer pathway. How does this sound? There is still a good chance this will not turn out to be cancer, but this way we would get you seen quickly and fully assessed. The specialist will likely examine you and may wish to perform a detailed scan (MRI) and, as you thought, a biopsy to make a firm diagnosis. Any questions so far?

Future ☐ I will ask reception to book your repeat test; I will give you a ring once the result is back.

Safety net ☐ If in future you have any problems passing urine, or any new pain, let a GP know.

Patient's Story

PSA Test Result

Doctor's notes Remigio Sanchez, 50 years. PMH: PSA 4.6 ng/mL, nil else. Medications: none.

Consultation: 3 weeks ago. Concerned about prostate cancer due to family history. No symptoms. Examination: prostate smooth, normal size. Abdomen soft, non-tender. PSA in 2 weeks then review.

How to act Eager to know what will happen to you.

PC *'I'm calling for my PSA result.'*

History You asked for the test as your brother has been diagnosed with prostate cancer, despite having no symptoms yourself. Your father also had prostate cancer, treated with a total prostatectomy.

You saw a GP who said your prostate felt fine but agreed to do a PSA. The GP had been running behind so didn't explain much about the test itself. You have never had any problems with your health.

You attended the gym prior to the test being taken.

You understand the PSA test will tell you if you have prostate cancer.

Social *'I haven't got time to be ill.'*

You moved from Argentina 6 years ago for work on oil rigs. You spend a lot of time away from home. Your work would not be sympathetic if you needed time off. They often make people redundant. You feel the pressure of finances at the moment with three children who want to go to university.

ICE You assume you have prostate cancer too and want to catch it early. You are worried that you will need chemotherapy.

You couldn't sleep last night because of fear of the result.

You expect the doctor to send you for a biopsy. You have had no UTI symptoms.

Learning Points

Assessment for prostate cancer is usually a two-part process – examination of the prostate and a PSA test.

Prostate cells adjacent to the urethra (transitional zone of the prostate) commonly change to become hyperplastic (BPH) whereas prostate cancer arises in the peripheral zone of the prostate – the part you can feel on DRE. Hence, men with early prostate cancer are usually asymptomatic. Men who present with LUTS due to prostate cancer often have locally advanced disease. However, BPH and prostate cancer can coexist.[1] Occasionally, tumours arise from the anterior portion of the gland and are impalpable.

NICE CKS prostate cancer diagnosis[2]

The aim of PSA testing is to detect localised prostate cancer when treatment can be offered that may cure cancer or extend life. It is not usually recommended for asymptomatic men with less than 10 years' life expectancy. Most men will have a PSA level less than 3 ng/mL. About 3 in 4 men with a raised PSA level (3 ng/mL or higher) will not have cancer. Around 15% of men with a normal PSA do have cancer. A PSA test will not distinguish between aggressive tumours (which are at an early stage but will develop quickly) and those which are not. Further tests may provide valuable information. 75% of patients with a high PSA have a normal biopsy.

PSA testing should be:

- Considered in men with suspected prostate cancer.
- Offered to men older than 50 years of age who request a PSA test.

Before a PSA test, people should **not** have:

- An active urinary infection or had one within the previous 6 weeks.
- Ejaculated in previous 48 hours.
- Exercised vigorously, for example cycling, in the previous 48 hours.
- Had a urological intervention such as prostate biopsy in previous 6 weeks.

After taking blood for PSA testing, the specimen must reach the laboratory within 16 hours.

Age (years)	PSA level of concern
Below 40	Use clinical judgement
40–49	More than 2.5 ng/mL
50–59	More than 3.5 ng/mL
60–69	More than 4.5 ng/mL
70–79	More than 6.5 ng/mL
Above 79	Use clinical judgement

Consider prostate cancer if there is LUTS, low back pain/bone pain, lethargy, erectile dysfunction, visible haematuria or anorexia/weight loss.

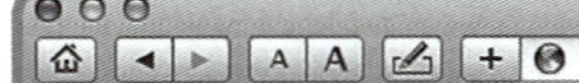

Doctor's Notes

Patient	Janet Harrison	78 years	F
PMH	Hypertension		
Medications	Amlodipine 10 mg once daily		
	Atorvastatin 20 mg once daily		
Allergies	No known drug allergies		
Consultations	Attended for annual BP review yesterday with chronic disease nurse. BP 132/70, pulse felt irregular. Briefly seen by duty doctor. Well, no signs of heart failure, heart sounds normal. Advised by duty doctor to do an ECG and book a review Weight 66 kg. BMI 24. Blood results for hypertension review: FBC normal, U&E – eGFR 64 mL/min/1.73 m^2, creatinine clearance 57 µmol/L. LFTs normal, HbA1c 38 mmol/mol. Lipids: TC 3.8 mmol/L, non-HDLC 2.1 mmol/L. Thyroid function normal. ECG – atrial fibrillation. HR 82 bpm		

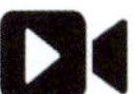

Example Consultation

Open ☐ Nothing too serious; your heart has gone into an irregular rhythm, which is common, but I'd like to talk to you about it as you may need treatment. Please tell me what led up to you having the heart tracing done.

History ☐ How have you been feeling? Any fluttering in your chest. Any breathlessness?

Impact ☐ Has breathlessness stopped you from doing anything? Does it affect your sleep?

ICE1 ☐ When the nurse mentioned a problem with your heart, what did you think?

Curious ☐ Would you mind sharing what happened to your husband? I'm sorry to hear that.

Flags ☐ Have you ever had any chest pains? Any dizziness or fainting episodes? Any ankle swelling?

ICE2 ☐ Has this been a worry to you? What did you fear may happen?

Risk ☐ It seems your blood pressure is well controlled: do you have any other health problems? Do you drink much caffeine? Or alcohol? Have you ever smoked?

ICE3 ☐ Given the experience you've had in the past with your husband's heart attack, were you expecting me to do anything particular today?

SummarICE ☐ Overall you're pretty well, so this abnormal heart tracing has come as a shock. You have been worried that it may lead to a heart problem and thought I may give you medication or refer you to a heart specialist.

Empathy ☐ I appreciate this has come out of the blue and is worrying for you.

Impression ☐ This irregular heart rhythm is called atrial fibrillation or AF for short.

Experience ☐ Have you heard of this before?

Explanation ☐ AF is a common heart problem. It is more common in people with a history of high BP and with age. The heart has four chambers: two at the top called the atria which collect blood arriving in the heart and two at the bottom called the ventricles which are the pumping chambers. In AF, the top chambers can start to beat quickly and out of sync with the bottom of the heart. The irregular beating of the atria is not dangerous, but it can cause two main problems. First, the heart can start to beat too fast, so it can't fill properly between squeezes, leading to dizziness or breathlessness. Second, due to turbulence in the atria as they jiggle about, small clots can form.

InCludE ☐ This is a different type of problem from your husband's. Heart attacks are caused by plumbing issues. This is more of an electrical fault. Having AF doesn't generally put you at increased risk of a heart attack, but because little clots may form, it does increase stroke risk. AF is a common problem, so GPs can usually manage it without specialist help.

Recommend ☐ To manage your heart running too fast, I would suggest a medication called a beta-blocker which slows the heart. To reduce your risk of a stroke – which is also higher because of your age and your hypertension – I would recommend a blood thinning medication to prevent clots forming. This medication does increase your risk of bleeding, e.g. a stomach bleed or one in your head. However, the potential benefit of preventing a life-limiting or life-altering stroke would likely outweigh the risk, particularly as you are otherwise well and your background risk of bleeding is low. What do you think?

Empower ☐ It's unlikely to be the main cause of your AF, but cutting down on caffeine may help prevent your heart becoming too fast. Could you switch to decaf tea? AF shouldn't stop you from doing anything; in fact, I would encourage you to remain physically active.

Future ☐ If you agree, I'd like you to start bisoprolol, a beta-blocker, 1.25 mg once daily and apixaban, a blood thinner, 5 mg twice a day. May I see you in a week to check your heart rate and BP to ensure the medicines are working well and that you're not having any side effects? We may need to adjust the bisoprolol dose to ensure your heart rate is well controlled.

Safety net ☐ If at any time you start to feel unwell, such as with dizziness or breathlessness, please contact us straight away.

Investigation/Results – 12.5

Patient's Story

Atrial Fibrillation

Doctor's notes Janet Harrison, 78 years. PMH: hypertension. Medications: amlodipine 10 mg, atorvastatin 20 mg, both once daily.

Last consultation: attended for annual BP review yesterday with chronic disease nurse. BP 132/70, pulse felt irregular. Briefly seen by duty doctor. Well, no signs of heart failure, heart sounds normal. Advised by duty doctor to do an ECG and book a review.

Weight 60 kg. BMI 24. Blood results for hypertension review: FBC normal, U&E – eGFR 64 mL/min/1.73 m^2, creatinine clearance 57 μmol/L. LFTs normal, HbA1c 38 mmol/mol. Lipids: TC 3.8 mmol/L, non-HDLC 2.1 mmol/L. ECG – AF. HR 82 bpm.

How to act Concerned.

PC ***'The nurse said there was something wrong with my heart – is it serious?'***

History You attended for your annual hypertension review. Your BP has been well controlled, so you weren't expecting any problems. You have not had any symptoms other than feeling a bit more breathless when you have been working in the garden. You had put this down to getting older. You are still able to get the work done, but have to rest if pushing a full wheelbarrow or if you need to do digging/raking. No chest pain, no palpitations, no dizziness, no syncope. No ankle oedema. No orthopnoea or PND. You generally feel pretty fit.

Social You are a retired primary school teacher. Your husband passed away suddenly from a heart attack 6 years ago so you live alone. You have two grown-up children you see a couple of times a month. You enjoy gardening and take pride in your beautiful garden. You are involved in village life, have friends in the village and are on several committees. You like to keep busy. You are helping to organise the annual village 'Open Garden' event. This is important to you so you hope the doctor won't tell you that you must rest; there is so much to do!

You are fond of a cup of tea, usually drinking 5–6 cups per day. Never smoked. Minimal alcohol; a couple of gin and tonics per week when with friends.

ICE You were worried when you heard there was a problem with your heart and feared you would have a heart attack like your husband. You expect the doctor will want you to take more medication; you wonder if you need to see a specialist.

Investigation/Results – 12.5

Learning Points

Atrial Fibrillation[1]

Always refer to the full text of the latest version of NICE guidance on AF management (March 2025).[1]

Suspect in patients with irregular pulse ± breathlessness, palpitations, chest discomfort, dizziness, syncope, reduced exercise tolerance. Look for AF in patients with potential complications, e.g. stroke/TIA.

Risk factors
Existing CVD (ischaemic heart disease, valvular disease, hypertension, pericarditis, cardiomyopathy, recent cardiothoracic surgery) or non-cardiac or lifestyle conditions, e.g. acute illness (pneumonia or PE), COPD, CKD, electrolyte disturbance, cancer, thyroid disease, DM, OSA, alcohol, obesity, smoking.

Diagnosis
12 lead ECG. If paroxysmal AF (intermittent symptoms lasting <48 hours) is suspected, 24-hour ambulatory ECG or event recorder may be required to capture the arrhythmia.

Differential irregular pulse
Atrial flutter, atrial or ventricular ectopics, SVT, sinus tachycardia.

Management
Admit if haemodynamically unstable, e.g. HR >150 or HR <40 or severe symptoms of breathlessness, dizziness/syncope, chest pain, LOC. Or if signs of complication, e.g. decompensated heart failure, stroke. Or if serious life-threatening cause/complication, or if acute reversible cause.

If stable and does not need admission, manage in primary care.

Refer for an ECHO/cardiology if valvular heart disease, heart failure or pre-excitation (e.g. Wolffe–Parkinson–White syndrome) are suspected.

Rate control
Beta-blocker (usually bisoprolol or atenolol) is first line. Rate-limiting calcium channel blocker (diltiazem or verapamil) can also be used. Digoxin is second line. Follow-up recommended after 7 days.

Rhythm control
This can be considered if acute onset (i.e. <48 hours) with reversible cause, e.g. chest infection, AF causing/worsening heart failure, young patient who is symptomatic.

Anticoagulation
Assess using CHA_2DS_2VASc for stroke risk and ORBIT score for bleeding risk.

- CHA_2DS_2VASc ≥2 – offer anticoagulation: first-line DOAC (apixaban, edoxaban, rivaroxaban or dabigatran). Remember to check CrCl and weight for dose determination.
- CHA_2DS_2VASc 1 in men – consider DOAC.
- CHA_2DS_2VASc 0 (or 1 in women) – anticoagulation not usually required.

Do not withhold anticoagulation based on age or falls risk alone. There is no cut-off of ORBIT score which would prevent use of anticoagulation but the ORBIT score can help frame risk discussions.

CHA_2DS_2VASc scoring

- Congestive heart failure/LV dysfunction – 1
- Hypertension (raised BP, systolic >140, ± diastolic >90, 2 occasions or controlled on meds) – 1
- Age ≥75 years – 2
- Diabetes – 1
- Stroke/TIA – 2
- Vascular disease (IHD, PVD) – 1
- Age 65–74 years – 1
- Female sex – 1

Easy to remember: anyone ≥75 years + all females aged 65 or over will automatically score 2 or higher.

Investigation/Results – 12.5

CHAPTER 13

PROFESSIONAL CONVERSATION/ PROFESSIONAL DILEMMA

	Cases in this chapter	RCGP 2025 curriculum	Learning points
13.1	Discussion with an ANP – Adult Safeguarding and Domestic Violence	**Smoking, alcohol and substance misuse** 'Be aware of wider social issues, including the need to protect children and family members … and respond to any safeguarding concerns' **Older adults (life stage)** 'Dementia'	Adult safeguarding
13.2	Discussion with a Social Worker – Self-Neglect	**Smoking, alcohol and substance misuse** 'Behavioural changes such as neglecting other activities, poor hygiene, secrecy, self-neglect and social withdrawal'	Self-neglect The Care Act 2014
13.3	Discussion with a Paramedic – Community-Acquired Pneumonia	**Respiratory health** 'Common and important conditions … lower respiratory tract infection' **Urgent and unscheduled care** 'Coordinate care with other services and professionals (for example ambulance service, community nurses and secondary care) and follow agreed protocols where appropriate, ensuring appropriate referral or follow up where necessary'	Community-acquired pneumonia: assessment, investigation and treatment CRB-65 score Treatment based on CRB-65 score AMTS assessment
13.4	Discussion with a Hospital Consultant – Cervical Cancer/ End of Life	**Gynaecology and breast health** 'Common and important conditions – cervical cancer' **End of life (life stage)** 'Holistically assess and support the needs of the patient, family and carer'	Medical complexity – EOL considerations
13.5	Discussion with a Physician Associate – Retinal Detachment	**Eyes and vision** 'Common and important conditions … retinal problems including retinal detachment' **Urgent and unscheduled care** 'Coordinate care with other services and professionals (for example ambulance service, community nurses and secondary care) and follow agreed protocols where appropriate, ensuring appropriate referral or follow up where necessary'	Retinal detachment

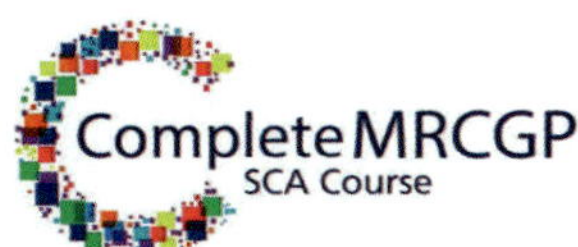

Links to the RCGP Curriculum

This broad blueprint group may feature clinical topics from throughout the curriculum and all life stages. In this chapter, the cases are drawn from the following clinical topic guides:

- Smoking, alcohol and substance misuse
- Respiratory health
- Gynaecology and breast health
- Eyes and vision
- Urgent and unscheduled care

Professional conversation

As GPs we work with many different professional colleagues and need to understand their roles and responsibilities. In your exam, you are likely to have to discuss a case with or supervise a colleague which may include:

- Staff member in your own practice, e.g. practice nurse, ANP, physician associate, paramedic practitioner, student nurse, medical student or doctor in training.
- Staff member from the community, e.g. community nurse, paramedic, social worker.
- Staff member from secondary care, e.g. specialist nurse, doctor or consultant.

Specifically, within the mark scheme, consider in relating to others (RTO):

- 'Works collaboratively, understanding the context within which different team members work.'
- 'Shows respect for colleagues, treating them fairly and without discrimination.'

Professional dilemma

Dilemmas may arise when discussing a complex case with a colleague or relative, or in the consultation. Ethical dilemmas may include respecting autonomy vs acting in the patient's best interests. Legal dimensions include confidentiality, consent and Gillick competence. Clinical dilemmas may mean that the usual guidelines aren't in the patient's best interest, e.g. urgent cancer referral for a frail, housebound patient. We explore these themes within this chapter's cases.

Skills and Pitfalls

In addition to the information in Chapter 1 'How to Demonstrate Skills: The Marking Scheme Made Easy' consider the following challenges for this blueprint group:

- Practise taking a history from a third person. As a general rule, take your history as if taking it from the patient themselves with slight adjustments to the questions. You'll need the same amount of information to come to a conclusion so normal consultation structure can help.
- These cases will often need 'double ICE' – What does your colleague/relative think? And their concerns and expected outcome? But also find out about the patient's ICE – this is where the dilemma may lie.
- Remember when consulting with a colleague you can ask them about their clinical findings; they may have examined the patient for you and may have observations, etc., they can share.
- Summarising the situation/problem/dilemma can be a helpful step prior to your impression; there may be multiple issues you need to tackle.
- Don't forget to give your impression. What is your conclusion from the information given? Do you agree or disagree with your colleague's assessment?

Skills and Pitfalls

- Management plans can be difficult to structure in these cases so perhaps consider working through each individual problem. For example, in a case of an elderly, housebound patient who has a history of mild dementia but who is now more confused with a urinary tract infection:
  - *'To treat the urinary tract infection, we would suggest ...'*
  - *'To help with the new problem of incontinence shall we ...'*
  - *'To keep the patient safe whilst they recover, we could ...'*

Medical Complexity in Working with Colleagues

Professional dilemma

As with prescribing, this is another important area with the potential for significant medical complexity and again offering the opportunity for you to earn great marks across the three domains. Remember that you can showcase your skills not just by what you do but, even more significantly, HOW you do it. You can demonstrate this through how you relate to the professional colleague, listening to them, respecting them, politely challenging them if needed, negotiating and together coming up with a safe, effective plan. Your colleague may be speaking to you about themselves or a patient. Consider if there are:

Ethical dilemmas – e.g. where respecting autonomy or acting in best interests is important.

Legal dimensions – e.g. confidentiality, consent or Gillick competence.

Clinical dilemmas – e.g. normal guidelines aren't necessarily in the patient's best interest.

Colleagues speaking about themselves

Here are some examples and the possible complexities, which include issues of professional boundaries as well as safety and wellbeing:

Example. The practice nurse, who is registered as a patient with the practice, asks to speak to you because the nurse manager, who is also your employee, is bullying her.

Possible complexity:

- Is the staff member consulting you as their doctor or as their professional colleague?
- What behaviour has she experienced that she is calling 'bullying'?
- Is 'bullying' part of a wider pattern? How would you find out and who would you involve in a wider discussion? (e.g. hearing the nurse manager's side of the story, GP partners, employers).
- Does the staff member need to take time off work for their health or wellbeing?
- Who is going to support the staff member and how?

Example. The practice's FY2 doctor, who is registered elsewhere as a patient, asks you if they could take a few days off work because they feel depressed.

Possible complexity:

- You are being approached as a 'GP' but you are not the GP to this F2 doctor. Avoid colluding and falling into the familiar role of GP, instead encouraging them to approach their own registered GP for help.
- Is there an immediate safety issue – e.g. do they have intrusive thoughts of self-harm or suicidal ideation? If so, what do you need to do right now to keep them safe?

Professional Conversation/Professional Dilemma

Medical Complexity in Working with Colleagues

- Have patients been put at risk during any recent consultations with a doctor who may be unwell? How would you determine this and who would you work with to find out?
- Which other colleagues could help the FY2 doctor? As well as their GP, perhaps their educational and clinical supervisors and any mental health and wellbeing services for doctors in training.

Example. The HCA asks if she could have advice as she has, in error, given a flu vaccine to a patient instead of a COVID vaccination. The patient already received the flu vaccination a week previously.

Possible complexity:

- Patient safety issues – Who will tell the patient about the error, with an apology and explanation, warn that they are not protected against COVID and offer them the correct vaccination, and how?
- How did the error happen? Human error? Is there a systems issue? Might other patients have experienced the same error? What steps could you and practice colleagues take to avoid a recurrence?
- Wellbeing of the HCA who may be upset or distraught that this has happened.
- Colluding with unprofessional behaviour, e.g. – if the HCA asks if it is OK to do nothing.

Colleagues speaking about a patient

Reading the patient notes prior to the case will alert you to the fact that you will be speaking to a third party, not directly to the patient.

Example. The district nurse phones to speak to you from the home of William Anderson, aged 80.

Possible complexity:

- Older person – issues about safety at home, social care and support. Ensure you are familiar with local services that support physical and mental health for patients and of your practice.
- Medical complexity from co-morbidities and polypharmacy.
- Mental capacity of the patient to make decisions about their care. Do you know how to assess capacity?

Example. The HV calls about Ben Tomson, 3, failing to thrive with bruises on his back.

Possible complexity:

- What might underlie 'failure to thrive'? Could there be a serious and urgent clinical condition such as leukaemia and how would you find out? Or could this be neglect or abuse from Ben's caregivers?
- Safeguarding issues – do you know who to involve and how to do this?

Example. The palliative care nurse calls about Ada Wood, 88, terminally ill with lung cancer.

Possible complexity:

- Physical or mental health needs. Appropriate/anticipatory medication available in the house.
- End-of-life issues such as ReSPECT form, DNACPR, advance directives.
- Possible need for admission for symptom control.
- Carer strain.

Conclusion

As with all cases, reading the notes carefully will enable you to anticipate some of the complex issues you may experience in the forthcoming consultation. Jot down any important details on your whiteboard. Think ahead about the colleague that you will be speaking to and how you relate to them (are they part of your PHCT or someone else, e.g. a hospital consultant?). At all times remember the need to act in the best interests of patients, ensuring they receive safe, high-quality care, but also remember to look after your colleague, being professional and respecting boundaries, signposting them to additional sources of help if appropriate.

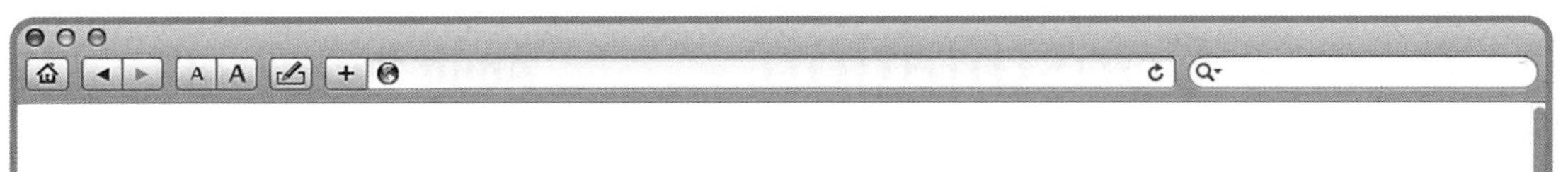

Doctor's Notes

Patient	Doris Jenkinson	79 years	F
PMH	None		
Medications	None		
Allergies	None		
Consultations	None		
Investigations	None		
Household	Arthur Jenkinson	84 years	M

Please speak to Suzanne, advanced nurse practitioner, about Doris.

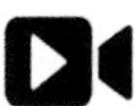

Example Consultation

Adult Safeguarding and Domestic Violence

Open ☐ Hi, Suzanne, how can I help?

ICE1 ☐ What's on your mind?

Flags ☐ What do you think she meant about not knowing how to handle Arthur? What's been happening at home? How does Doris appear? How was her mood? Does she feel unsafe at home? Has he threatened to kill her? Does Arthur wander out of the house alone, for example at night? Are there any other safety risks at home, e.g. gas being turned on?

History ☐ What is the background? What did Arthur do when he was working? And how about family? Do they live close by? Is Doris aware of financial benefits she might be entitled to?

Risk ☐ Sometimes farmers legally own shotguns. Do you know if there is a gun in the house? That's a relief. And, with family being far away, does Doris have any local support? Are there extended family or friends nearby who help? How long has this been getting worse? Are there any significant injuries you're worried about? Any signs of serious infection such as a high temperature? And how was the house? Did it appear reasonably clean or neglected?

ICE2 ☐ What worries you most about this situation? What is Doris' biggest fear?

ICE3 ☐ What were you thinking might need to happen? Have you mentioned any of this to Doris yet? How did she react? Did she state that she wanted help?

Impression ☐ From what you have described, there seem to be a couple of issues. First, Doris is experiencing domestic violence, albeit from someone who doesn't necessarily know what he is doing. Also, Arthur's condition is deteriorating and he needs a review and support.

InCLudE ☐ I share your worry that this is a difficult and unsafe situation. Given Arthur has dementia, it is unlikely that the police would want to act.

Empathy ☐ These situations are always difficult, so I'm not surprised you were unsure what to do.

Recommend ☐ Regarding the safeguarding concern, I suggest speaking to Doris about referring to social services. This would help her to get extra support. She is clearly doing all she can, but the current situation is unsafe for them both. You could also flag this couple to our safeguarding lead for discussion at the next meeting. I suspect social services will offer carer support or it may be that Arthur needs to be in a specialist care home to support his needs. If Doris prefers to have Arthur at home, we should refer him urgently to the older people's mental health team who may be able to offer medication which can calm him. I suggest we contact our dementia outreach team for an urgent review. One possibility is that they admit him to a mental health ward to assess and treat. I wonder if she is getting all the benefits she may be entitled to, for example attendance allowance, carer's allowance and council tax reduction due to severe mental impairment? These might make a real difference and enable her to employ extra support at home. Do you feel able to speak to Doris about what we have discussed? She can access telephone support from charities such as Dementia UK and contact her local Admiral nurse team to discuss other sources of help. With Arthur's condition getting worse, we should also arrange blood tests, a urine dipstick and an ECG to see if there is a treatable cause for the deterioration. For the wound, I agree regarding antibiotics; could you book her back in for a review later in the week?

Safety net ☐ Please let Doris know that, if she is worried, she can contact us or, if she is feeling threatened, she can call the police.

Future ☐ I think it would be helpful for you or me to meet up with Doris again in a couple of weeks to see how she is doing and see what's happening with social services, mental health services and Arthur's situation. Please could you ask her to book in with reception before she leaves?

Patient's Story **Adult Safeguarding and Domestic Violence**

Doctor's notes Doris Jenkinson, 79 years. Household: Arthur Jenkinson, 84 years. No PMH/DH/investigations/consultations.

'Please speak to Suzanne, advanced nurse practitioner, about Doris.'

How to act Professional but concerned.

PC *Hi, Doctor, I just wanted your advice as I'm a bit worried about Doris who I've just seen.'*

History You are Suzanne, a new advanced nurse practitioner in primary care. Previously, you had worked in a pre-op assessment clinic so you are a little unsure regarding processes around safeguarding and domestic violence. You have just seen Doris for a wound assessment. She has a nasty skin tear on her elbow which has become infected, hence she booked the appointment. When you asked how it happened, she initially stated she fell. However, you noticed multiple bruises on her arms and chest as well as a fading bruise on her cheek. You were worried she may need a referral to the clinic so you asked more about what is happening. Doris broke down in tears saying she didn't know how to handle Arthur any more.

Social Doris lives with her husband, Arthur; they are both patients in the practice. Arthur has mixed dementia (vascular and Alzheimer's). He was diagnosed 7 years ago and the couple have been coping until recently. Arthur's confusion has increased; he is often paranoid and has begun lashing out. He is a retired farmer so is still physically strong. He used to legally own a shotgun with a licence but his licence was rescinded when he was diagnosed with dementia and there is no gun in the house.

He was always such a kind and gentle man; it is upsetting for Doris that his dementia is affecting his behaviour in this way. Their grown-up children live a 2-hour drive away and visit when they can, which is not often. Their neighbour will sometimes watch Arthur whilst Doris goes to the shops but she has been put off helping due to the violent outbursts. Arthur does not wander out of the house and there have been no safety risks such as the gas being turned on.

Doris and Arthur are not in receipt of any benefits and Doris is not aware that she is entitled to anything.

Examination Doris has a fading bruise on her cheek and a skin tear on her elbow from a fall following a push from Arthur. Multiple bruises on her arms and upper chest. Elbow wound has minor infection, systemically well. Not depressed but tearful about situation.

ICE You are concerned that Doris is at risk but don't know what to do as the problem is caused by Arthur's dementia. You didn't know if the police should be involved or not. Doris would like Arthur to stay at home as that is what he would have wanted but she feels they now need help.

You think the elbow wound needs a prescription for antibiotics.

Learning Points — Safeguarding and Domestic Violence

As a general rule, if you find yourself wondering whether a safeguarding referral is required, it probably is. Safeguarding is certainly a consideration when there is any suggestion of domestic violence, drug and alcohol abuse or significant mental illness in the home. This is particularly relevant when children are involved, even when a parent assures you that the child/children have not been directly involved, because there is still significant risk of emotional abuse and neglect due to the environment they are living in. As professionals we need to acknowledge this and explain it to the parent/guardian. Remember that not every referral automatically results in action being taken or children being removed from the family, which is often the main fear when safeguarding concerns are raised. It's important to be able to speak about this to patients in a supportive way, rather than in an accusatory manner.

When discussing safeguarding with colleagues, try to ascertain all the information you would have asked had you been the clinician, so you can help the colleague determine if a referral is necessary. If the next steps are unclear, you may wish to signpost them to your practice safeguarding lead for further advice. Consider whether the person/family should be added to the agenda for discussion at your practice's next safeguarding meeting. As anyone can make a safeguarding referral, the colleague is likely to be able to do this themselves but may ask for your advice and support in doing so. This may include advice about what to say to the person/family about why the referral is being made and any likely outcomes.

It would be easy in this example case to focus entirely on the safeguarding/domestic violence aspects of the case. However, don't forget that Arthur is also your patient, and helping him with his dementia will help Doris as well.

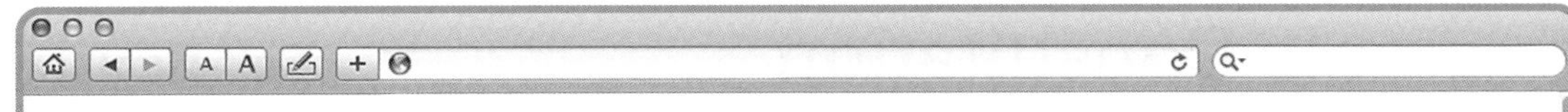

Doctor's Notes

Patient Brian Fielding 69 years M

PMH None

Medications None

Allergies No information

Consultations Last appointment 2019, came with dental abscess. Analgesia given and signposted to emergency dental services. BP 151/90 at this appointment. Advised to follow-up with nurse for repeat BP but no appointment made

Investigations No recent investigation

Household No household members registered

Telephone call to discuss patient Brian Fielding (69 years) with social worker (Zoe Marshall).

Example Consultation

Open ☐ Hi, Zoe, how can I help? Can you tell me a little about the current situation?

ICE2 ☐ When you saw Brian, what worries did you have?

Flags ☐ Any indicators of why Brian isn't looking after himself well? Did you see any evidence of drug or alcohol misuse such as bottles being left around or him smelling of alcohol? How did he seem in himself? Did his mood seem low? Did he make any comments about not wanting to be here/suicide? Does he seem confused at all? Was there anything about his physical health which concerned you, or has Brian mentioned any pain/health problems? Can he remember how he fell? Were the paramedics worried about any health issue when they saw him? Did you ask Brian about the skin lesion? Did he say how long it had been there? Any changes in size? Or bleeding/irritation?

ICE1☐ What do you think is going on?

Risk ☐ Does Brian have anyone supporting him? Any family or friends? Are you aware of any significant life events recently such as bereavement? Does he have any way of getting help, for example if he fell again? Have you managed to get any help in place so far?

ICE3 ☐ When you spoke to Brian about his social situation, what was his perspective? Has he given any indication that he would like some help from his GP? Is he aware of this conversation? Did you discuss any outcome you were hoping for with him?

InCLudE ☐ Unfortunately, we haven't seen Brian for some time, so I agree a review would be helpful.

Impression ☐ There seems to be a few things to consider. I agree, it sounds like Brian is neglecting himself so it's important we consider his social situation. But we also need to consider his physical health regarding his skin lesion, which could potentially be a type of skin cancer, and his slightly raised blood pressure. From what you have told me, it doesn't seem that there is any reason to doubt his capacity so if he declines help there may not be much we can do. However, if we can gain Brian's trust, he may allow us to help him. It sounds like you've already made a start there which is great.

Recommend ☐ I would like to assess his skin and recheck his blood pressure. If he's willing, a set of blood tests would be helpful to assess his health and check for any problems caused by untreated high blood pressure. Do you think he would agree to this? I'm also wondering whether he would be happy to meet our social prescriber? Our social prescriber is able to spend more time with patients than clinicians so can often get to the route of the concern more easily. They can talk to him about local support which may help with loneliness and can advise him regarding any extra benefits/support he may be entitled to. What do you think?

Future ☐ I'll task our social prescriber and ask them to make contact. I will ask our reception team to ring Brian to book him in with me later this week to look at his skin lesion and to discuss his blood pressure.

Safety net ☐ Please let Brian know the plan and reassure him he can contact us anytime if he has any concerns.

Patient's Story

Self-Neglect

Doctor's notes Brian Fielding, 69 years. No PMH/DH/allergies. Last appointment 2019, came with dental abscess. Analgesia given and signposted to emergency dental services. BP 151/90 at this appointment. Advised to follow-up with nurse for repeat BP but no appointment made.

No household members registered.

Telephone call to discuss patient with social worker (Zoe Marshall).

How to act Concerned.

PC *'Hi, Doctor, I'd like to discuss a patient of yours I'm concerned about.'*

History You are a social worker (Zoe Marshall) who wishes to discuss a patient, Brian Fielding (69 years), with his GP. You became involved in the case after Brian's neighbour phoned an ambulance when he witnessed Brian trip and fall in his garden 3 days ago. The paramedics came and checked him over, found no injury or acute medical problem, but noted his house was cluttered and dirty. Brian's observations were normal, other than a slightly raised BP at 149/85. He had a normal ECG. Brian stated that he just tripped over a loose paving stone and lost his balance. No dizziness. No head injury. They also felt that Brian had been struggling with his personal hygiene and were concerned that a lot of food in the fridge was out of date.

PMH Brian has no chronic medical problems that you are aware of; however, you noted a skin lesion on his face which you are worried about.

Brian has stated he's fine and doesn't wish to bother the doctors. The skin lesion has been there for a couple of months; Brian thought it was just a wart or something due to ageing. However, he is a little concerned that it has grown quite quickly. No bleeding or itching.

Mental state You're not sure about his mood; he does seem a little low but you're not sure if that is significant enough to be depression. He hasn't given any signs of self-harm or suicidal thoughts. You did not see any evidence of drug or alcohol misuse when you visited him.

If asked about confusion/capacity when you have spoken to Brian, you haven't had any concerns about his memory. He knows where he is and the time. If specifically asked about capacity, you believe Brian has capacity.

Brian's ICE He seemed to be happy living how he is and just wants to be left alone. However, he did mention that he would see the GP about his skin and does wonder if he ought to have had a check-up of his general health in the last year or two.

Social Brian lives alone. He is divorced; his ex-wife Janet occasionally calls in on him. His neighbour keeps a vague eye out for him, but Brian generally keeps to himself. Brian lost contact with his children during the divorce; he thinks they live in London.

The social work team have offered carers; Brian does not want this. He has agreed for the social work team to get someone to help him clean up his house and for the fire service to do an assessment.

ICE You would like to know if the GP has any useful information regarding Brian and to highlight the current issues. Brian is aware that you are going to speak to his GP and he is happy for you to do so. You would like the GP to review him.

Learning Points

Self-Neglect[1]

Self-neglect can take many forms, from personal hygiene issues and hoarding disorders to neglect of one's health or environment. It is a recognised category of abuse and neglect (Care Act 2014)[2] so should trigger safeguarding processes when identified by a health professional.

Examples of indicators of self-neglect:

- Pressure ulcers.
- Malnutrition or unexplained weight loss.
- Stockpiles of untaken medication.
- Inappropriate clothing or clothing in poor condition.
- Limited movement at home, e.g. spending long periods in a chair.
- Lack of food or out-of-date food.
- Appearing regularly intoxicated.
- Unkempt pets.
- Consider their environment – warm, clean, safe?

When assessing someone suspected of self-neglect there are often several factors to consider. Start by considering if there is an obvious cause for the self-neglect. For example, is the person physically incapable of caring for themselves? Do they have mobility or pain issues? Do they have the cognitive ability to look after themselves? Do they have dementia or serious mental illness? Do they have a learning disability or impairment from significant neurodiversity? Are they suffering from a lack of motivation after a life event such as bereavement or loss of employment? Are they struggling financially? Have they lost their support network or a key person who was caring for them before?

Secondly, if the individual is actively choosing to live in a particular way, do they have capacity? An understanding of the Mental Capacity Act is essential when considering self-neglect. Everyone is free to make unwise decisions. However, repeated and significant unwise decisions should provoke an assessment of mental capacity. It is important to acknowledge that patients with capacity can refuse help, and often do so, which can make it difficult for professionals to intervene. Taking time to build trust with the individual is vital to encouraging their engagement with support processes. Taking a soft approach, avoiding being overbearing and demanding of the person, encouraging small positive steps and taking a person-centred approach can help increase engagement.

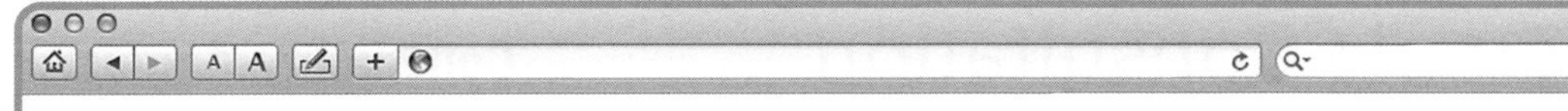

Doctor's Notes

Patient	Lionel Morgan	82 years	M
PMH	Parkinson's disease		
Medications	Co-careldopa 25/100, 2 tablets TDS		
	Entacapone 200 mg twice a day		
Allergies	No information		
Consultations	None recent		
Investigations	No information		
Household	Betty Morgan	80 years	F

Telephone call with paramedic – Ahmed. He is with Lionel Morgan, 82 years.

Example Consultation

Community-Acquired Pneumonia

Open ☐ Hi, Ahmed, how can I help?

History ☐ Can you tell me any more about your assessment? How long has he been coughing for? Any sputum?

ICE1 ☐ From your assessment what do you think is going on? What did Lionel say when you told him what you thought?

Impact ☐ How is this illness affecting Lionel? Is he very different from his usual self?

Flags ☐ How does Lionel seem in himself? Does he have any abnormal observations? Does he seem confused? Has he coughed up any blood? Has he lost any weight recently? Does he have any chest pain or leg swelling? What does his chest sound like?

ICE2 ☐ What worries you most about Lionel's situation?

Empathy ☐ Does he have a ReSPECT form in place?

Risk ☐ Have you discussed with him the risks of staying at home? What did he say? Did he say why he doesn't wish to go to hospital? How much support does he have at home? Is he mobilising okay? Has he been remembering to take his medication? Is he swallowing okay?

ICE3 ☐ What outcome had you hoped for?

SummarICE ☐ So in summary, you suspect Lionel has community-acquired pneumonia and his CRB-65 score is 1. As he is frail and his Sats are a bit low, you felt admission was necessary; however, Lionel disagrees. He agrees he probably has an infection but worries most about dying in hospital and would prefer to be treated at home.

Impression ☐ I agree this sounds like CAP and given the overall situation a hospital review may be helpful; however, if this is not what Lionel wishes we'll need to think of an alternative plan.

Experience ☐ From your experience, do you think Lionel has capacity and understands the risks of staying at home?

InCludE ☐ As Lionel understands this, I think it would be reasonable to follow Lionel's wishes and treat him with antibiotics at home.

Recommend ☐ I recommend using a combination of antibiotics to give best cover as he is quite poorly and frail. I will send a prescription for amoxicillin and clarithromycin to his chemist. Please could you just check with him that he has no allergies to antibiotics? Could one of his relatives pick this up for him?

Future ☐ I would like to review him in 48 hours to see how he is getting on. We can then discuss his options further. If he is recovering, great; if not we could revisit his thoughts about possible hospital care. Is this okay with Lionel?

Empower ☐ Either way, it will give us an opportunity to talk about his future wishes and put these on paper, if he wants us to. We can also review if there is anything we can do to make his life easier regarding his Parkinson's disease as well. Could you mention this to him please?

Specifics ☐ I have booked a visit for 2 days' time. I'll give him a call before coming to check it's still appropriate to visit.

Safety net ☐ If he deteriorates in the meantime, please could you ask him or Betty to ring us or 999 straight away?

Patient's Story

Community-Acquired Pneumonia

Doctor's notes	Lionel Morgan, 82 years. Parkinson's disease. Medications: co-careldopa 25/100, 2 tablets TDS, entacapone 200 mg twice a day. No information on allergies or investigations; no recent consultations. Household: Betty Morgan, 80 years. Telephone call with paramedic – Ahmed. He is with Lionel Morgan, 82 years.
How to act	Professional but concerned.
PC	***'Hi, Doctor, I'm after some advice about Lionel.'***
History	Paramedic attending Lionel Morgan, who is an 82-year-old gentleman. His wife, Betty, phoned an ambulance this morning as Lionel looked breathless. He has struggled to get out of bed more than usual today. Betty thinks Lionel has a chest infection.
History obtained from Betty	Lionel has been coughing green phlegm for 4 days. He looks breathless but isn't wheezy. He is not choking on his food. No blood seen. No other viral URTI symptoms. Temperature 102°F.
History obtained from Lionel	No pain. Green sputum.
Social	Lionel lives with his wife, Betty, who does all of his ADL and takes care of his medicines. Lionel is well looked after at home, and his three children live close by. He has never smoked. He does not drink alcohol. No asbestos exposure.
Examination	Bronchial breathing and crackles in the left base. Temperature 38.2°C. HR 90 bpm regular. Sats 94%. RR 24. BP 120/68. Not done formal AMTS but is orientated to person, place and time. Mobilising slowly with four-wheeled walker.
Paramedic's impression	You think Lionel has pneumonia and would benefit from transfer to hospital for further assessment. Lionel has stated that he really does not wish to go to hospital. You feel this is risky as he could get worse if not treated properly.
Lionel's ICE	He does not wish to go to hospital because he is afraid he won't come out again. If he is going to die, he would rather be at home. He feels his Parkinson's disease affects his enjoyment of life and the deterioration in his condition is difficult, though expected. He will accept antibiotics and any care he can be given at home. He is willing to revisit the discussion in 48 hours; however, if he is worsening he thinks he would prefer to be kept comfortable. No ReSPECT form in place.

Learning Points

Community-Acquired Pneumonia[1]

Pneumonia Pneumonia is an infection of the lung parenchyma (alveoli). It can be difficult to differentiate acute bronchitis/LRTI and CAP. NICE states 'clinical judgement must always be used to diagnose CAP because no combination of symptoms or signs is clearly diagnostic.'[1]

Calculate CRB-65 score 1 point each for: confusion (AMTS ≤8/10, or new disorientation to person, place or time), RR ≥30/min, systolic BP <90 or diastolic BP ≤60, age ≥65 years.

Mortality risk from CRB-65 scores

Score = 0	'Low risk'[2]	<1% mortality risk[2,3]
Score = 1–2	'Intermediate risk'[2]	1–10% mortality risk[2,3]
Score = 3–4	'High risk'[2]	>10% mortality risk[2,3]

Sputum culture 'Do not routinely recommend microbiological tests for people with low-severity community-acquired pneumonia.'[1]

CRP testing Consider if clinically a diagnosis of pneumonia is not clear or there is uncertainty about whether antibiotics are indicated.[1]

<20 mg/L	'Do not routinely offer antibiotic therapy.'[1]
20–100 mg/L	'Consider a delayed antibiotic prescription.'[1]
>100 mg/L	Antibiotics indicated.

NB: A fever is 100°F (= 37.8°C). Many older patients still use Fahrenheit.

AMTS[4] To save time, ask the hard questions first; once they have got >2 wrong then move on. Scored out of 10 with 1 point for each correct answer. Score <8 is significant.

Address to remember (42 West Street), age, time, year, where are we, two persons, DOB, king, First World War dates, 20–1 backwards, ?recall address correct.

Treatment of pneumonia based on CRB score

Score = 0 5 days antibiotics. See your local guidance. E.g. amoxicillin 500 mg TDS or doxycycline 200 mg day 1 then 100 mg daily or clarithromycin 500 mg BD (erythromycin in pregnancy if penicillin allergy).

Score = 1–2 Consider hospital admission, particularly if score 2. 5 days amoxicillin + 5 days clarithromycin (erythromycin if pregnant). If penicillin allergy, doxycycline or clarithromycin alone.

Score = 3–4 Admit urgently to hospital.

Clinical judgement is important, not just CRB-65 score. Consider oxygen levels, person's wishes, co-morbidities, frailty and social situation.

Recovery and safety net

Useful to explain to patients that the recovery can take a long time. Fever usually resolves within 1 week, chest pain and sputum should settle by 4 weeks, cough and breathlessness by 6 weeks, fatigue by 3 months, with full resolution by 6 months.[1] See GP if no response within 3 days, and sooner if worsening symptoms.

Practising holistically

In this scenario, asking about swallowing demonstrates you have considered the chronic co-morbidities in this acute situation and thought about aspiration pneumonia. When a carer is present, acknowledge them and their role. If there is no time to discuss the impact of a chronic disease (Parkinson's) in this first consultation then signpost that you will do so later.

Doctor's Notes

Patient	Louise Barker	33 years	F
PMH	Metastatic cervical cancer diagnosed 5 months ago, previous hysterectomy		
	NVD 2 years ago		
Medications	Cyclizine 50 mg TDS PRN		
	Co-codamol 30/500 QDS PRN		
Allergies	No information		
Consultations	Cancer care review with GP 4 weeks ago: trying to remain positive, feeling OK, pain and nausea well controlled. Has consultant follow-up in 4 weeks following blood tests and scans. Review after this		
Investigations	No information		
Household	Nick Barker	36 years	M
	Megan Barker	2 years	F

Please discuss Louise with Dr Lim, locum consultant oncologist at your local hospital.

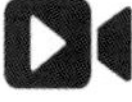

Example Consultation

Cervical Cancer/End of Life

Open ☐ Hello, Dr Lim, how can I help?

History ☐ I've got some information from her records, but please could you summarise where we are up to with Louise's condition so I'm sure I understand the situation fully?

Sense ☐ I sense this was a particularly difficult conversation and one you hadn't wished to do over the phone.

ICE1/2 ☐ You've mentioned Louise now has multiorgan failure and sadly little time left; other than this being a really awful situation, was there anything that is particularly troubling you?

Impact ☐ Did you get a feel for how they are coping at home?

Risk ☐ Did you get a sense of how Mr Barker is managing emotionally? It sounds like he has lots of questions and fears on his mind.

ICE3 ☐ Following your discussion with Louise and then Nick, did you have any particular action in mind? Do Louise/Nick know you are phoning me?

SummarICE ☐ So, sadly Louise is likely to pass away soon and you're concerned about how this young family will cope and believe that the usual end-of-life discussions and support may not have taken place. You were hoping we could visit Louise to further assess.

Options ☐ I can certainly arrange an urgent visit to assess the situation further. We can get the palliative care team involved and potentially the hospice team. If Mr Barker is worried about the final days and finding Louise dead, he may prefer her final days to be in the local hospice. Or perhaps they may prefer to have carers at home? Other thoughts I am having are that we need to discuss anticipatory medications and prescribe these so they are available in the house and ensure that a ReSPECT form has been discussed with Louise. For Nick, we could provide a Fit note to let him have some much needed time off work, and get him some carers' support. It may be that all his anxiety and distress is entirely due to his understandable reaction to the situation but I'd like to screen him for any underlying mental health problem as well.

InCludE ☐ Given what Mr Barker has said about it being his fault, I will see if there is an opportunity to discuss this and explain that the virus is common and Louise has just been very unlucky.

Empower ☐ I'll suggest he opens up to family and friends to get support and perhaps create a memory box for Megan. Some families find these helpful.

Future ☐ I will give the family a call shortly to offer a visit.

Safety net ☐ Do you know if the family have any numbers for the urgent care services? If not, I'll make sure they get these.

Patient's Story

Cervical Cancer/End of Life

Doctor's notes Louise Barker, 33 years. Metastatic cervical cancer diagnosed 5 months ago, previous hysterectomy. NVD 2 years ago.

Medications: cyclizine 50 mg TDS PRN, co-codamol 30/500 QDS PRN.

Consultations: cancer care review with GP 4 weeks ago: trying to remain positive, feeling OK, pain and nausea well controlled. Has consultant follow-up in 4 weeks following blood tests and scans. Review after this.

Investigations/allergies: no information.

Household: Nick Barker, 36 years; Megan Barker, 2 years.

How to act Professional and concerned, but also a little upset.

PC ***'I just thought I should talk to you, Doctor.'***

History You are a locum oncology consultant from the local hospital. You have just had to give Louise and her husband, Nick, difficult news over the phone. She was due to attend clinic today but didn't as she felt too tired and unwell. You have only met Louise and her husband once before, 6 weeks ago. She has metastatic cervical cancer. When the cancer was first diagnosed, she underwent a hysterectomy followed by chemotherapy but, unfortunately, she didn't respond to the chemotherapy and she was referred back to the MDT for a decision. The decision was made for best supportive care. She did have bloods 4 days ago which show she has renal failure, liver failure and anaemia. Her most recent scan shows advanced disease. You had hoped to speak to her in person today to explain her body was showing signs of multiorgan failure and sadly there is nothing more that can be offered.

Social You're also concerned about Louise's husband. After Louise had handed him the phone back he had started to say that he didn't know how he would cope without Louise and that he was frightened of finding her dead. They have a 2-year-old daughter, Megan. Nick mentioned not having time to go to work and felt too distracted but didn't know what to do so he phoned in sick last week. He had said, ***'It's all my fault'***. You think he was referring to the fact that cervical cancer is caused by a sexually transmitted infection, which had come up in a previous appointment when they asked the cause. You wanted to ask him some more questions, but he changed the subject and said he needed to take Louise to the toilet then ended the call.

ICE You don't think she will have long to live. You don't believe she has any pre-emptives in place as she had been managing pretty well until the last few days. You get the impression that end-of-life discussions have been put off as neither Louise nor her husband were ready to accept she would die. You hope the doctor will visit Louise and her husband to talk to them in person. You expect the GP to offer palliative care support, pre-emptive medication and potentially hospice support but as you're a locum you're not entirely certain of the local primary care set up. (Don't give this information too freely; allow GP to suggest these actions but prompt if not suggested.)

Points to consider in medically complex cases

When a patient presents with a condition which is usually treated by a specialist, or has been under specialist care but the hospital team has run out of options, it can be easy to feel 'so what can I do?'

If you get such a case in your SCA, focus on answering questions the patient may have, impact and symptom palliation. In doing so, you will soon realise that there is lots you can do. This may involve information giving, emotional support, treatment of symptoms or practical advice such as support around work, difficulties at home (e.g. ADLs), finance, carer support or signposting to other sources of support (e.g. charities or community services).

End-of-life/medically complex cases may also present as a discussion with a relative. Try not to get too worried about confidentiality. You can discuss information given to you by the relative and speak in general or hypothetical terms. Below is some advice about how you can manage cases where you are speaking to a relative or other individual who is not the patient, or a health professional directly involved in their care.

Confidentiality

Unless the patient has given consent, no information can be given to the NOK. However, you can speak in general terms about a condition or likely outcome, e.g. 'often in similar situations the hospice can offer support'.

You cannot give new information to the relative but can discuss what they already know. Again, be general to avoid any confidentiality issues, e.g. in this case you could discuss cervical cancer in general (such as links to HPV) but not the specifics of Louise's case.

Do not	Do not presume you understand their concerns. Explore their thoughts.
Do	Ensure the relative feels understood – summarise their ICE!
	Reassure them that they will receive the help they need specifically related to their concerns.
	Allow the person to do the majority of the talking, be flexible with what they hope to discuss.

Example consultation structure when discussing end-of-life care

1. Silences, exploring thoughts or stating what you sense can help initiate a sensitive conversation.
2. Check their understanding of the situation.
3. Collect all thoughts, concerns, fears, anxieties and expectations.
4. Be curious. Explore any cues they may have hinted. Silences or repeating words to encourage further discussion may be useful here.
5. Consider the carer; are they well? Their mood, their responsibilities as a carer, other stressors in their life, the impact of the situation?
6. Summarise the ICE. This is a powerful way to help the person feel understood and also focuses the management plan.
7. Enquire about communication between the relatives and patient.
8. Provide options/suggestions to manage each concern in turn.
9. Consider if other professionals or support groups may be helpful.
10. Empower with regard to their concerns.
11. Plan future meetings. Is anything required in the meantime?
12. Safety net: rescue treatment and contact numbers in the event of sudden deterioration.

If appropriate – in the event of death, do they know who to call? Usually, it is the GP or OOH GP to certify death, followed by the undertaker.

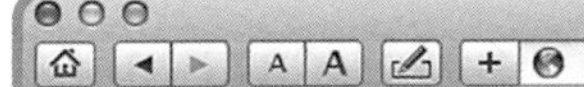

Doctor's Notes

Patient	Eric Johnson	61 years	M
PMH	Type 2 diabetes – diagnosed 10 years ago		
Medications	Metformin 500 mg TDS		
	Gliclazide 160 mg daily		
	Blood glucose testing strips		
Allergies	No information		
Consultations	Annual diabetes review with practice nurse 1 month ago. Foot check normal. Compliant with medications, no issues, diabetic eye check done by hospital 3 months ago, mild non-proliferative diabetic retinopathy. Discussed checking BM before driving, managing with this		
Investigations	HbA1c 59 mmol/L		
Household	Kath Johnson	62 years	F

Please discuss Eric with your practice physician associate (Simon) following an appointment in his minor illness clinic.

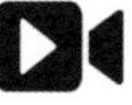

Example Consultation

Retinal Detachment

Open ☐ Hello, Simon, how can I help? Did he say how he first noticed it?

History ☐ Does the vision fluctuate or is it just as bad all the time? Any pain in the eyeball? Any redness? Any other eye symptoms? Has it affected his driving? Is he working at present? Any issues with computers?

Flags ☐ Any floaters? Anything that appears to be like a curtain coming across his vision? Any flashes?

Curious ☐ You mentioned him being stressed. What is stressing him?

ICE1 ☐ What thoughts have you had about this? What about Eric? Did he say what he thought it was?

Risk ☐ Does Eric wear glasses? Is he short-sighted or long-sighted? Does he ever wear contact lenses? Did he have any eye problems when he was a baby? Has anyone in the family had anything similar? Has he been hit in the eye recently?

ICE2 ☐ What worries you most? Has Eric expressed any concerns?

Impact ☐ Sight is really important and he needs to be able to drive safely to do his job. With diabetes, he needs to be able to see well to check his blood sugars so that he can monitor his control. Diabetes, as you know, can affect eyesight so it is especially important to get blood sugars under control so we do need to take this problem seriously.

Examination ☐ What have you found on examination?

ICE3 ☐ Have you formulated a plan for him? Has Eric expressed any thoughts about treatment options?

SummarICE ☐ To summarise, for the last couple of weeks the sight in his right eye has got worse – it is now blurred and he had a near miss in the car. He has had some understandable stress at work and he feels it is very important to fly to the USA next week.

InCludE ☐ I don't think it's likely this is caused by the diabetes, but the squash ball may possibly have had a role.

Impression ☐ I suspect retinal detachment, which means the membrane at the back of the eye (the retina) has become unstuck. Being very short-sighted is a risk factor, as is recent trauma to the eye. The flashers and floaters you described can be a sign of this condition.

Explanation ☐ Another possibility is bleeding into the jelly part of his eye called vitreous haemorrhage – this can also cause floaters.

Options ☐ I recommend Eric is referred to the urgent eye clinic as if left untreated it could get worse. Could you speak to Eric about this and arrange the referral via contacting the switchboard at the hospital? They may treat it today either with laser treatment or by putting a gas or oil bubble into the eye to help hold the retina back in place.

InCludE ☐ Unfortunately, I think it is unlikely that he will be able to fly to the USA next week as this could prevent healing of the retinal problem and could be very risky for his eyesight. You can advise him to inform the eye specialist in case there is a way of managing this which won't affect his air travel. He must not drive while his vision is a concern. Can someone drive him to the hospital?

Future ☐ Less urgent for today, but please could you ask him to arrange follow-up for his BP and diabetes control? Both could be better and he may have underlying hypertension which needs treatment.

Safety net ☐ If for any reason he can't make it to hospital, please let me know.

Patient's Story

Retinal Detachment

Doctor's notes Eric Johnson, 61 years. Type 2 diabetes – diagnosed 10 years ago.

Medications: metformin 500 mg TDS, gliclazide 160 mg daily, blood glucose testing strips.

Consultations: annual diabetes review with practice nurse 1 month ago. Foot check normal. Compliant with medications, no issues, diabetic eye check done by hospital 3 months ago, mild non-proliferative diabetic retinopathy. Discussed checking BM before driving, managing with this.

Investigations: HbA1c 59 mmol/L.

Household: Kath Johnson, 62 years.

Please discuss Eric with your practice physician associate (Simon) following an appointment in his minor illness clinic.

How to act Unsure.

PC ***'I've just seen a patient with blurred vision; eyes aren't my strong point, but it seems serious.'***

History Eric is a 61-year-old businessman with diabetes that is not optimally managed. Over the last couple of weeks, he has noticed a slight reduction in VA in his right eye. He put this down to stress at work (financial viability of his company – selling tractors) or the diabetes not being well controlled. But last week he realised he couldn't see a car that was on his right-hand side when driving and had a near miss. This was very scary. He has also noticed a few flashes and floaters in his right eye over the last couple of weeks. He has always been short-sighted and wears quite thick lenses and contact lenses for sport. Eric tries to keep fit by playing squash and he was hit in the eye by a ball a few weeks ago. The eye was a bit sore for a few hours but then okay. He did not seek help at the time because he was busy.

Social Married, with grown-up children. Businessman, working long hours. Important business meeting in the USA next week – crucial he gets to this as there is potential for a big order that could make or break the company.

Eric's ICE He is unsure what is causing it but wonders if it was the eye injury with the ball. He suspects his diabetes may be another possibility. He expected the doctor to tell him off about his diabetes or tell him not to get so stressed (and this would annoy him). He is worried that either his vision is deteriorating or the doctor will say he can't fly.

Simon's ICE Also wonders if the problem is related to diabetes but wasn't sure what non-proliferative diabetic retinopathy is. Concerned as there seems to be a big difference between the right and left eye but not sure if this is to do with the diabetes. Would like advice from GP. Unable to answer questions about flying.

You've learnt the basics of eye examination and have managed to check VA and found the reduced vision in the right eye but couldn't see much with fundoscopy.

Examination No redness or bruising seen. Eye movements normal. Pupils equal and react to light.

VA left eye – 6/9, right eye – 6/60. Reduced visual field – lateral vision right eye.

Fundoscopy –difficult and retina not seen clearly.

BP today 147/84.

Learning Points

Retinal Detachment[1]

Epidemiology 1 to 1.5/10,000 people per year.

(One or two new cases per year in a medium-sized practice of 10,000 patients.)

Risk increases with increasing age: lifetime risk = 3% at 85 years.

Average age of occurrence = 60 years.

Male = female.

Risk factors Short-sightedness, FH, eye trauma, previous cataract surgery, diabetes (proliferative retinopathy), inflammatory eye problems (e.g. uveitis, scleritis), malignancy (secondary deposit or ocular melanoma primary), congenital eye disease (glaucoma, prematurity, cataract).

Symptoms New onset of floaters (lines, haze, dots).

New onset flashes of light.

Sudden onset loss of vision – starts at edge of vision and progresses to centre.

Often described as a 'curtain'.

Reduced visual acuity – blurred vision.

Contralateral eye affected in 10%.

Examination Visual acuity – may be reduced to 'counting fingers'.

Management of new-onset floaters/flashing lights

- Urgent (same-day ophthalmology) – if 'curtain', visual field loss, blurred vision, abnormal fundoscopy.
- Less urgent (slit lamp within 24 hours) – if no reduction in VA, no field loss, fundoscopy normal.
- Either case: PIL produced by RNIB – 'Understanding retinal detachment'.[2]

Hospital treatment

There are various ways of closing the hole and holding the retina against the eye wall. Surgeons often use a gas or oil bubble, then laser or cryotherapy to 'stick' it in place. The patient has to lie in a particular 'posture' to get the bubble in the right place. No air travel is permitted if gas has been used as the gas could expand and cause glaucoma and/or blindness.

Managing medical complexity – acute on chronic

When a patient has a chronic illness as well as the acute presentation (diabetes in this case), think about how the new problem will impact on their ability to manage their chronic illness and how the new problem will interact with the pre-existing condition (e.g. drug interactions, competing management priorities). In this case, problems with sight could make it difficult to use and read a blood sugar monitor, with implications for diabetic control, ultimately risking further sight damage.

APPENDIX 1

CASE MAPPING ACROSS THE GP CURRICULUM

The table below shows how the cases in the book map to the clinical curriculum areas. Some cases cover more than one area and these are marked with*.

Clinical curriculum area	Name, age and gender of patient	Chapter and case number	Problem
Allergy and clinical immunology	Lacey Archer 21 F*	9.4	Occupational allergy
Cardiovascular health	Hibiki Hayashi 75 M	5.3	Angina
	Mary Jones 45 F*	7.1	Chest pain of recent onset
	Vincent Riley 60 M	11.3	High cholesterol
	Richard Turner 57 M	11.4	Hypertension
	Jason Wright 26 M	12.1	Hypertrophic cardiomyopathy
	Janet Harrison 78 F*	12.5	Atrial fibrillation
Dermatology	Arthur Miller 13 M	2.2	Eczema
	Maureen Staples 70 F	4.4	Psoriasis
	Francesca Reece 32 F	9.2	Melasma
	Lacey Archer 21 F*	9.4	Occupational allergy
	Paul Haydock 21 M*	10.3	Rash – Lyme disease
ENT, speech and hearing	Anthony Warren 72 M	5.1	Deafness and tinnitus
	Doran O'Brian 39 M	9.5	Sinusitis
Eyes and vision	Fred Scott 81 M	5.2	AMD and cataract
	Daniela Adamovich 4 F	9.1	Squint
	Eric Johnson 61 M*	13.5	Retinal detachment
Gastroenterology	Hamza Khan 19 M	10.5	Bowel symptoms – IBS
	Daniel Hernandez 38 M	11.1	Dyspepsia/reflux
Genomic medicine	Olivia Wales 29 F*	3.3	Genetic testing
	Jason Wright 26 M	12.1	Hypertrophic cardiomyopathy
Gynaecology and breast health	Hilda Rowland 53 F	3.2	Post-menopausal bleeding
	Louise Barker 33 F	13.4	Cervical cancer/end of life

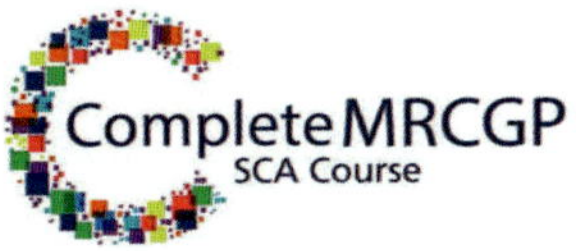

Clinical curriculum area	Name, age and gender of patient	Chapter and case number	Problem
Haematology	Connor McGowen 12 M	2.1	Anaemia
	Raymond Styles 86 M	8.3	Suspected DVT
	William Jefferies 65 M	12.2	Myeloma
Infectious diseases and travel health	Jennifer Adeyemi 27 F	3.1	Varicella in pregnancy
	Paul Haydock 21 M*	10.3	Rash – Lyme disease
Learning disability	Matthew Dalton 24 M*	4.1	Down syndrome
	Janine Paton 33 F*	8.2	Mental health and learning disability
Maternity and reproductive health	Olivia Wales 29 F*	3.3	Genetic testing
	Chloe Livingstone-Smith 28 F*	6.4	Postnatal psychosis
Mental health	Eleanor Cartwright 15 F	2.4	Eating disorder
	Stephen Harper 42 M	6.1	Anxiety
	Jessica Miller 24 F	6.2	Depression review
	Andrea Lockwood 36 F	6.3	Personality disorder
	Chloe Livingstone-Smith 28 F*	6.4	Postnatal psychosis
	Janine Paton 33 F*	8.2	Mental health and learning disability
	Doris Jenkinson 79 F*	13.1	Adult safeguarding and domestic violence
Metabolic problems and endocrinology	Fatima Sayed 47 F	4.2	Hyperthyroidism
	Mary Owen 35 F*	7.3	Hyperglycaemia
	Jayne Fitzpatrick 56 F	10.4	Tired all the time
Musculoskeletal health	Robert Hayes 32 M*	7.4	Knee pain
	Selina Richards 31 F	10.1	Foot pain – plantar fasciitis
	Rachel West 43 F	11.2	Chronic pain
Neurodevelopmental conditions and neurodiversity	Matthew Dalton 24 M*	4.1	Down syndrome
	Janine Paton 33 F*	8.2	Mental health and learning disability
	Sara Azmeh 28 F	9.3	Education about services
Neurology	Maggie Freestone 72 F	5.5	Peripheral neuropathy
	Lydia Cooper 25 F	10.2	Neurological symptoms – multiple sclerosis
	Yasmin Small 23 F	11.5	Migraine
Renal and urology	Kalpesh Khan 6 M	2.3	Recurrent UTI
	Arthur Smalling 49 M	4.3	Prostatitis
	Rosie Carpenter 40 F*	7.2	Abdominal pain
	Alexander Dickens 78 M	12.3	Acute kidney injury
	Remigio Sanchez 50 M	12.4	PSA test result
Respiratory health	Peter Atkins 9 M	2.5	Asthma diagnosis
	Chao Lin 82 M	4.5	COPD

Clinical curriculum area	Name, age and gender of patient	Chapter and case number	Problem
	Doris Ripley 76 F	5.4	Lung cancer/end of life
	Daisy Fitton 24 F*	7.5	Acute asthma
	Lionel Morgan 82 M*	13.3	Community-acquired pneumonia
Sexual health	Kevin Barton 57 M	3.4	Erectile dysfunction
	Florence Wriggley 15 F	3.5	Gender dysphoria
	Fedora Baros 38 F	8.5	LARC and sterilisation
Smoking, alcohol and substance misuse	Katherine Knight 68 F	6.5	Harmful drinking
	Isabel Forster 33 F	8.1	Domestic violence
	Kirsty West 38 F	8.4	Alcohol and safeguarding
	Doris Jenkinson 79 F*	13.1	Adult safeguarding and domestic violence
	Brian Fielding 69 M	13.2	Self-neglect
Urgent and unscheduled care	Mary Jones 45 F*	7.1	Chest pain of recent onset
	Rosie Carpenter 40 F*	7.2	Abdominal pain
	Mary Owen 35 F*	7.3	Hyperglycaemia
	Robert Hayes 32 M*	7.4	Knee pain
	Daisy Fitton 24 F*	7.5	Acute asthma
	Janet Harrison 78 F*	12.5	Atrial fibrillation
	Lionel Morgan 82 M*	13.3	Community-acquired pneumonia
	Eric Johnson 61 M*	13.5	Retinal detachment

APPENDIX 2

USEFUL WEBSITES AND RESOURCES

Chapter 1 Introduction and Background to the Exam

GP curriculum	**RCGP GP curriculum**	https://www.rcgp.org.uk/mrcgp-exams/gp-curriculum
	SCA preparation course	www.completemrcgp.co.uk
	Consultation skills	Moulton L. *The Naked Consultation: A Practical Guide to Primary Care Consultation Skills*, 2nd edn. London: CRC Press, 2016.
Information for GPs	**Patient.info**	https://patient.info/doctor
	GP Notebook	https://gpnotebook.com/en-GB
	CKS	Clinical Knowledge Summaries: https://cks.nice.org.uk/. 'Providing primary care practitioners with a readily accessible summary of the current evidence base and practical advice on best practice'
	SIGN	Scottish Intercollegiate Guidelines Network: http://sign.ac.uk/
	NICE	National Institute for Health and Care Excellence: https://www.nice.org.uk/guidance
	RCGP eLearning	http://elearning.rcgp.org.uk/

Keeping up to date	http://www.pulse-learning.co.uk/
	http://www.gponline.com/education
Courses not to miss	https://www.redwhale.co.uk/courses/
	https://www.nbmedical.com/courses/subject/hot-topics-gp-update
	http://www.rcgp.org.uk/learning/one-day-essentials/
	www.completemrcgp.co.uk
Conference not to miss	https://www.rcgpac.org.uk/
Time out from revision	Watch a TED Talk for inspiration!

Chapter 2 Patient Less Than 19 Years Old

Parent advice	https://www.what0-18.nhs.uk/parentscarers/worried-your-child-unwell
	Wester-Stratton C. *The Incredible Years. A Trouble-Shooting Guide for Parents of Children Aged 3–8 Years*, 3rd edn. Atlanta, GA: The Incredible Years, 2019.
Vitamin D guidelines for children	https://www.nuh.nhs.uk/vitamin-d-deficiency-in-children/

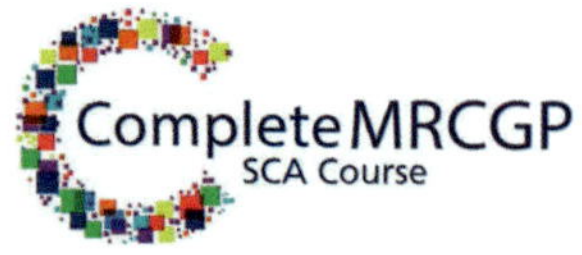

Chapter 3 Gender, Reproductive and Sexual Heath, Including Women's, Men's, LGBTQ+, Gynae and Breast

Medicines in pregnancy	http://www.medicinesinpregnancy.org/
Medicines in breastfeeding	https://www.ncbi.nlm.nih.gov/books/NBK501922/
Contraception	www.fsrh.org
RCOG Green-top Guidelines	https://www.rcog.org.uk/guidelines

Chapter 4 Long-Term Conditions, Including Cancer, Multi-Morbidity and Disability

Cancer	https://www.macmillan.org.uk/
Dementia	https://www.dementiauk.org/
Epilepsy	https://www.epilepsy.org.uk/
Rheumatoid arthritis	https://www.arthritis.org/diseases/rheumatoid-arthritis
Stroke	https://www.stroke.org.uk/resources

Chapter 5 Older Adults, Including Frailty and People at the End of Life

Age UK	https://www.ageuk.org.uk/information-advice/care/
Frailty resources	https://www.england.nhs.uk/ourwork/clinical-policy/older-people/frailty/frailty-resources/
Osteoporosis assessment	https://www.sheffield.ac.uk/FRAX/
Vitamin D guidelines for adults	https://ods.od.nih.gov/factsheets/VitaminD-HealthProfessional/

Chapter 6 Mental Health, Including Addiction, Smoking, Alcohol and Substance Misuse

Mental health resources for patients	**Patient leaflets**	https://selfhelp.cntw.nhs.uk/
	Mental health resources	https://www.mind.org.uk/
	Mindfulness	https://www.oxfordmindfulness.org/learn-mindfulness/
	Online programme	https://moodgym.com.au
Antidepressant switches	https://www.mims.co.uk/table-antidepressants-guide-switchingwithdrawing/mental-health/article/1415768	
CBT books	**For the keen reader**	Williams M., Penman D. *Mindfulness: A Practical Guide to Finding Peace in a Frantic World.* London: Piatkus Books, 2011.
	If struggling to concentrate	Black A. *Living in the Moment: With Mindfulness Meditations*. London: Ryland, Peters & Small, 2012.
Alcohol – useful information	https://www.who.int/health-topics/alcohol#tab=tab_1	
Substance misuse resources	https://www.mind.org.uk/information-support/types-of-mental-health-problems/recreational-drugs-alcohol-and-addiction/drug-and-alcohol-addiction-useful-contacts/	

Prescribing in psychiatry Taylor D.M., Paton C., Kapur S. *The Maudsley Prescribing Guidelines in Psychiatry,* 14th edn. Oxford: Wiley-Blackwell, 2021.

Chapter 7 Urgent and Unscheduled Care

Joint exercises https://www.versusarthritis.org/about-arthritis/exercising-with-arthritis/

STarT Back screening tool https://www.physio-pedia.com/STarT_Back_Screening_Tool

Physiotherapy website http://www.sheffieldachesandpains.com/

Chapter 8 Health Disadvantage and Vulnerabilities, Including Veterans, Mental Capacity, Safeguarding and Communication Difficulties

Learning disability PILs https://www.nhsinform.scot/translations/formats/easy-read

Royal National Institute of Blind People https://rnib.org.uk/

British Deaf Association https://bda.org.uk/

Chapter 9 Ethnicity, Culture, Diversity and Inclusivity

Homelessness https://www.shelter.org.uk/

Sex workers https://basisyorkshire.org.uk

PILs in different languages https://www.cntw.nhs.uk/resource-library/

Chapter 10 New Presentation of Undifferentiated Disease

Chest problems https://www.brit-thoracic.org.uk/quality-improvement/guidelines/

Cardiovascular risk http://qrisk.org/

BMJ's Easily Missed series http://www.bmj.com/specialties/easily-missed

We recommend this exercise – for each 'easily missed' condition:
(i) consider what symptoms the patient may have presented with and
(ii) then for each symptom think about what the most likely diagnoses are (common things are common!) and what is 'easily missed'.

Chapter 11 Prescribing

Antidepressant switches https://www.mims.co.uk/table-antidepressants-guide-switchingwithdrawing/mental-health/article/1415768

Antimicrobial guidelines https://elearning.rcgp.org.uk/mod/book/view.php?id=14887

Drug monitoring requirements http://www.bucksformulary.nhs.uk/docs/sc/

Vitamin D guidelines for adults https://ods.od.nih.gov/factsheets/VitaminD-HealthProfessional/

Chapter 12 Investigation/Results

Interpreting liver blood tests	https://britishlivertrust.org.uk/health-professionals/primary-care-resources/
Interpreting kidney blood tests	https://www.nhs.uk/conditions/kidney-disease/diagnosis/
Interpreting PSA results	https://www.cancerresearchuk.org/about-cancer/tests-and-scans/prostate-specific-antigen-psa-test

Chapter 13 Professional Conversation/Professional Dilemma

Fitness to drive or travel	**DVLA at a glance**	https://www.gov.uk/guidance/assessing-fitness-to-drive-a-guide-for-medical-professionals
	Fitness to fly	https://www.caa.co.uk/passengers/before-you-fly/am-i-fit-to-fly/guidance-for-health-professionals/assessing-fitness-to-fly/
	Travel clinic	http://www.fitfortravel.nhs.uk/home.aspx
Resources for people with dementia	**Age UK** **Dementia UK**	https://www.ageuk.org.uk/ https://www.dementiauk.org/

All websites last accessed May 2025.

APPENDIX 3

FEVER IN THE UNDER 5s

This traffic light table should be used in conjunction with the recommendations in NICE Guideline NG143 'Fever in under 5s: assessment and initial management'.[1]

Other	Green – low risk	Amber – intermediate risk	Red – high risk
Colour (of skin, lips or tongue)	• Normal colour	• Pallor reported by parent/carer	• Pale/mottled/ashen/blue
Activity	• Responds normally to social cues • Content/smiles • Stays awake or awakens quickly • Strong normal cry/not crying	• Not responding normally to social cues • No smile • Wakes only with prolonged stimulation • Decreased activity	• No response to social cues • Appears ill to a healthcare professional • Does not wake or if roused does not stay awake • Weak, high-pitched or continuous cry

Respiratory		• Nasal flaring
		• Tachypnoea:
		  • RR >50 breaths/min, age 6–12 months
		  • RR >40 breaths/min, age >12 months
		• Oxygen saturation ≤95% in air
		• Crackles in the chest
			• Grunting
			• Tachypnoea: RR >60 breaths/min
			• Moderate or severe chest indrawing

Circulation and hydration	• Normal skin and eyes
	• Moist mucous membranes
		• Tachycardia:
		  • >160 beats/min, age <12 months
		  • >150 beats/min, age 12–24 months
		  • >140 beats/min, age 2–5 years
		• CRT ≥3 seconds
		• Dry mucous membranes
		• Poor feeding in infants
		• Reduced urine output
			• Reduced skin turgor

Other	• None of the amber or red symptoms or signs	• Age 3–6 months, temperature ≥39°C • Fever for ≥5 days • Rigors • Swelling of a limb or joint • Non-weight-bearing limb/not using an extremity	• Age <3 months, temperature ≥38°C* • Non-blanching rash • Bulging fontanelle • Neck stiffness • Status epilepticus • Focal neurological signs • Focal seizures

Abbreviations: CRT, capillary refill time; RR, respiratory rate.

* Some vaccinations have been found to induce fever in children aged under 3 months.

Please remember that guidelines are constantly updated. Always refer to the latest guidance and remember that information from NICE is only applicable to patients in the UK.

REFERENCES

Information taken from NICE guidelines with kind permission. Please note the guidelines change frequently and you should **always** check for the latest updated guidance. Remember that NICE guidance is only applicable to patients in the UK.

Chapter 1 Introduction and Background to the Exam

MRCGP simulated consultation assessment

1. Royal College of General Practioners. MRCGP: simulated consultation assessment (SCA). https://www.rcgp.org.uk/mrcgp-exams/simulated-consultation-assessment.

Blueprint groups

2. Royal College of General Practioners. Preparing for the SCA. https://www.rcgp.org.uk/mrcgp-exams/simulated-consultation-assessment/preparing.

RCGP capabilities

3. Royal College of General Practioners. WPBA capabilities framework with IPUs. https://www.rcgp.org.uk/mrcgp-exams/wpba/capability-framework.

Consultation models

4. Pendleton D., Schofield T., Tate P. *The Consultation: An Approach to Learning and Teaching.* Oxford: Oxford University Press, 1984.
5. Helman C.G. Disease versus illness in general practice. *J R Coll. Gen Pract* 1981; 31: 548–52.
6. Neighbour R. *The Inner Consultation*. London: CRC Press, 1987.
7. Silverman J., Kurtz S., Draper J. *Skills for Communicating with Patients.* London: CRC Press, 2013.
8. Watson A., Gillespie D. *The Modern Guide to GP Consulting: 6S for Success.* London: CRC Press, 2013.

Chapter 2 Patient Less Than 19 Years Old

Anaemia

1. WHO. Anaemia. https://www.who.int/publications/i/item/9789240088542. Mar 2024.
2. NICE. British National Formulary for Children (BNFc). https://bnfc.nice.org.uk/. Apr 2025.

Atopic eczema

1. PCDS. Eczema: atopic eczema. https://www.pcds.org.uk/clinical-guidance/atopic-eczema. Nov 2024.

UTIs in children

1. NICE Guideline NG224. Urinary tract infection in under 16s: diagnosis and management. July 2022.
2. NICE Guideline NG143. Fever in under 5s: assessment and initial management. Nov 2021.

Eating disorder

1. NICE Guideline NG69. Eating disorders: recognition and treatment. Dec 2020.

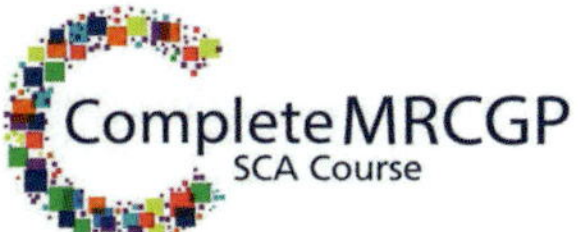

Asthma diagnosis

1. Pellegrino R., Viegi G., Brusasco V. et al. Interpretive strategies for lung function tests. *Eur Respir J* 2005; 26: 948.
2. NICE CKS. Health topics. Asthma. https://cks.nice.org.uk/topics/asthma/. Apr 2025.
3. GINA. 2024 GINA main report. https://ginasthma.org/2024-report/.

Chapter 3 Gender, Reproductive and Sexual Health

Varicella in pregnancy

1. NICE CKS. Health topics. Chickenpox. https://cks.nice.org.uk/chickenpox#!management. Nov 2023.
2. RCOG Green-top Guideline No. 13. Chickenpox in pregnancy. https://www.rcog.org.uk/guidance/browse-all-guidance/green-top-guidelines/chickenpox-in-pregnancy-green-top-guideline-no-13/. Aug 2024.

Suspected gynaecological cancer

1. NICE Guideline NG12. Suspected cancer: recognition and referral. Apr 2025.

Cystic fibrosis

1. Patient. Cystic fibrosis. https://patient.info/doctor/cystic-fibrosis-pro. Aug 2024.
2. NICE Guideline NG78. Cystic fibrosis: diagnosis and management. Oct 2017, reviewed by NICE Dec 2024.

Erectile dysfunction

1. British Association of Urological Surgeons. Sexual health inventory for men (SHIM). https://www.baus.org.uk/patients/information_leaflets/214/sexual_health_inventory_for_men_shim.
2. Patient. Erectile dysfunction. http://patient.info/doctor/erectile-dysfunction. Mar 2022.
3. Relate. https://www.relate.org.uk/.
4. NICE Guideline NG12. Suspected cancer: recognition and referral. Apr 2025.
5. NICE CKS. Health topics. How should I assess a man with erectile dysfunction? https://cks.nice.org.uk/topics/erectile-dysfunction/diagnosis/assessment/. Oct 2024.

Gender dysphoria

1. Stonewall. List of LGBTQ+ terms. https://www.stonewall.org.uk/help-advice/glossary-terms.
2. NHS. Body dysmorphic disorder (BDD). https://www.nhs.uk/conditions/body-dysmorphia/. Oct 2023.
3. Arden & GEM. National Referral Support Service for the NHS Gender Incongruence Service for Children and Young People. https://www.ardengemcsu.nhs.uk/services/clinical-support/national-referral-support-service-for-the-nhs-gender-incongruence-service-for-children-and-young-people/. Oct 2024. (This site also has very useful links to support services for young people who are distressed.)
4. NHS. Coping with your teenager. https://www.nhs.uk/mental-health/children-and-young-adults/advice-for-parents/cope-with-your-teenager/.

Chapter 4 Long-Term Conditions, Including Cancer, Multi-Morbidity and Disability

Down syndrome

1. Holland T. Ageing and its consequences for people with Down's syndrome. https://www.intellectualdisability.info/life-stages/articles/ageing-and-its-consequences-for-people-with-downs-syndrome. 2006.

2. Trumble T. People with Down's syndrome at all ages: some tips for family physicians. https://www.intellectualdisability.info/life-stages/articles/people-with-downs-syndrome-at-all-ages-some-tips-for-family-physicians. 2002.
3. Hoghton M., RCGP Learning Disabilities Group. A step by step guide for GP practices. Annual health checks for people with a learning disability. https://www.choiceforum.org/docs/circ.pdf. 2010.

Hyperthyroidism

1. NICE CKS. Health topics. Hyperthyroidism. https://cks.nice.org.uk/topics/hyperthyroidism/. Jan 2025.
2. British Thyroid Foundation. Patient leaflets: 'Your guide to hyperthyroidism' and 'Your guide to antithyroid drug treatment to treat hyperthyroidism'. https://www.btf-thyroid.org/pages/category/patient-leaflets.

Prostatitis

1. NICE CKS. Health topics. Prostatitis – acute. http://cks.nice.org.uk/prostatitis-acute. June 2024.
2. NICE CKS. Health topics. Prostatitis – chronic. http://cks.nice.org.uk/prostatitis-chronic. June 2024.

Psoriasis

1. RCGP Curriculum. Clinical topics guides. Dermatology. https://www.rcgp.org.uk/mrcgp-exams/gp-curriculum/clinical-topic-guides#dermatology.
2. PCDS. Psoriasis: an overview and chronic plaque psoriasis. https://www.pcds.org.uk/clinical-guidance/psoriasis-an-overview. Jan 2025.
3. NICE CKS. Health topics. Psoriasis, management. https://cks.nice.org.uk/topics/psoriasis/management/. Dec 2024.

COPD

1. GOLD. 2020 Global Strategy for Prevention, Diagnosis and Management of COPD. https://goldcopd.org/gold-reports/.
2. NICE CKS. Health topics. Chronic obstructive pulmonary disease. https://cks.nice.org.uk/topics/chronic-obstructive-pulmonary-disease/management/stable-copd/. Feb 2025.

Chapter 5 Older Adults, Including Frailty and People at the End of Life

Deafness and tinnitus

1. NICE Guideline NG98. Hearing loss in adults: assessment and management. https://www.nice.org.uk/guidance/ng98. Oct 2023.
2. NICE CKS. Health topics. Tinnitus. https://cks.nice.org.uk/tinnitus#!scenario. Apr 2022.
3. Zhang Y.P., Gao Q.Y., Gao J.W. et al. The association between tinnitus and risk of cardiovascular events and all-cause mortality: insight from the UK Biobank. *Acta Cardiol* 2024; 79(3): 374–82.

AMD and cataract

1. NICE CKS. Health topics. Cataracts. http://cks.nice.org.uk/cataracts. Mar 2025.
2. NICE CKS. Health topics. Macular degeneration degeneration. https://cks.nice.org.uk/macular-degeneration-age-related. Aug 2022.
3. Patient. Age-related macular degeneration. http://patient.info/doctor/age-related-macular-degeneration-pro. Nov 2023.

Additional useful resources

NIH. Age-related macular degeneration. https://www.nei.nih.gov/learn-about-eye-health/eye-conditions-and-diseases/age-related-macular-degeneration. (Patient information leaflet available in auditory form and large text.)

RNIB. Cataracts. https://www.rnib.org.uk/your-eyes/eye-conditions-az/cataracts/. (Patient information leaflet.) Apr 2025.

Angina

1. NICE Guideline CG126. Stable angina: management. Aug 2016.
2. Patient. Stable angina. https://patient.info/doctor/stable-angina-2. Mar 2022.
3. NICE CKS. Health topics. Angina. https://cks.nice.org.uk/topics/angina/. Mar 2025.
4. Bosch J., Lonn E., Pogue J. et al. Long-term effects of ramipril on cardiovascular events and on diabetes: results of the HOPE study extension. *Circulation* 2005; 112: 1339.

Lung cancer

1. Radiopaedia. Coin lesion. https://radiopaedia.org/articles/coin-lesion-lung?lang=gb. June 2022.
2. NICE Guideline NG12. Suspected cancer: recognition and referral. Apr 2025.
3. NICE CKS. Health topic. Lung and pleural cancers – recognition and referral. https://cks.nice.org.uk/lung-and-pleural-cancers-recognition-and-referral#!scenario. Apr 2025.

Peripheral neuropathy

1. Patient. Peripheral neuropathy. https://patient.info/brain-nerves/peripheral-neuropathy-leaflet#nav-2. Jan 2024.

Chapter 6 Mental Health, Including Addiction, Smoking, Alcohol and Substance Misuse

Anxiety

1. NICE Clinical Guideline CG113. Generalised anxiety disorder and panic disorder in adults: management. June 2020.
2. Williams C.J. *Overcoming Depression: A Five Areas Approach.* London: Arnold, 2001.
3. Williams C., Garland A. A cognitive–behavioural therapy assessment model for use in everyday clinical practice. *Adv Psychiatr Treat* 2002; 8: 172–9.

Depression review

1. Black, A. *Living in the Moment: Don't Dwell on the Past or Worry about the Future. Simply BE in the Present with Mindfulness Meditations.* CICO Books. 2012.
2. NICE Guideline NG222. Depression in adults: treatment and management. Sept 2024.

Personality disorder

1. https://patient.info/doctor/emotionally-unstable-personality-disorder. Jan 2022.
2. NICE Clinical Guideline CG78. Borderline personality disorder: recognition and management. Jul 2024.
3. NHS. Symptoms – borderline personality disorder. https://www.nhs.uk/mental-health/conditions/borderline-personality-disorder/symptoms/. Nov 2022.

Postnatal psychosis

1. RCPsych. Postnatal depression. https://www.rcpsych.ac.uk/mental-health/mental-illnesses-and-mental-health-problems/postnatal-depression-key-facts.

2. NICE Clinical Guideline CG192. Antenatal and postnatal mental health: clinical management and service guidance. Jul 2024.
3. Patient. Postpartum psychosis. http://patient.info/doctor/postpartum-psychosis-pro. July 2023.

Harmful drinking

1. NICE Clinical Guideline CG115. Alcohol-use disorders: diagnosis, assessment and management of harmful drinking (high-risk drinking) and alcohol dependence. Jul 2019.

Chapter 7 Urgent and Unscheduled Care

Chest pain of recent onset

1. NICE CKS. Health topics. Chest pain. https://cks.nice.org.uk/topics/chest-pain/. Aug 2022.

Abdominal pain

1. Patient. Acute abdomen. https://patient.info/doctor/acute-abdomen. June 2024.

Hyperglycaemia

1. NHS. Diabetic ketoacidosis. https://www.nhs.uk/conditions/diabetic-ketoacidosis/. June 2023.

Knee pain

1. NICE CKS. Health topics. Osteoarthritis: scenario: management. https://cks.nice.org.uk/topics/osteo arthritis. Dec 2023.
2. Kobayashi H. Kanamura T., Koshida S. Mechanisms of the anterior cruciate ligament injury in sports activities: a twenty-year clinical research of 1,700 athletes. *J Sports Sci Med* 2010; 9: 669–75.

Acute asthma

1. NICE CKS. Health topics. Asthma: scenario: acute exacerbation of asthma. https://cks.nice.org.uk/topics/asthma/management/acute-exacerbation-of-asthma/. Apr 2025.
2. Global Initiative for Asthma. https://ginasthma.org/.
3. NICE CKS. Health topics. Chronic obstructive pulmonary disease. https://cks.nice.org.uk/topics/chronic-obstructive-pulmonary-disease/management/acute-exacerbation/. Feb 2025.

Chapter 8 Health Disadvantage and Vulnerabilities, Including Veterans, Mental Capacity, Safeguarding and Communication Difficulties

Violence

1. Women's Aid. What is coercive control? https://www.womensaid.org.uk/information-support/what-is-domestic-abuse/coercive-control/.
2. Stark E. *Coercive Control: How Men Entrap Women in Personal Life*. New York: Oxford University Press, 2009.

Mental health and learning disability

1. Department of Health. *Valuing People: A New Strategy for Learning Disability for the 21st Century*. Cm 5086. 2001.
2. RCGP Curriculum. Clinical topic guides. 2025. Learning disability.

Suspected DVT

1. NICE Guideline NG158. Venous thromboembolic diseases: diagnosis, management and thrombophilia testing. Aug 2023.

References

2. NICE CKS. Health topics. Anticoagulation – oral. https://cks.nice.org.uk/topics/anticoagulation-oral/. Mar 2025.
3. NICE CKS. Health topics. Deep vein thrombosis: scenario: management of deep vein thrombosis. https://cks.nice.org.uk/topics/deep-vein-thrombosis/management/management/. Feb 2025. (Includes Wells score.)

Alcohol and safeguarding

1. NICE Public Health Guideline PH24. Alcohol-use disorders: prevention. June 2010.
2. American Psychiatric Association. *Diagnostic and Statistical Manual of Mental Disorders*, Fifth edition. DSM-5-TR. APA, 2023.
3. WHO. *International Classification of Diseases*, 11th Revision. ICD-11. WHO, 2022.

LARC and sterilisation

1. FSRH. Progestogen only implants. https://www.fsrh.org/Public/Documents/clinical-guidance-progestogen-only-implants.aspx. Jul 2023.
2. FSRH. Progesterone-only injectables. https://www.fsrh.org/Public/Public/Standards-and-Guidance/Progestogen-only-Injectables.aspx. July 2023.
3. FSRH. FSRH guideline. https://www.fsrh.org/Public/Documents/ceu-guidance-intrauterine-contraception.aspx. Jan 2025.

Chapter 9 Ethnicity, Culture, Diversity and Inclusivity

Squint

1. Patient. Strabismus (squint) classification and management. https://patient.info/doctor/strabismus-squint. Oct 2021.
2. Patient. Amblyopia. https://patient.info/doctor/strabismus-squint. June 2023.
3. NHS. Squint. http://www.nhs.uk/conditions/Squint/. May 2023. (Includes a video of an ophthalmologist describing squint and its treatment for patients/carers.)
4. Moorfields Eye Hospital. Atropine treatment for amblyopia (lazy eye). https://www.moorfields.nhs.uk/mediaLocal/csznky3h/atropine-treatment-for-amblyopia.pdf. Aug 2021.

Melasma

1. DermNet. Melasma. https://www.dermnetnz.org/colour/melasma.html. Oct 2020.
2. British Skin Foundation. Melasma. https://knowyourskin.britishskinfoundation.org.uk/condition/melasma/.
3. Pandya A., Hynan L., Bhore R. Reliability assessment and validation of the Melasma Area and Severity Index (MASI) and a new modified MASI scoring method. *J Am Acad Dermatol* 2011; 64: 78–83.

Occupational allergy

1. NICE CKS. Health topics. Dermatitis – contact. https://cks.nice.org.uk/dermatitis-contact/. Jan 2024.

Sinusitis

1. NICE CKS. Health topics. Sinusitis. http://cks.nice.org.uk/sinusitis/. Aug 2024.

Chapter 10 New Presentation of Undifferentiated Disease

Foot pain

1. Cooper A., Blythe J., Wise E. *BMJ Masterclass for GPs. Musculoskeletal Medicine. Course Materials*. 2013.
2. MDCalc. Ottawa ankle rule. http://www.mdcalc.com/ottawa-ankle-rule/.

3. NICE CKS. Health topic. Gout. http://cks.nice.org.uk/gout#!scenario. June 2023.

Neurological symptoms – Multiple sclerosis

1. Patient. Multiple sclerosis. https://patient.info/doctor/multiple-sclerosis-pro. July 2022.
2. NICE CKS. Clinical topic. Multiple sclerosis. https://cks.nice.org.uk/topics/multiple-sclerosis/. May 2024.

Rash – Lyme disease

1. Patient. Lyme disease. https://patient.info/doctor/lyme-disease-pro. Apr 2022.
2. NICE CKS. Clinical topic. Lyme disease: scenario: management of Lyme disease. https://cks.nice.org.uk/topics/lyme-disease/management/management/. Mar 2024.
3. NICE Guidance NG95. Lyme disease – guidance. Oct 2018.

Bowel symptoms – IBS

1. NICE CKS. Clinical topic. Irritable bowel syndrome. https://cks.nice.org.uk/topics/irritable-bowel-syndrome/. Aug 2023.

Chapter 11 Prescribing

Dyspepsia/Reflux

1. NICE CKS. Health topic. Dyspepsia – unidentified cause. https://cks.nice.org.uk/topics/dyspepsia-unidentified-cause/. May 2024.
2. NICE Guideline NG12. Suspected cancer: recognition and referral. April 2025.
3. NICE CKS. Health topic. Gastrointestinal tract (upper) cancers – recognition and referral. https://cks.nice.org.uk/topics/gastrointestinal-tract-upper-cancers-recognition-referral/. Apr 2025.

Chronic pain

1. NICE CKS. Health topic. Chronic pain. https://cks.nice.org.uk/topics/chronic-pain/. Jan 2025.
2. Understanding pain in less than 5 minutes. https://www.youtube.com/watch?v=C_3phB93rvI.

High cholesterol

1. NICE CKS. Health topic. CVD risk assessment and management: scenario: assessing cardiovascular risk. https://cks.nice.org.uk/topics/cvd-risk-assessment-management/management/cvd-risk-assessment. Sept 2024.

Hypertension

1. NICE Guideline NG136. Hypertension in adults: diagnosis and management. Nov 2023.

Migraine

1. NICE CKS. Health topic. Migraine. https://cks.nice.org.uk/topics/migraine/. Feb 2024.

Chapter 12 Investigation/Results

Hypertrophic cardiomyopathy

1. British Heart Foundation. Hypertrophic cardiomyopathy (HCM). https://www.bhf.org.uk/informationsupport/conditions/hypertrophic-cardiomyopathy.
2. Liao Y.W., Redfern J., Somauroo J.D., Cooper R.M. Hypertrophic cardiomyopathy and exercise restrictions: time to let the shackles off? *Br J Cardiol* 2020; 27: 64–6.
3. American Heart Association. AHA HCM SCD calculator. https://professional.heart.org/en/guidelines-and-statements/hcm-risk-calculator.

Myeloma

1. Myeloma UK. What is myeloma? https://www.myeloma.org.uk/understanding-myeloma/what-is-myeloma/.
2. NICE CKS. Health topics. Multiple myeloma. https://cks.nice.org.uk/multiple-myeloma/. Apr 2022.

Acute kidney injury

1. NICE CKS. Health topics. Acute kidney injury. https://cks.nice.org.uk/topics/chronic-kidney-disease/. Sept 2024.
2. NHS Scotland. Effective prescribing and therapeutics. Medicines and dehydration. https://www.therapeutics.scot.nhs.uk/polypharmacy/sick-day-rules/. (Medicine sick day rules.)
3. 'Think kidneys' Acute kidney injury, potential problematic drugs and actions to take in primary care. www.thinkkidneys.nhs.uk/aki.

PSA test result

1. Fred Hutch Cancer Center. Facts about prostate cancer. https://www.fredhutch.org/en/diseases/prostate-cancer/facts-resources.html.
2. NICE CKS. Health topics. Prostate cancer: PSA testing. https://cks.nice.org.uk/topics/prostate-cancer/diagnosis/assessment/#psa-testing. Apr 2025.

Atrial fibrillation

1. NICE CKS. Health topics. Atrial fibrillation: management. https://cks.nice.org.uk/topics/atrial-fibrilla tion/management/. Mar 2025.

Chapter 13 Professional Conversation/Professional Dilemma

Self-neglect

1. Nottingham and Nottinghamshire Multi-Agency Safeguarding Adults at Risk. Self-neglect advice and toolkit. https://nsab.nottinghamshire.gov.uk/media/er1jskhb/selfneglectadviceandtoolkit.pdf. 2019.
2. GOV.UK. Care Act 2014. https://www.legislation.gov.uk/ukpga/2014/23/contents.

Community-acquired pneumonia

1. NICE Guideline NG138. Pneumonia (community-acquired): antimicrobial prescribing. Jul 2022.
2. BMJ Best Practice. Community-acquired pneumonia in adults (non COVID-19). https://bestpractice.bmj.com/topics/en-gb/3000108/management-recommendations.
3. Lim W.S., van der Eerden M.M., Laing R. et al. Defining community-acquired pneumonia severity on presentation to hospital: an international derivation and validation study. *Thorax* 2003; 58: 377.
4. Hodkinson H.M. Evaluation of a mental test score for assessment of mental impairment in the elderly. *Age Ageing* 1972; 1: 233.

Retinal detachment

1. NICE CKS. Health topics. Retinal detachment. http://cks.nice.org.uk/retinal-detachment/. Aug 2024.
2. RNIB. Understanding retinal detachment. https://media.rnib.org.uk/documents/Understanding-Retinal-Detachment-2020_e4bdzwe.pdf. June 2023.

Appendix 3 Fever in the under 5s

1. NICE Guideline NG143. Fever in under 5s: assessment and initial management. https://www.nice.org.uk/guidance/ng143. Nov 2021.

All websites last accessed May 2025.

INDEX

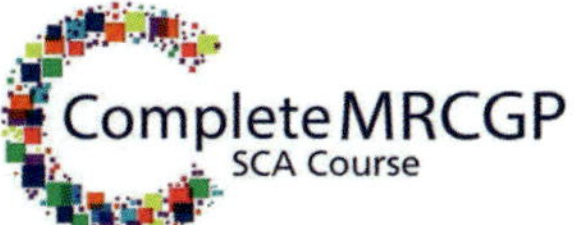
Complete MRCGP
SCA Course

D

E

F

G

P

Q

R

S

T

U

V

W